COGNITIVE-BEHAVIORAL MANAGEMENT OF TIC DISORDERS

COGNITIVE-BEHAVIORAL MANAGEMENT OF TIC DISORDERS

Kieron O'Connor

Fernand-Seguin Research Centre, Louis-H. Lafontaine Hospital,
Department of Psychiatry, University of Montreal, Quebec

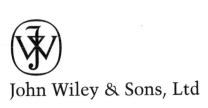

John Wiley & Sons, Ltd

Other Wiley Editorial Offices

John Wiley & Sons Inc., 111 River Street, Hoboken, NJ 07030, USA

Jossey-Bass, 989 Market Street, San Francisco, CA 94103-1741, USA

Wiley-VCH Verlag GmbH, Boschstr. 12, D-69469 Weinheim, Germany

John Wiley & Sons Australia Ltd, 33 Park Road, Milton, Queensland 4064, Australia

John Wiley & Sons (Asia) Pte Ltd, 2 Clementi Loop #02-01, Jin Xing Distripark, Singapore 129809

John Wiley & Sons Canada Ltd, 22 Worcester Road, Etobicoke, Ontario, Canada M9W 1L1

Wiley also publishes its books in a variety of electronic formats. Some content that appears in print may
not be available in electronic books.

Library of Congress Cataloging-in-Publication Data

O'Connor, Kieron Philip.
   Cognitive-behavioral management of tic disorders / Kieron O'Connor.
      p.   cm.
   Includes bibliographical references and index.
   ISBN-13 978-0-470-09379-5 – ISBN-13 978-0-470-09380-1
   ISBN-10 0-470-09379-X – ISBN-10 0-470-09380-3
   1. Tic disorders.   2. Tic disorders – Treatment.   3. Cognitive therapy.   I. Title.

   RC552 .T5027   2005
   616.8'3 – dc22   2004028130

British Library Cataloguing in Publication Data

A catalogue record for this book is available from the British Library

ISBN-13 978-0-470-09379-5 (hbk) 978-0-470-09380-1 (pbk)
ISBN-10 0-470-09379-X (hbk)   0-470-09380-3 (pbk)

Typeset in 10/12pt Palatino by TechBooks, New Delhi, India

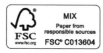

CONTENTS

ABOUT THE AUTHOR

Kieron O'Connor began his research career working as a research officer at the Medical Research Council (UK) Clinical Psychiatry Unit at Graylingwell Hospital, Chichester, Sussex. In 1979, he was awarded a Master of Philosophy (MPhil) by thesis in experimental psychology from the University of Sussex, and in 1984 a doctorate degree (PhD) in research psychology at the Institute of Psychiatry, University of London. He completed the British Psychology Society clinical diploma training course in 1986, and transferred to the University College, Institute of Laryngology and Otology, working partly as a research lecturer, investigating psychological aspects of vertigo and dizziness, and also as a clinical psychologist at Bloomsbury Health Authority.

In 1988, he was awarded the first of a series of fellowships by the Fonds de la Recherche en Santé du Québec, and established a clinical research program at the Fernand-Seguin Research Center, Louis-H. Lafontaine Hospital, University of Montreal, Canada. The multidisciplinary research program, which focuses on obsessive-compulsive disorder (OCD), Tourette and tic disorder and delusional disorder, is currently funded by the Canadian Institutes of Health Research. He is actively involved in several community-based initiatives to provide support and information to people with OCD and Tourette's syndrome and their families, and is scientific advisor to the Quebec OCD Foundation.

He is currently associate research professor at the Psychiatry Department of University of Montreal, and also holds an honorary cross appointment as associate professor in the Department of Psychology, University of Quebec at Montreal. He is author or co-author on over 100 scientific publications. He is also co-author with Frederick Aardema and Marie-Claude Pélissier of *Beyond Reasonable Doubt: Reasoning Processes in OCD Disorder and Related Disorders*, published in 2005 by Wiley.

PREFACE

The focus in this text is on cognitive-behavioral approaches and related psychoeducational and psychophysiological methods, to aid the management of tics in people with Gilles de la Tourette's syndrome and chronic tic disorder. The initial section of the book reviews the relevant literature and research work in this area. The middle section presents a cognitive–psychophysiological model of tics, together with an outline of empirical studies testing the model. The final section and appendices provide a therapist and client manual for use in tic management, with four case illustrations.

Cognitive-behavior therapy (CBT) will probably be familiar to professional and non-professional readers alike as a recently developed evidence-based psychological intervention that has been successfully applied to anxiety, affective and, lately, psychotic disorders. In practice, the CBT approach often complements other more medical approaches, but it nonetheless follows a distinct case conceptualization of psychiatric disorder based on CBT principles. It views symptoms as behavior, actively maintained by thought and behavior patterns in the here and now, rather than as the result of more remote hypothetical intrapsychic processes. Consequently, treatment follows a learning model, where control over symptoms depends on the active collaboration of the client in successful acquisition and application of new ways of thinking and behaving. In this tradition, behavioral and learning principles have been applied in several recent attempts to understand and treat tic and habit disorders. The term "habit disorder" has an uncertain diagnostic status in psychiatric nosology, but covers a range of usually manual habits such as nail biting, skin picking, scratching, rubbing, hair pulling, teeth grinding, neck and knuckle cracking.

A habit disorder generally seems to be under some degree of voluntary control but which the person, nonetheless, is unable to stop, unlike tics which appear more like neurological reflexes. There is debate as to whether tics and habits form a continuum. However, habit disorders, in particular trichotillomania, have already formed the subject of a number of comprehensive manualized CBT treatments emphasizing, in addition to behavioral control, the emotional, interpersonal and cognitive dimensions of the habitual behavior (e.g., Mansuetto et al., 1999). There is a less extensive CBT literature on treating tics, but tics as found in Tourette's syndrome and other tic disorders have, however, formed the target for a behavioral approach termed "habit reversal" (Azrin & Nunn, 1973; Woods & Miltenberger, 2001). There is a growing body of clinical evidence supporting the effectiveness of habit reversal in reducing tics, but there have been few large-scale studies of its efficacy, and since habit reversal is a multicomponent program, it is unclear which are its crucial elements. Also, habit reversal procedures are inspired by behavioral principles rather than a specific model of tic phenomenology. But tics are not just conditioned responses. Consequently, the clinical success of behavior therapy has not been accompanied by an improved and more comprehensive cognitive-behavioral conceptualization of tic maintenance or genesis. Also, the habit reversal view of tics as isolated behavioral events, and the failure to explicitly address cognitive variables, can limit its consideration of the wider everyday cognitive-behavioral context relevant to tic management.

The gap between behavior and cognition is, to some extent, an artificial one, and even in a strictly behavioral approach, the clients must understand the model, and articulate their motivation and reasons for changing the habit and be able mentally to link cause and effect in their application of techniques. Although seldom explicitly measured, it is clear from case studies reporting behavior therapy for tics that, as in other psychiatric disorders, behavioral change can be accompanied by a change in thinking about the disorder. However, in our own work, we realized that cognitive factors were not only a useful adjunct to behavior therapy but were often central to the occurrence of the tic. For example, anticipation can provoke tics or even just thinking about ticcing can provoke tics, and negative evaluation of high-risk situations can lead to increased levels of tension and ticcing.

Previous models of tics have focused either on the role of central brain structures or on localized social or behavioral operants reinforcing the tic, but there is also a vast and largely untapped literature on the intermediate processes between brain and behavior relating to the psychology and psychophysiology of motor behavior. Motor psychophysiology can shed light on how central commands control the intricacies of preparation and muscle tension, and how such preparation and tension can produce unwanted voluntary and involuntary movements. This approach views cognition and behavior, voluntary and non-voluntary action as different stages in the same motor action sequence. Thought-action, cognitive-motor coupling can be accommodated by a cognitive–psychophysiological model which takes account of forward planning and feedback correction as a part of motor control, and views even non-voluntary actions as occurring against a background behavioral action plan.

As the motor theorist Bernstein (1967) pointed out, no individual contraction can be considered independent of the wider intentional actions of the motor program, and this motor program, in turn, has to be understood in terms of an ecological adaptation to the environment. Hence, it may be towards the overall telic activity of the person that we need to look for clues about tic onset rather than to just neurobiological structures or situational operants. The cognitive–psychophysiological model led to the development of a CBT approach that, although complementing and building on previous behavioral interventions, placed cognitive factors center stage. In effect, isolated habit reversal strategies are integrated into a wider cognitive-motor restructuring of behavior preceding tic onset in order to prevent the tic occurrence rather than resist it once it has appeared. Inevitably, such cognitive and motor restructuring addresses the wider behavioral context surrounding the person's style of action.

The major claims of the model have been empirically tested through psychometric, experimental and clinical studies discussed in Chapters 3 and 4. The program itself has been validated as an effective treatment for adults and adolescents with Tourette's, chronic tic and habit disorder. It is designed to be implemented in conjunction with a professionaly trained therapist, and both client and therapist manuals are provided. Issues about its future application to other client groups and disorders are discussed in Chapter 5.

Kieron O'Connor
Montreal, September 2004

There is a dedicated website for this book at www.wiley.com/go/tic containing the forms from Appendices 1, 2, 6, 7 and 8 and the client manual. These are available to readers to view and download.

ACKNOWLEDGMENTS

Thanks go to the following:

- Annette Maillet for typing the manuscript.
- Danielle Gareau for her collaboration in the development and translation of the first version of the program published in French, *Tics et problèmes de tension musculaire*. Montreal: Sogides, Édition de l'Homme, 1994.
- Dr Emmanuel Stip and his residents for invaluable help in psychiatric evaluations.
- Caroline Berthiaume and Jeremy Dohan for providing the four case studies in Chapter 6.
- Julie Leclerc for help with Table 6.1.
- Marie-Claude Pélissier for help with Table 2.1.
- Marc Lavoic for his collaboration with neurobiological aspects.
- Genevieve Thibault for providing neurophysiological information.
- Edith St-Jean, Sophie Robillard, Vicky Leblanc, Jeremy Dohan, Caroline Berthiaume, Pascale Doucet, Stéphanie Lévesque, Mathilde Brault, Julie Charette, Andréa Leduc, Frederick Aardema, Marie-Claude Pélissier, Genevieve Paradis, Annick Rouleau, Julie Leclerc, Josée Loiselle, Denise Pitre, all of whom contributed to the realization of the current clinical program.
- The Canadian Institute of Health Research, the Fonds de la Recherche en Santé du Québec for research funding permitting validation of the program.
- The direction and personnel of the Fernand-Seguin Research Center, Louis-H. Lafontaine Hospital, Department of Psychiatry, University of Montreal for providing infrastructure support and other resources to facilitate the research program.
- All clients who have participated in our clinical projects, without whom this book would not be possible.
- Claire Ruston, Ruth Graham, and Vivien Ward of the Wiley editorial team for their help with the publishing process.

Chapter 1

THE NATURE OF TIC DISORDERS

▶ DEFINITION

Tics are defined, rather vaguely, in the *Diagnostic and Statistical Manual of Mental Disorders* (DSM-IV; American Psychiatric Association, 1994) nosology as a recurrent, non-rhythmic series of movements (of a non-voluntary nature) in one or several muscle groups. Tics are usually divided into simple and complex tics of a motor, sensory, phonic or cognitive nature. In practice, simple tics have to be differentiated from behaviors such as routines, automatisms and stereotypes; from spasms of neurological or neurochemical origin, and from dystonias and torticollis of a possibly psychoneurological origin. Also, complex tics, which are complex if they involve sequences of several distinct muscle movements, can visibly resemble the ritualized compulsions of obsessive-compulsive disorder (OCD).

▶ DIAGNOSIS

Tics occur over all cultures, and have been reported anecdotally since classical times. The first clinical descriptions, however, were provided in the nineteenth century by Itard (1825), who reported a case of an aristocrat exhibiting tics, barking and obscenities, and later Gilles de la Tourette (1885), who gave a detailed description of eight additional cases. Currently, the DSM-IV distinguishes transitory tics from chronic tic disorders (TD) and Gilles de la Tourette's syndrome (TS). Transitory tics are those occurring for a short period, usually in early childhood, which slowly disappear or show spontaneous remission later in adolescence. In TD, typically, one or several simple or complex tics are present. Often the tics are stable over a period of years since childhood. The tics occur daily and cause distress. Although the diagnostic criterion specifies onset prior to age 18, tics may develop in adulthood. TS is recognized in the DSM-III and DSM-IV as a distinct diagnostic category with multiple tics including at least one phonic tic occurring several times a day, every day, throughout a period of more than one year and whose location, number, frequency and severity can change over time with onset before the age of 18 years. Although clinician consensus tends to view TD as a milder form of TS, diagnosis of TS is categorical not dimensional. Kraemer et al. (2004) point well to the pitfalls of using categorical instead of dimensional approaches to classification, and although both have uses in different settings, the reliance entirely on

Cognitive-Behavioral Management of Tic Disorders by K. O'Connor.
Copyright © 2005 John Wiley & Sons, Ltd.

categorization of TS and TD in the complete absence of a dimensional model could be problematic. There seems to be a consensus among researchers that TD and TS share enough common aspects to be considered on a continuum of severity (e.g., Spencer et al., 1995). But the diagnosis of TS is currently dichotomous, not dimensional, and depends crucially on the existence of a vocal tic, although there has been controversy about current criteria for TS (e.g., First et al., 1995; Tourette Syndrome Classification Study Group, 1993). Some current assessment instruments do adopt a dimensional approach (see Table 6.1).

Tics may be simple or complex. A *simple* tic involves one principal muscle group. Simple tics include blinking, cheek twitches, head or knee jerks and shoulder shrugs. Tics are mainly confined to the upper body and the most common occur in the eye, head, shoulders and face, and follow a rostral–caudal development. Tics can also be vocal and include coughs, tongue clacking, sniffing, whistling, throat clearing, hiccing, barking and growling. Some recurrent involuntary somatic sensations are classified as sensory tics. These are identified as heavy, warm or tingling premonitory sensations, often muscle focused and leading to muscle tension (Lohr & Wisniewski, 1987; Shapiro & Shapiro, 1986; Shapiro et al., 1988) but the term "premonitory sensation" is now preferred over sensory tic (Cath et al., 2001a). Table 1.1 gives examples of common tics.

Tics are classified as *complex* if there is a contraction in more than one group of muscles (Comings & Comings, 1984). Complex tics may involve sequences of movements, and may take the form of bizarre mannerisms involving several limbs or extremities. J's complex tic begins with a turn of the head towards the right, his hand comes up across his forehead and descends over his head, while his head makes a full semi-circle rotation, and he exhales at the same time. M's complex tic begins with an extension of the shoulder and then a contraction back to the center while his left shoulder repeats the same action. He repeats this back and forth until he "feels right". Complex tics may also take the form of self-inflicted repetitive injurious actions such as head or face slapping, face scratching, teeth grinding, neck cracking, tense–release hand-gripping cycles, or finger twiddling. In neck cracking, the person may manually lift, turn and replace the head on the cervical vertebrae, producing a clicking or grinding sound. Similarly, in knuckle cracking, the person will force the fingers down onto the knuckle joints.

Complex vocal or, more precisely, phonic tics (Jankovic, 1997) take the form of repeated sounds, words or phrases or swear words, and, in rare cases, coprolalia (swearing). Normal actions and words of the person may also be repeated or exaggerated, and copying others can itself evolve into a complex repetitive movement either by echopraxia (motor mimicry) or by echolalia (repeating others' words, phrases or sounds). Complex tics can resemble habit disorders (HD) such as trichotillomania (hair pulling), bruxism (teeth grinding), scabiomania (skin scratching or picking), onychophagia (nail biting), which are, however, classified among the impulse control disorders. There is a covariation between tics and HD and among different types of HD (Woods et al., 1996a). So a person with tics is more likely, than normal, to suffer also from HD. Although complex tics by their semi-voluntary nature may have some intentional aim even if the intention is

Table 1.1 Examples of simple/complex tics

Parts of body	Involuntary repetitive movement habits
Vocal	Coughing, burping, throat clearing, humming, making noises, swallowing, repeating phrases or tunes
Hands	Rubbing fingers together, waggling or clinching fingers or cracking fingers or knuckles, scratching, twiddling, doodling, tapping, fidgeting, stroking (earlobes, chin, etc.), playing with objects, clenching/unclenching the fist
Eyes	Winking, excessive blinking, eyelid tremor squinting, straining eye muscles
Face	Nose wrinkling, ear tics, cheek tics, forehead and temple tension
Mouth	Lip movements, chewing, teeth grinding, tongue ducking, parsing, pouting, forcing tongue against palate, biting tongue, biting fingernails
Head	Head tic to the side, front or back
Shoulders	Movement shrug up and down or forwards or backwards or on one side
Abdomen	Tensing stomach or abdomen into a knot
Legs	Moving legs repetitively up and down or towards and away from each other
Torso	Tensing, twisting or gyrating movements involving legs, arms or trunk
Mental	Playing a tune or phrase over and over in the head, mentally counting for no reason

sensory adjustment (making symmetrical movements to feel "just right"), simple tics seem to serve no purpose.

Tics generally appear in the superior part of the body, including eyes, forehead, mouth, face, neck, shoulders, and can occur anywhere between one and 200 times per minute. Simple facial tics generally have a higher frequency. The onset of simple tics generally precedes complex tics, and simple tics can develop at any time in childhood from 0 to 5 years. Vocal tics develop after motor tics and it is rare for tics to develop post-adolescence, although they can develop in adults (Cohen et al., 1992), often following trauma or surgery. For example, eye blinks may develop as a defensive reaction to light following eye surgery. However, tics seem to wax and wane in severity throughout life and may in the case of TS be substituted by completely different tics or may even spontaneously remit (Nomoto, 1989).

Technically speaking, complex tics are distinguishable from stereotypies and compulsive rituals, routines and habits, since tics are neither completely conscious purposeful rituals, nor totally non-sensical repetitions. In fact, the term "behavioral stereotypy" is usually applied to abnormal repetitive actions associated with organic loss and mental deficiency. In practice, however, it is sometimes difficult to distinguish tics, routines, habits and repetitive movements. The relationship between these three is puzzling since some movements have impulsive as well as compulsive elements. Shapiro and Shapiro (1986) referred to "impulsive compulsions" to highlight the confusion, and Rasmussen and Eisen (1992) and other authors have equally underlined the importance of understanding the relationship between impulsion and compulsion for clarifying diagnosis. In normal automated routines, there may be little awareness but there is overall volitional control. In rituals, there may be awareness but no control. In reflexes and tics, there may be neither awareness nor control.

▶ WHAT COUNTS AS A TIC?

People themselves often refer to a number of movements and habits as tics. They may consider playing with a paper clip or toying with an object as a tic, but obviously to qualify as a clinical problem, a tic must produce distress and be sufficiently uncontrollable. Playing with a paper clip can be stopped by focusing attention on it. Similarly, routines of the day such as tying shoe laces, driving to work, the way we walk or eat a sandwich are automated habits and may even become endearing or irritating personal characteristics, but they are essentially under voluntary control and we can change them with practice in the same way that we can learn other motor skills (eg., sport activities) through practice. Of course, where habits are motivated by fear or strongly held self-interest or are tied to pleasurable sensory states, they may be more difficult to change.

The paradox of tics is that they take place in voluntary muscles. The muscles concerned with regulating heart rate, breathing or other autonomic functions are not considered to produce tics. So tics occur in muscles used usually for voluntary control, and yet they appear non-voluntary; not only non-voluntary but often undetected by the person. Here again we have another paradox since although at the time they occur, tics are non-voluntary and often non-conscious, the urge to tic can be wilfully mentally suppressed or physically held in for often considerable periods of time. Although some simple tics resemble neurological spasms, more complex tics can resemble complex, willful actions. A man feels compelled to stand up and adjust his shoulders back and forth for five minutes to an exact frequency and symmetry in order to feel just right. Is this a tic, a habit or a compulsion? It is not surprising that tics have caused diagnostic problems.

De Groot, Janus and Bornstein (1995), in a study of 20 symptoms in 92 children and adolescents, extracted five factors accounting for 63% of the variance and which were labeled in order of importance "aggressive movements", "oro-facial contractions", "body movements", "peripheral movements and simple phonic tics", and finally "complex motor and phonic tics". Alsobrook and Pauls (2002) conducted a factor analysis of 29 symptoms in 85 cases of TS and found a four-factor solution adequate to account for 61% of the variance. The factors grouped symptoms respectively into "temper fits and aggression", "motor and phonic tics", "compulsive behaviors" and "absence of grunting and the presence of tapping". However, the clusters in both these studies may reflect the peculiar diversity of the sample and not be stable clusters of symptoms for TS in general. In vocal tics, it is usually the content which determines complexity – a repeated sentence or phrase being considered complex, whereas a single sound or word, even if lasting a long time, would be simple. The status of sensory tics is more controversial, with some arguing that they are precursors to motor tics rather than a sensory phenomenon in themselves. One form of tic, mental or cognitive, is often underdiagnosed and poorly understood. These tics are frequently confused with obsessions or ruminations since the person repeats a song or a phrase or a scene over and over mentally. But in fact they have more in common with other tics than with obsessions.

► COMORBIDITY AND COVARIATION

One problem with subtyping by symptoms is that there is often a lot of covariation between simple and complex tics and also habit disorders. In TS, multiple tics are frequently found together with other behavioral and attentional problems, such as attention deficit and hyperactivity disorder (ADHD) (Knell & Comings, 1993).

The comorbidity of a tic disorder with OCD varies across studies between 25 and 63%. But where OCD occurs with either TS or TD, the tics and obsessions seem to develop independently (Swedo & Leonard, 1994). In the case of tic-related OCD, the compulsions seem to resemble more sensory-based rituals, and raises the question as to whether such rituals are better classified as impulsive than compulsive (see Table 1.2). George et al. (1990) have developed a clinical questionnaire with some clinical face validity to distinguish the sensory-based types from other compulsions. Although TDs do not seem to have any greater psychiatric comorbidity than normal, there is considerable concern over concurrent behavioral disorders. Indeed, for many patients and their families, it is the accompanying behavioral disorders such as ADHD that cause many of the apparent deficits in TS. In particular, severity of tic symptoms has been positively related to behavioral problems. There have also been tentative suggestions that TS may share comorbidity with

Table 1.2   Sensory compulsions

- Touching objects
- Touching self
- Stroking surfaces
- Repeated handling/fondling of objects or material
- Saying something to shock
- Imitating others' actions/words/sounds
- Self-stimulation/self-injury
- Impulsive sexual gestures
- Repeating an action just for the feel
- Running a violent scene or act repeatedly over in the head to be excited
- Crumpling up or destroying objects for the feel or sound
- Adjusting body parts to produce sensations/stimulation or to "feel" right

Source: Inspired by George et al. (1990). Obsessions in obsessive-compulsive disorder with and without Gilles de la Tourette's syndrome. *American Journal of Psychiatry,* **150** (1), 93–97.

bipolar disorder and schizophrenia. This comorbidity issue is particularly important in children where the presence of both TS and OCD may initiate behavioral disturbances such as rage syndrome. The relationship between childhood and adult comorbidities also remains uncertain. For example, the literature on adult manifestations of hyperactivity is sparse (Lamberg, 2003).

▶ SECONDARY DISTRESS

Tics are rarely life-threatening except in rare cases where they may provoke auto-mutilation. Some complex tics can be quite severe and self-mutilating and involve head banging, eye gouging, neck dislocation. Even in the absence of mutilation, psychosocial distress in TD and TS can be considerable and can involve secondary phobias, depressions and social anxieties and worries over self-image, very low self-esteem and relationship problems. In our assessment of the interference of TD and HD in daily activities (see Appendix 1d), we found cases of unemployment, marital conflict, interpersonal difficulties, strained work relations, self-imposed travel restrictions, anxiety attending social or public functions, performance worries (e.g., about driving, speaking, teaching, dancing, sport), all of which were perceived (by the affected person) to be a result of the tic habit (O'Connor et al., 2001b). People with tics often experience low self-esteem and are (or become) hyperattentive to the judgment of others with consequent low self-satisfaction (Thibert et al., 1995). In TD, ironically, the very anticipation of experiencing a negative self-evaluation can provoke the tic (see later section).

▶ PREVALENCE

The incidence of TS in adults is about 0.1–1%. Estimates of TS in children have been as high as 3% with an increase to 28% in special needs group (see Robertson, 2000, for review). The lifetime prevalence of TD is not known but estimates vary between 5% and 10% of the population, with estimates of 18% in child populations (Mason et al., 1998). In an epidemiological study of the Quebec population, O'Connor et al. (1998) found a self-report rate of 8% lifetime prevalence. Other recent estimates have placed the prevalence of TS at 1% and TD at 10% of the population (Robertson, 2001; Robertson & Stern, 2000). There are, however, problems with clinical estimates of prevalence. Fallon and Schwab-Stone (1992) pinpointed several methodological shortcomings in evaluating comorbidity studies of TD, in particular sample selection bias (e.g., the clinician's illusion springing from the use of clinical, not community, samples). Identifying cases through self-report can also be problematic, especially if people are misinformed about tics, or employ a commonsense definition.

Tics develop in childhood and simple tics usually precede more complex tics, with phonic tics usually developing which will often begin as breathing or sniffing noises subsequent to motor and sensory tics. The most notorious TS vocal tic, coprolalia (swearing), is rare. In our adult TS samples, only 5.4% show any such verbalizations.

Goldenberg et al. (1994) reported a prevalence of 8%. Kurlan (1992) estimates that coprolalia or copropraxia (obscene gestures) are maximal during adolescence and decline with age. Interestingly, one of our TS clients in Quebec with coprolalia, who was perfectly bilingual (English, French), would swear in whatever language he was speaking at the time. Since the lexical content of swear words is very different in English (bodily parts or functions) and French (religious symbols), clearly it is the act of swearing, and not the words, that is important. There is some evidence that TS with coprolalia have easier or less inhibited access to scatological vocabulary (Stip et al., 1999).

Leckman et al. (1998) note a 10-fold higher prevalence of TS in children than in adults, with a peak of the worst period even at age 10 with mean onset at age 5.6 years. Of their sample of 42 TS patients, they note that, at age 18, over half were tic-free. They also suggest that the course of tics can be modeled to fit normal maturational processes. Approximately 15% of children develop transitory tics, of which 80% show spontaneous remission. Tics can develop as learned habits or by mimicry, and often in TS they will displace themselves around the body.

Although the type of tics may not differ between children and adults, associated problems differ. Learning difficulties in children and adolescents seem predictive of peripheral tics and phonic tics, and in children tics are frequently associated with rage and aggressive movements. Robertson et al. (1989) noted that 33% of TS patients showed automutilating behaviors such as head hitting, self-wounding and fist beating and this mostly in adolescents. Gilles de la Tourette (1885), in his original case series, reported a case of automutilation in a boy of 14 who chewed his lips.

► RELATIONSHIP OF TICS WITH OTHER DISRUPTIVE BEHAVIORS

Several clinical studies have reported an association of tic severity and behavioral disturbance but others fail to find a connection. The reason for the discrepancy may be that other conditions such as ADHD are not taken into account. Sukhodolosky et al. (2003), for example, reported that while TS did not differ from controls on gestures of aggression and disruption, those with TS + ADHD were significantly higher on measures of aggression and disruption. ADHD is a controversial diagnosis and needs to be distinguished from simple motor restlessness. Zapella (2002) reported a series of cases with early onset TS and reversible autistic behavior, where the initially autistic-type behavior reversed as a result of emotional and behavioral interaction and shared emotional experience with parents, while the tics developed into full-blown TS. The authors note that the children were over-sensitive and the parents also had tics. Kerbeshian and Burd (2003) reported that TS is a positive prognostic indicator in autism. Other have suggested evidence of comorbidity of TS with bipolar disorder (Kent & Craddock, 2003).

Coffey et al. (2000) tried to distinguish the impact of tic severity versus illness severity in children and adolescents with TS. Subjects were 156 consecutively referred children. Twelve per cent were hospitalized and though tic severity was a marginal predictor of hospitalization, major depression and bipolar disorder were more robust predictors even after adjustment for all other sociodemographic and clinical variables. Previous studies have shown that anxiety is strongly associated with tic severity. Depression is associated with greater dysfunction in TD. Although only a few reports have recognized the presence of bipolar disorder and TD, this comorbidity signals very poor prognosis.

Wilkinson et al. (2001) examined the impact of TS with and without comorbid disorder on family life, using the family impact scale (FIS). There was significant positive correlation between the number of comorbid behavior disorders and FIS. Other studies have examined comorbidity of TS and schizophrenia. Müller et al. (2002) point to an overlap of symptoms between schizophrenia and TS, including motor/vocal symptoms, echolalia, echopraxia and repetitive stereotypical movements or bizarre gestures and grimaces. They describe five cases, mainly delusional, where the initial presence of TD was associated in later life, mainly with psychotic anxiety. Of course tics can arise as a consequence of neuroleptic administration (Tardive Tourette Syndrome).

▶ DISTINGUISHING IMPULSIONS AND COMPULSIONS: SENSORY TICS, COGNITIVE TICS AND OBSESSIONS

Shapiro and Shapiro (1992) have argued that sensory preoccupations are not to be confused with obsessions since there seems to be no logic to the preoccupation. Cognitive content would appear to be a key distinguishing feature of tics and rituals. On the face of it, tics are involuntary impulsive purposeless movements whereas OCD is characterized by the presence of intrusive thoughts. Miguel et al. (1995), in a study of intentions preceding OCD and TD, reported that whereas all 15 adults with OCD reported thoughts preceding rituals, only two out of 12 with TS reported thoughts, the remainder of the sample reporting sensations. The assumption implicit in this voluntary/non-voluntary, cognitive/non-cognitive distinction between tics and rituals is that no cognitive activity precedes tic onset, but tics do not occur in a void and a sensory sensation or premonitory urge frequently precipitates the tic. This sensation is frequently associated with tension in the surrounding muscle area. Leckman et al. (1993) reported that 93% of a sample of 135 people with tics aged 8–71 reported premonitory urges prior to the tic and this, according to the authors, challenged the conventional wisdom that tics are involuntary. Chee and Sachdev (1997) studied 50 TS patients, 50 OCD patients and 50 healthy controls to determine the prevalence and phenomenology of sensory tics. The authors attempted to distinguish sensory tics (experienced as transient, recurrent, localizable and close to the skin) from urges (experiences as a drive preceding a behavioral response, conscious, not localizable and suppressible). The sensory tics in both the TS and OCD groups were predominantly located in rostral anatomical sites. The lifetime prevalence of sensory tics in the TS group was 28%, compared to 10% in the OCD group and 8% in the controls. The authors conclude that sensory tics are a separate tic phenomena independent of motor tics and seem to be a common feature of TS and a subgroup of OCD predisposed to tics. It is not clear if this sensation serves as a warning, a precipitator or is, in fact, part of the tic, since the sensation can persist even when treatment alleviates the actual tic movement. One possible interpretation of sensory tics is that they represent the subjectively experienced component of neural dysfunction below the threshold for motor or vocal tic production (Chee & Sachdev, 1997). Kane (1994) has suggested that the urges represent a heightened attention to physical sensations, and that a particularly heightened sensitivity of the person with tics to somatic sensation produces an attentional focus which provokes the tic. O'Connor (2002) has suggested that the premonitory sensation may be a product of both cognitive and sensory factors (see Figure 2.2).

Cath et al. (1992a) have introduced the notion of a "cognitive tic" as a means of clarifying some of the confusion between intrusive mental impulses and obsessional ruminations. The distinguishing factor between "cognitive tics" and "ruminations", according to Cath et al. (1992a), is that the latter are impulsive with no rationale behind them, whereas ruminations are driven by an aversive ego-dystonic content. So apparent meaningful thought or rational self-statements may be examples of mental or "cognitive" tics, rather than obsessions. Even if intrusive thoughts are complex, their unwanted appearance may still be impulsive rather than intentional, and some intrusions may be a more complex version of cognitive tics. Both cognitive tics and obsessions need also to be distinguished from cognitive rituals. These are mental operations such as wiping away or suppressing or substituting intrusive thoughts as a way of neutralizing their impact. Mental neutralization is equivalent to the overt neutralization of compulsive rituals.

The "just right" phenomenon is a label applied to compulsions such as arranging books, or performing symmetrical movements, which seem to lack an obsessional precursor other than the need for everything to be "just right". According to Leckman et al. (1994/1995), it is a complex mix of high activation, sensory-perceptual sensitivity, doubting and repetitive action. This phenomenon could fall into the category of "cognitive tic" in the sense that the content is cognitive but the relief is experienced predominantly as a sensory fulfillment, and there are no external consequences. However, a careful psychological evaluation is necessary to effect such a differential diagnosis since although there may not be observable physical consequences to the "just right" ritual, there may be consequences for self-image and how the person feels about themselves if things are not "just right".

The notion of impulsivity and compulsivity as separate and opposing parts of a spectrum have come under close scrutiny. Firstly, the terms are vaguely defined and may be confusing states with traits. A trait of impulsivity includes a range of antisocial behaviors, not just a single impulsive action. Generally speaking, people with TS or TD do not have higher impulsivity than normal (Summerfeldt et al., 2004). The distinction between impulsive and compulsive actions might profit from an alternative division into automated (fast responses with minimal thinking) versus more controlled responses, which comprise in different degrees different stages of all actions. Here an impulsive act might be an automatic action, and a compulsive act more carefully controlled, but the difference is at the level of the act, not the personality trait (Table 1.3).

Table 1.3   Cognitive-behavioral differences between TS and OCD

Tics in Tourette's syndrome	OCD rituals
Action not goal-directed and regulates "feel" and sensery release	Action goal-directed and aims to neutralize obsessional doubt and anxiety
High chronic level of peripheral and central motor activation (e.g., muscle tension)	Normal arousal except under conditions of stress hyperfunctionality in cognitive/attentional systems
Distinct tics can substitute for each other	Distinct rituals rarely substitute for one another
Onset linked to behavioral activity and tension	Onset linked to intrusive thoughts
Predominant emotion at tic onset is frustration/impatience/dissatisfaction	Predominant emotion preceding compulsive activity is anxiety
Perfectionism in personal organization and personal standards	Perfectionism concerns doubts about actions, concern over mistakes
Over-active style of planning action	Normal style of planning action but more effortful
Respond to awareness training and relaxation therapy	Do not respond to relaxation and awareness training

Source: Adapted from O'Connor (in press) Contrasting Tourette's Syndrome and tic disorders with OCD. In: Abramowitz & Moats (eds), *Handbook of Controversial Issues in Obsessive-Compulsive Disorder*. Kluwer Academic Press.

Shapiro and Shapiro (1986) argued that it is precisely the confusion between impulsion and compulsion that results in erroneous rates of comorbidity between OCD and TD. Impulsions, according to Shapiro and Shapiro (1986), give pleasure – feelings of guilt and regret only arising later – whereas compulsions cause anxiety and tension. Shapiro's distinction between the impulsive-type rituals found in TS and the "genuine" compulsions of OCD has been incorporated into the clinical questionnaire mentioned earlier and designed to distinguish TS-type compulsions from OCD compulsions (George et al., 1990). The TS rituals, according to George et al. (1990), tend to be ego-syntonic, impulsive and directed to the self, whereas obsessional compulsions are more elaborate, ego-dystonic and world-directed actions like cleaning or checking (see Table 1.2 on p. 5).

Cath et al. (2001a, 2001d) have carried out a series of studies aimed to distinguish TS/TD from OCD symptoms. A factor analysis ($n = 92$) of TS/TD, OCD ± TD and OCD only revealed distinct compulsive and impulsive factors. The OCD group scored higher on the compulsive factor, and the TS/TD group scored higher on the impulsive factor. When OCD − TD were compared to OCD + TD, the former scored higher on obsessionality. TS/TD patients reported more echophenomena, trichotillomania, touching, symmetry behavior, self-injurious behaviors, but less checking, repeating and rumination. Self-injurious or aggressive thoughts were experienced as non-anxiety-related. The OCD patients reported more washing behavior. Müller et al. (1997) reported echophenomena to be predictive of TS in 56%

of cases when compared to OCD. Cath et al. (2001a) found that the presence of touching behaviors accurately predicted diagnosis of TS in 77% of cases and echophenomena predicted 83% of TS. OCD and TS groups may have similar thoughts but TS patients show more playfulness with their thoughts, while those with OC show more anxiety. Shapiro et al. (1988) have argued that repetitive thoughts and actions in TS patients are performed automatically as a consequence of a failure to restrain impulses and are not anxiety-related. A questionnaire designed by George et al. (1990) explicitly distinguishes the sensory-based overt and covert rituals of TS patients from the more intentional obsessions of OCD patients. Cath et al. (2001d) also note the importance of distinguishing cognitive tics from mental obsessions. Cognitive tics are playful and are usually aimed at tension reduction rather than harm avoidance.

► EMOTIONAL ASSOCIATIONS

Tics in common parlance are considered "nervous" tics, but the associated emotions at the time of tic onset are mainly frustration, impatience and dissatisfaction rather than anxiety (O'Connor et al., 1993). Although a recent study did report a correlation between the number of tics and self-reported anxiety level (Woods et al., 1996b), people with TD are not more neurotic as measured by the *Eysenck Personality Inventory* (O'Connor et al., 1997a).

Although the literature specifically addressing self-esteem is sparse, one speculative hypothesis may be that clients with TD are preoccupied by how they are perceived by others, and clients with OCD have a more pervasive lack of self-confidence and are preoccupied more by their performance in general in the world. The difference noted above in the type of OCD rituals experienced in those with TS + OCD and those with just OCD suggests less fear of consequences in TS. The TS + OCD group seem to experience less contamination and washing rituals and more symmetry and ordering.

The client with TD rarely has concerns about performance efficacy, but seems overly preoccupied by the judgment of others about his or her appearance and self-image (O'Connor et al., 1993). Christensen et al. (1993) have noted that in other impulsive disorders (e.g., compulsive buying), the person's self-esteem seems to depend unduly on the response of others.

Thibert et al. (1995) reported that clients with TS and OCD had a higher degree of self-consciousness coupled with social anxiety than clients with TS without OCD. But both groups had low self-satisfaction and self-esteem. In TD, unlike in OCD, the very thought of experiencing a negative self-evaluation can provoke the tic. Watson and Sterling (1998) note in the functional analysis of a case of a vocal tic that social attention was a precipitating factor. On the other hand, in OCD, it is often the self-oriented interpretations placed on the obsession, e.g., that the person should control it or should not have such thoughts, that may maintain the obsession (Clark, 2004).

A key distinction between tics and OCD compulsions is the emotional experience at the time of doing the tic or OCD ritual. A person with an impulsion experiences pleasure from the deed (Hoogduin, 1986), whereas someone committing a compulsive act experiences anxiety and tension which is temporarily relieved by the neutralization. Shapiro and Shapiro (1986) originally noted that impulsions give pleasure, with feelings of guilt and regret only arising later. Cath et al. (1992a) found that the key differentiator between OCD and TS was indeed "felt emotion". Clients with OCD, according to these authors, always found thoughts unpleasant, whereas clients with TS often felt a relief from tension, and even a neutrally affective playfulness after the tic. The evolution of emotion in simple tics tends to follow the pattern of immediate frustration and tension, with the tic inducing temporary short-term relief from tension but leading finally to renewed tension.

In a habit disorder, clients can report a clear sense of activation during the hair pulling (King et al., 1995). There may be a neurochemical basis for suggesting that tic movements affect the person in a milder but similar way to stimulants, such as nicotine, and may both act on the catecholamine system (O'Connor, 1989; Peterson et al., 1994). There is some evidence of substitution between cigarette smoking and tics. Tics *can* become more intense after smoking cessation (Peterson et al., 1994) and nicotine procalix has been found somewhat effective in reducing tic frequency (McConville & Norman, 1992; Richards, 1992). Sanberg et al. (1997) suggest that transdermal nicotine could serve as an effective aid to neuroleptic medication in TS.

Miele et al. (1990) have argued that a number of behavioral syndromes, especially compulsive and impulsive disorders, appear to share descriptive similarities with chemical dependence. Availability of alternative rewards to replace the tic-induced stimulation seems crucial to success in relapse prevention and even more so in the treatment of HD such as hair pulling (Azrin & Peterson, 1988a, 1988b). The next sections discuss, in more detail, differences in psychological management strategies.

▶ SELF-MANAGEMENT STRATEGIES

The problem behavior is self-managed and resisted in TD. Self-management strategies employed in TD serve the same purpose of suppression, delaying or disguising the problem behavior and are counterproductive in producing both increased tension and desire to perform the tic/ritual. Clients with TD are capable of suppressing tics completely for shorter or longer intervals. The most common strategies adopted are: tensing of muscles antagonistic to the tic muscles which can block the movement; tensing of the general area where the tic takes place; changing posture, suppressing or delaying onset; attempting to hide the tic by disguising it with another movement (see Wojcieszek & Lang, 1995). The result of these strategies is often extreme discomfort and an increased desire to tic, but the tic is temporarily impeded and so the outward impression is one of normality. Although the difficulty of suppression varies between clients in TD, the counterproductive effect is similar. If, instead of suppression, the person is encouraged to step back and let the urge flow by unimpeded and without censure, some of the associated sensation is alleviated. Relaxing muscles instead of tensing them to resist the tic can alleviate tension in TD (O'Connor et al., 1995, 1997b). Awareness training by itself can be an effective self-management strategy in TD (Woods et al., 1996a; Wright & Miltenberger, 1987). The person with tics *may* be able to carry on daily life unaware of the tic (Rosenberg et al., 1994). Successful management also depends on the situations in which the problem occurs, as revealed by functional analysis.

▶ COPING STRATEGIES MAINTAINING THE TIC CYCLE

The person's own model of tic development, management and consequences is an important influence on the anticipations and coping reactions to the tic. Clients may subscribe to a hydraulic model of tic management (for example, "If I keep it in, it will build up and I'll have to let it out later one way or another since I can't contain it"). The person then adopts behavioral strategies which amplify this hydraulic sentiment and so confirm its validity by, for example, accepting the interpretation that detection of the premonitory urge means that a tic is imminent (Leckman et al., 1993, p. 102). As discussed earlier, it is not clear if this premonitory urge precedes or follows the anticipation of a tic, and hence whether the urge results from an attempt to deal with the tic, or is an independent warning sign. Other appraisals relate to how the person feels the tic will be received and appraised by others in the situation. These appraisals may raise arousal and may explain how, in some cases, just the anticipation of ticcing can raise tension and frustration and hence, by itself, provoke a tic.

Behavioral strategies adopted to cope with tic behavior divide into: *containment, correction* and *concealment*. *Containment* would include tensing, holding in or adopting a posture to contain the tic, such as lying down, or contracting the muscle to attempt an informal competing response. *Correction* includes actively occupying the muscle by integrating the tic into an action, or trying to normalize the tic action by modifying its course, or actively converting it into another movement. *Concealment* would include disguising the tic by wearing baggy clothes, carrying a bag over the shoulder, masking the tic through performing a larger act (e.g., sneezing), or finally by avoidance of tic-evoking situations (see Appendix 1h). These gestures fulfill the same role as neutralization, avoidance or coping strategies in other anxiety disorders and effectively reinforce apprehensions about ticcing and so maintain the tension level (see Figure 1.1).

▶ FUNCTIONAL ANALYSIS AND SITUATIONAL VARIABILITY

The circumstances eliciting tics and habits are the overall state, or mood, or situations (or anticipations about situations) in which people find themselves. Christensen et al. (1993) noted a series of emotional precursors to onset of hair pulling. Azrin and Nunn (1977) recognized that different strategies need to be applied in habit reversal depending on different situations. Several authors have

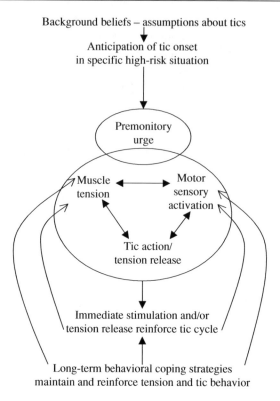

Figure 1.1   Self-reinforcing cognitive-behavioral tic cycle

noted that tics and habits are elicited by negative states, including depression, lack of self-worth and boredom (Dean et al., 1992). In a clinical context, functional analysis is frequently employed to clarify the antecedents and consequences reinforcing tic behavior (e.g., Carr et al., 1996; Fuata & Griffiths, 1992; Scotti et al., 1994). However, few studies have systematically examined situational factors.

In a series of studies examining situational variables, O'Connor et al. (1993, 1994) initially monitored high-, medium- and low-risk situations in 13 clients with tics and found that the clients showed idiosyncratic situation profiles, *but* that these profiles showed little consistency across clients (Table 1.4). All subjects identified situations when the tic occurred and when it did not occur. High-risk situations could be either high- or low-arousal situations – for example, one client was most likely to tic when active at work, another when relaxing at home. However, this situational blurring was clarified when considering cognitive constructs underlying the situations, since whatever the physical activity level, the accompanying thoughts and feelings most frequently concerned impatience and frustration and not performing as desired. These findings of a cognitive and situational profile have been replicated in subsequent studies (O'Connor et al., 1997a, 1997b) (see Chapter 4). Anticipation of a high-risk tic situation can by itself elicit the tic, suggesting a strong potential role of cognitions (and cognitive appraisal processes) in tic production.

Table 1.4   Examples of low- and high-risk situations for tic onset plus associated construct dimensions in 10 people with chronic TD

	Low-risk situations	High-risk situations	Principal personal construct dimension
1	Occupied, working, cooking	Preparing for bed, passenger in car	Mobility versus immobility
2	Lying down/relaxing	Arguing or expressing disagreement	Self-image projected as unimportant versus fear of being rejected or judged in bad light
3	Singing, housework	Driving, speaking to people	Bored-automatic tasks versus stimulated concentration
4	Typing, reading at home	A busy day when there are lots of meetings with a tight agenda	Free choice, time for herself versus obligations required by others
5	Speaking with friends, shopping	Reading, watching TV, reflecting on preoccupations	Well occupied versus wasting time
6	Listening to music, drawing	Searching for an idea, waiting for something/someone	Feeling valued and reassured versus fear of judgment, making error in public
7	Reading, watching TV	When hands are occupied, when teaching	One thing at a time, undemanding, relaxed, versus over-stimulated, too many activities
8	Reading, being massaged	As a passenger in a car, arguing with spouse	Secure, relaxed versus concentrated, tense
9	Working, shopping with friends	Watching TV or reading alone in the house, getting ready for work	Active with others versus inactive alone
10	Cooking, knitting	Unexpected guests, thinking of financial difficulties	Self-image important versus self-image unimportant

Source: From O'Connor et al. (1994). Personal constructs amongst chronic tic sufferers. *British Journal of Clinical Psychology* **13**(2), 151–158.

Several studies have suggested that phonic tics in particular might be contingent on activities rather than stimulus conditions. Roane et al. (2002), in an insightful functional analysis of a young man's vocal tics, examined a number of reinforcement contingencies that might reveal cues for the verbal tic. These included environmental factors: when alone, task demand, play, automatic reinforcement, preference objects, tangible, musical, auditory, oral stimulation. However, none seemed consistently related to tic onset. Naturalistic observation revealed that posture was more related, as tics were absent when lying down but more present in an upright position. The authors conclude that the tic was autoreinforcing but do not explore the significance of lying down as a strategy for the patient. The authors report they were unable to determine the mechanism behind the attenuation of the tic when lying down, but they emphasize the limitations of analyses restricted to environmental analysis and preference analysis of stimulation cues.

Carr et al. (1996) found no stimulus contingency for a vocal tic in an 11-year-old male student. However, it seemed exacerbated when he was spoken to disapprovingly or when he was allowed to escape academic study. Watson and Sterling (1998) found a vocal tic related to eating and social activity. Woods et al. (2001) reported a controlled study showing that talking, in particular about tics, increased the likelihood of vocal but not motor tics.

► CONCLUSIONS

In this chapter, we have defined tics and described the difficulties in differential diagnosis, their clinical phenomenology and associations. Tics can cause very serious impediments in everyday functioning and are not simply idiosyncratic eccentricities. TS is the most severe form of TD and includes phonic tics, but management problems for TS, particularly in children, seem mainly due to the presence of comorbidities which can provoke other problems in functioning. TD can be considered on a continuum from a single monosymptomatic tic to multiple complex and simple tics, but currently diagnosis is categorical, although tics can be assessed dimensionally and also be typed by their anatomical location or by their form and content. Tics are paradoxical in that they affect voluntary muscles, yet appear non-voluntary. Indeed, it appears that tics cannot really be considered as non-voluntary since they can be mentally and physically controlled. They are impulsive, often non-conscious productions which can also be resisted and withheld. They can change location or stay the same over many years, yet clearly they peak in childhood and in some cases seem related to the maturational cycle and disappear during adolescence. Tics are clearly distinct from OCD rituals and HD and yet there is covariation and comorbidity among these disorders. Although the tic does look and feel like an uncontrollable impulse, the relation between TD and other impulsive traits is uncertain and behavioral and cognitive factors play a role in onset. In the next chapter, we examine in more detail theories about the origins of tics.

Chapter 2

UNDERSTANDING TIC DISORDERS: ETIOLOGICAL MODELS

▶ OVERVIEW OF NEUROBIOLOGICAL MODELS

Current clinician consensus is that TS and, by implication, TD are neurobiological disorders (Leckman & Cohen, 1999). The nature of these disorders is either a difficulty inhibiting sensory urges or a difficulty inhibiting behavior due to problems in neurochemical modulation affecting cortical–subcortical areas.

One hypothesis, that of a structural deficit, is mostly derived from lesions studies and from studies of actual basal ganglia dysfunction which produce motor impairment (see Peterson et al., 1999). Parallels have been drawn between TD and basal ganglia dysfunction disorders such as Huntington's chorea, but there is no firm evidence of common structural deficit. Judith Rapoport, in a 1990 editorial, pursues the hypothesis that Parkinson's disease, Sydenham's chorea, OCD and other movement disorders are traceable to basal ganglia dysfunction. The evidence for the argument is drawn largely from studies where direct lesions of the basal ganglia produce behavior that resembles TS or OCD. But, as she notes, much clinical information contradicts the hypothesis including the efficacy of behavior therapy. Casey et al. (2002) present a model of neurocognitive control, whereby the basal ganglia are involved in the inhibition of competing actions, while the frontal cortex represents the relevant thoughts guiding selective behavior. Casey et al. (2002) suggest that the ability to support information against competing sources increases with age as a result of development of the thalamocortical loops, so explaining the maturational trend of tics to diminish with age. Another hypothesis, that tics result from increased motor neuron firing which induces clonus-like activity (e.g., Smith & Lees, 1989), remains speculative, and in any case lacks specificity to TS/TD. An alternative speculation that tic behavior (and OCD) may result from an abnormality in the neural basis of innate motor routines (e.g., Knowlton et al., 1996) relies overly on linking tics and rituals to species-specific innate behavior. There is no consistent evidence of any uniform structural deficit in TS. However, there is evidence of differences in brain functioning.

Functional magnetic resonance imaging (fMRI) studies (Biswal et al., 1998) have shown an over-activation of the sensorimotor and supplementary motor area and recruitment of larger portions of these areas in five patients with TS during the execution of a finger-tapping task. In a very comprehensive and well-controlled study of brain imaging in TS, Bradley Peterson and collaborators compared 154 TS patients with 130 controls (Peterson et al., 2003). They found the volume of the caudate nucleus decreased across all TS age groups. Neuroleptic medication seemed to reverse these decreases in volume. However, asymmetries reported in previous smaller case studies were not replicated. In addition, there was no relationship between decreased volume and tic symptom severity, and the authors note that it is possible that the findings may be due to chronic compensatory responses to the presence of tics. Peterson et al. (2003) also note that the basal ganglia cannot be considered independently of other brain regions in understanding symptom severity and diversity. Cortical functional differences may result from functional compensation of the brain to tic suppression. A plausible hypothesis, in this vein, is that the need to suppress tics produces striatal hypermetabolism, and that compensatory mechanisms may even lead to larger orbitofrontal and parietal brain adaptations (Peterson, 2001; Peterson et al., 1999). But longitudinal studies are necessary to establish this link. Electrophysiological studies support functional impairment in inhibition.

▶ NEUROPHYSIOLOGICAL STUDIES

In the few studies looking at electrophysiological indices from scalp-recorded EEG, the general finding when looking at early sensory-related evoked potential components to stimuli across modality is either: higher amplitude and faster latency than controls, hence implying heightened sensory reactivity; or no difference with controls (Johannes et al., 2001). The amplitude of responses seems exacerbated when the task is simple, and there seems less attention to relevant rare stimuli with lower accompanying amplitude of early attention-related negative components in auditory oddball or visual pop-out tasks (Johannes et al., 1997; van Woerkom et al., 1994). TS also seem to invest more additional attentional effort than controls to achieve the same results on simple tasks but make more errors on complex ones (Johannes et al., 1997, 2001).

Several electrophysiological studies have demonstrated that patients with TS have problems allocating attentional resources, using appropriate attentional effort and monitoring stimuli long enough and appropriately enough for successful error correction (e.g., Johannes et al., 2002). Clients with TS also seem disproportionately affected by dual task performance where the second task is a competing complex task. Johannes et al. (2001) reported that people with TS had more problem dividing attention between a visual and an auditory task, as shown in less difference in elicited cortical evoked potentials related to divided task evaluation. Interestingly, when the second task is a routine repetitive task, this may aid performance in TS. Frequently, people with TS report anecdotally that they pay attention better after sports activity, or when they are stimulated by other movement or distraction.

Several studies have shown an augmentation in frontal negativity during the later evoked potential components, perhaps delaying the later stages of inhibition and decision making. This frontal negativity reflects problems with inhibition and seems particularly present during sustained and focused attention (O'Connor, 1980). Inhibitory problems seem also to impede efficient action monitoring as reflected in difficulties terminating post-imperative frontal wave and bringing monitoring to resolution (Johannes et al., 2001).

It should be noted that in most of these evoked potential studies, the sampling confounded people with TS with other comorbidities such as ADHD. However, it is also of note that brain potential studies show for the most part that a negative going readiness potential signaling voluntary initiation of movement precedes tic onset (e.g. Karp et al., 1996), indicating that tics are at least semi-voluntary. Early excitatory components such as brain stem potentials are normal in TS, thus indicating few problems with sensory pathways. There is some evidence that people with TS and ADHD show less pre-pulse inhibition to an excitatory startle response, indicating difficulties in sensorimotor gating and sensory inhibition (Castellanos et al., 1996).

▶ **Cortical Inhibitory Functions**

Electrophysiological evidence suggests that patients with TS have no problems initiating GO reaction to stimuli but inhibit STOP signals in a different way. In particular, they seem to show a more anterior distribution of the readiness potential, suggesting less controlled preparation (Duggal & Haque Nizamie, 2002; Johannes et al., 2001; Karp et al., 1996).

O'Connor et al. (1999, 2000), using a countermanding [GO–STOP] paradigm, found no difference in psychomotor speed between TD groups and non-tic controls, but the authors did find that participants with TD showed more difficulty when inhibiting an automated than a controlled response and the tic group also showed no practice effect on performance over trial blocks. Ziemann et al. (1997) also reported evidence of normal motor threshold and excitability but a reduced or impaired motor inhibition in patients with TS, and likewise Georgiou et al. (1997) found no impairment in those with TS during fast, goal-directed movements. The presence of high activation could impact on movement inhibition.

These motor inhibition problems may themselves, however, be due to a strategy rather than deficit. For example, distraction from tics, or hyperactivity or tic suppression, could affect performance (Channon et al., 1992; Silverstein et al., 1995). Motor differences between adult TS/TD groups and controls, for example, on the Purdue Pegboard, can decrease following behavioral treatment (O'Connor et al., 2001c) (see Chapter 4).

Goh et al. (2002) studied the inhibition of expected movement in Tourette's syndrome. They examined responses under different states of attentional control, namely during attention focus, shift and sustained attention. In 10 age–sex matched TS patients and controls, the TS patients were slower at executing pre-programming of movements for both direction or distance. Goh et al. (2002) suggest that motor deficits in TS may lie at the level of movement preparation or initiation, not execution. The deficit in TS may not be one of "pure" simple inhibition since, in general,

TS patients are able to inhibit irrelevant distraction. Rather the problem may be a more subtle motor disorder exacerbated under increased task demand with perhaps a problem in the fine interplay between attentional and motor aspects of the task demand.

Although such problems with inhibition could be subserved by orbitofrontal–subcortical circuits, differences could indicate functional rather than structural deficit and spring from adoption of a particular information-processing style. Thibault et al. (2004) reported a more active early attentional component in TD but a smaller later memory updating component, so indicating that over-investment in attentional resources may impede later response resolution. The selective problems in inhibition in TD may be a result of deliberate over-preparation which subsequently makes inhibition more difficult. Feelings of over-competitiveness may inhibit as well as enhance motor performance (Stanne et al., 1999).

▶ NEUROBIOLOGICAL TREATMENTS

The disruption of movement and involuntary tremor has been linked to the dopamine (DA) system, so both TS and TD could involve dysregulation of dopamine system. Elevated DA could be consistent with the state of heightened activation, noted above, in TS (Muller-Vahl et al., 2000). The hypothesis of elevated DA in TS/TD would seem particularly plausible given the presence of DA receptors, in cortical projections to frontal areas, thus supporting the link between DA and motor activation. DA neurons are also found in mid-brain structures such as the subtantia nigra, and this system projects to a variety of brain structures including frontal areas. Also, the DA hypothesis would be consistent with a brain-imaging study which found that TS patients showed significantly elevated right frontal activity compared with controls (George et al., 1992). There is, however, no difference between controls and TD/TS groups in baseline DA levels or DA turnover (see Anderson et al., 1999, for review), which has led investigators to propose more elaborate DA deficits such as disturbance in the balance of D_1 to D_2 receptors and differences in the number of DA transport sites. In fact, support for a hyperfunctional DA system comes principally from the limited success of treatment protocols using DA antagonists. But clinically speaking, not all patients improve as a result of neuroleptic administration (Regeur et al., 1986), and DA antagonists are not the only drug family of choice.

The initial drug of choice for those with TS, a low dosage of haloperidol, had the potential for unwanted extrapyramidal effects and noradrenergic side-effects. Consequently, pimozide is now preferred in terms of efficacy and, apart from increase weight gain and risk for depression, shows a more acceptable side-effect profile and good clinical response in some studies, but is contested in others (Sallee et al., 1997). Pimozide antagonizes DA receptors with selectivity for the D_1 DA subtype. Other DA agents antagonistic to presynaptic D_2 receptors similar to pimozide, such as pergolide, have shown benefit in TS patients (Griesemer, 1997). However, some of these DA agents show "tardive Tourette's" (i.e., paradoxical worsening of TS), secondary to neuroleptics. Atypical neuroleptics such as olanzapine have shown more favourable outcome and less side-effects in comparison to the more typical neuroleptics such as pimozide (Robertson & Stern, 2000). But it produces sedation, flat affect, tardive dyskinesia, and pro-longation of heart period. However, trials of DA *agonists* such as deprenyl and clonidine have shown efficacy in TS clients and alpha-2 adrenergic agonists such as quanfacine have also been reported to improve tic management (Chappell et al., 1995). On the other hand, stimulants such as methylphenidate (MPH) or dextroamphetamine are controversial, often showing initial worsening of motor tics while improving ADHD and disruptive behavior. However, recent evidence suggests that eventually, after 18 weeks, even stimulants may lead to improve-ment and a combination of MPH + clonidine may give the optimal effect (Kurlan, 2001). Although, given the short half-life, repeated daily dosing is necessary. Butolin toxin (Botox), which essentially impairs functional innervation of the mus-cle leading to temporary atrophy, has been reported useful in some cases of vocal tics when injected into vocal cords (Jankovic, 1997; Scott & Jankovic, 1996), but in other case studies, the urge to tic was not reduced and the voice is often affected; the tic was more often than not replaced with another tic (Carpenter et al., 1999, p. 380). Other pharmacotherapies which in single cases seem to have produced temporary relief from tics include: cannabinoids, nicotine, opiates, lithium, benzodiazepines, calcium antagonists, hormone therapy. The neurochemical picture becomes more complex in the light of differences between TS/TD groups and controls in other neurotransmitter systems such as GABA, serotonin and glutamate (Anderson et al., 1999).

Benzodiazepines such as Rivotril, which act on the GABA system, can often act as muscle relaxant and reduce tic frequency, but there is a risk of dependence. Serotonin depletion and DA excess may be part of a dual mechanism regulating activation. Desipramine and imipramine, which are tricyclic antidepressants, have been used in TD, particularly to control hyperactivity (Dion, 2004), as have selective serotonin uptake inhibitors such as venlafaxine and others usually given in OCD. Their effect on tics can be relatively rapid (2–3 days) compared to OCD and depres-sion. Also, they are frequently given as potentiators or boosters to help the efficacy of neuroleptics. The selective serotonin reuptake inhibitors (SSRIs) may carry a risk of increased suicidal ideation in those under 18 years. Serotonin has a large concentration in frontal areas and has been linked with motivational and mood fac-tors, in particular during stress, whereas DA may be more involved in reward and stimulation. So, effectively, the neurochemistry of TD may implicate both cortical and subcortical neurochemical factors, and hence both excitatory and inhibitory motor processes, exhibiting characteristics of disinhibition in their activation and impulsive reflex-like nature together with inhibition in the form of tension resisting or suppressing activity at the same time. Cath et al. (2001b) have suggested that the TS spectrum as opposed to the OC spectrum are less responsive to SSRIs and more responsive to selective noradrenaline reuptake inhibitors (SNRIs).

Psychopharmacological treatment regimes produce variable treatment response and the tics themselves are rarely eliminated by neuroleptics or other types of medication (Regeur et al., 1986). Double-blind placebo-controlled designs have found tic frequency reduced by about 50% using haloperidol or pimozide (Shapiro et al., 1989) and unwanted side-effects occur in about 80% of individuals. More recent double-blind controlled trials with risperidone report decreases in symptoms of 35% (Dion et al., 2002), 42% (Gilbert et al., 2004) and 56% (Bruggeman et al., 2001) but with significant dropout and side effects. According to Peterson and Azrin (1992), only about 20–30% continue their medication for an extended period of time. Single cases have reported use of diverse stereotactic surgical procedures with beneficial results including: limbic and frontal leucotomies, bilateral cerebellar dentatomy, ventrolateral thalamotomy and gamma capsulotomy. But long-term outcome in these surgical cases is not well documented (Rauch et al., 1995).

In summary, the neurobiological and neurochemical findings are puzzling and inconclusive, with a range of neurotransmitter systems seemingly involved in at least one successful case study treatment of TD/TS, including medications which are both agonist and antagonistic to DA (e.g., MPH). Hence, for a DA model of tics, clinical psychopharmacological support is equivocal. Even within the family of DA antagonists there are wide individual differences in response and there is no coherent theory as to why some neuroleptics are effective and some are not.

▶ PANDAS Infections

The acronym "PANDAS" (pediatric autoimmune neuropsychiatric disorders associated with streptococcal infections) is used to describe neuropsychiatric symptoms resulting from autoimmune responses to streptococcal infection in vulnerable children (Kleinsasser et al., 1999). It has been hypothesized that such patients have an immune process initiated by infection that affects the basal ganglia and causes OCD-like symptoms. A PANDAS may arise when antibodies directed against invading bacteria cross-react with basal ganglia structures, resulting in exacerbation of OCD or TD (Giedd et al., 1996). The hypothesis of PANDAS is that OCD occurs via a process analogous to Sydenham's chorea through infections with group A beta-hemolytic streptococci (GABHS), among others, which trigger autoimmune responses and cause or exacerbate cases of childhood-onset of OCD or TD. Trifiletti and Packard (1999) supported the presence of immune abnormalities in several neuropsychiatric disorders (TS, OCD and PANDAS). According to these researchers, there is a consensus that about 10% of people with TS and OCD have a clear streptococcal trigger, so supporting the PANDAS hypothesis.

Swedo et al. (1998) described the clinical characteristics of a group of 50 patients with OCD and TD in which symptom onset was triggered by GABHS infection in 44% of the children and by pharyngitis in 28%. This study characterized a homogeneous patient group where symptom exacerbation was triggered by GABHS infections. Among the 50 children, there were 144 separate episodes relating infection to symptom exacerbation: 31% were associated with the GABHS infection, 42% with symptoms of pharyngitis or respiratory infection and 4% with GABHS exposure. Lougee et al. (2000) reported that the rates of OCD in first-degree relatives of pediatric probands with PANDAS are higher than those reported in the general population. This study revealed that 26% of the probands had at least one first-degree relative with OCD, including mothers (19%), fathers (11%) and siblings (5%).

Findings in conflict with the PANDAS hypothesis have been obtained by Black et al. (1998), who tested the serum from 13 adult patients with OCD for panels of autoantibody markers of autoimmunity. Black et al. (1998) also investigated the frequency of neuron-specific auto-antibodies to determine if any of these might serve as a serological marker for adult OCD. Although most of their subjects had onset of OCD before 19 years of age or before puberty, the study revealed no evidence of autoimmunity involving any of the assayed antibodies.

If the hypothesis of PANDAS is sound, then immunological treatments should lead to decreased symptoms at least in some cases of OCD. Allen et al. (1995) studied four cases with abrupt, severe onset or worsening of OCD or tics post-infection and all had a clinically significant response immediately after antibiotic treatment. Garvey et al. (1999) proposed penicillin prophylaxis to prevent exacerbation of streptococcal-triggered neuropsychiatric symptoms. Nevertheless, findings demonstrated that there were an equal number of infections in both the active and placebo phases of this study. Based on their results, no conclusions can be drawn from prophylactic treatment in preventing tic or OCD symptoms exacerbation.

These contradictory results demonstrate that more research is needed to better understand this PANDAS mechanism. As Snider and Swedo (2003) note, many questions remain unanswered. At best, the PANDAS hypothesis can only apply to a subcategory of TD, since it does not explain how the tic symptoms appear in adults and children who have never experienced PANDAS during their childhood.

▶ GENETIC FACTORS

Essentially, the genetic model holds that there is a genetic vulnerability for TS/TD patients and penetrance is probably by an autosomal dominant gene tic transmission (although recent gene mapping suggests it may be more complex and heterogeneous [Pauls, 2001]). Although there does seem evidence of family pedigree, the criteria for inclusion in pedigree studies is often subsyndromal caseness (Fallon & Schwab-Stone, 1992). Pauls (1992) suggests that OCD may be the female expression and tics the male expression of the same genetic disorder and finds support for the claim in studies of proband relatives which indicated that male relatives were more likely to have TS or TD while females were more likely to have an OCD (Eapen et al., 1993). Pauls (1992) has, however, noted that some forms of OCD may not be related to TS, but that the patterns of inheritance of TS and OCD within the same families are consistent with the transmission of an autosomal dominant genetic locus with high penetrance. Leonard et al. (1992), who examined the lifetime and current prevalence of TS in child probands diagnosed as OCD and in their first-degree relatives, found a greater incidence of OCD in male relatives so countering Pauls' (1992) assertion that OCD may be the female expression, and tics the male expression of the same genetic disorder. McMahon et al. (1996) found no sex differences, and also noted that the tic severity of descendants was minimal. These authors found no correlation between the presence of OCD in individual relatives, and the appearance of OCD in a given proband, supporting again the assertion that even in TS with OCD, the tics and the OCD rituals develop independently. De Groot and Bornstein (1994; de Groot et al., 1995) found a correlation between Leyton Obsessional Inventory (LOI) symptoms in parents and their expression in the offspring. But, interestingly, they reported an asymmetry in their findings. If the focus was on TS probands, a high LOI score did not predict a high LOI score in the parents, but (contrary to the Yale study), high LOI scores of the parents did predict high LOI scores in the probands.

In the Yale Child Study Center studies (Leckman & Chittenden, 1990), statistical modeling of genetic transmission using segregation analysis gave penetrance rates high enough for an autosomal dominant hypothesis only if OCD, TS and TD were all included. Robertson and Gourdie (1990) agreed with the Yale study that the TS phenotype has to be broadened to include TD and OCD criteria of "caseness" if an autosomal dominant penetrance is to be supported, and even then the inheritance is incomplete.

Shapiro and Shapiro (1992) reported no overlap between OCD and TD or TS, and are of the opinion that the association between OCD and TS is spurious. Shapiro and Shapiro (1992) point to methodological limitations in studies demonstrating epidemiological and genetic associations, such as: the inclusion of over-general phenotypes, inadequate sampling techniques, unreliable diagnostic criteria, lack of blind evaluation, definitional confusion of what constitutes a tic, and the use of inappropriate controls. Obviously a blurring of phenotype boundaries between TS and OCD compromises findings of genetic linkage between the disorders.

In TS itself, genetic studies seem to favour an autosomal dominant mode of transmission with incomplete penetrance and variable expression (Eapen et al., 1997; Müller et al., 1995). Although even here there is no consensus, Barr and Sandors (1998), for example, state there is no convincing evidence of genetic linkage. Robertson and Stern (1998) note that the "presumed" genetic substrate in TS has not been identified, and as many as 35% of TS patients may not acquire the disorder genetically (Parraga et al., 1998). Genetic transmission of OCD, by contrast, while possibly familial, is more heterogeneous and there seems no equivalent pedigree in OCD to support a direct genetic influence of parental incidence of OCD on proband OCD (Pauls et al., 1995). As regards non-TS TD, there are not currently enough studies available to draw any conclusion on the mode, if any, of genetic transmission. Evidence is so far equivocal with Hyde and Weinberger (1995), arguing for a common genetic basis for all TD, whereas Brett et al. (1995) reported no evidence of common genetic variation between TS and TD.

► PSYCHOSOCIAL FACTORS

Perfectionism has been associated with parental rearing practices, in particular parental criticism and lack of encouragement (e.g., Frost et al., 1990; Rachman & Hodgson, 1980). There has at present been no intensive study into the rearing style experienced by TS patients, but there is some clinical evidence that the style experienced by people with both phobia and obsessions may be characterized as "affectionless control" (Gerlsma et al., 1990). Hafner (1988) found that OCD self-help group members reported higher levels of parental over-protection as compared to normal controls. In another study, Hoekstra et al. (1989) found that people with OCD reported more rejection and less caring than normal controls, but findings were mixed for over-protection; those with excessive washing reported more parental over-protection than normals whereas those with excessive checking reported less over-protection than normals. Vogel et al. (1997) compared outpatients with OCD and healthy controls in their recalled parental styles of upbringing and found no differences between the two groups. However, the study by Vogel and collaborators did not test other anxious control groups. Turgeon et al. (1998) found no differences in parental protectiveness between patients with OCD, agoraphobia and a non-anxious control group.

These instruments rely on retrospective accounts of the (now adult) child and hence suffer from possible recall bias. The parenting questionnaires may not tap important incidental learning experiences in childhood of the more dynamic aspects of family interaction as measured by attachment profiles. For example, Zuellig et al. (1997) reported increased feelings of anger and vulnerability in generalized anxiety using an adult attachment interview. Schut et al. (1997) reported that individuals with trichotillomania tended to use hostile dominance as their primary interpersonal style and this related to perceived childhood experiences as measured by an Inventory of Adult Attachment. So far, no studies have examined these hypotheses in TS or TD.

▶ NEUROPSYCHOLOGICAL ASPECTS

Both tics and compulsive–perseverative-type symptoms can occur in a range of brain-damaged syndromes, which indicates that variants of both disorders can accompany neurological loss of coherent cognitive input (Berthier et al., 1996). In view of the automatic perseverative nature of TD, a common etiology might be traceable to frontal lobe deficit. However, there is little consistent evidence of such deficit, as measured directly by EEG or other brain-mapping procedures, or indirectly by tests of central faculties supposedly controlled by the frontal lobes (e.g., executive functioning).

Müller et al. (2003) investigated neuropsychological function in a group of 14 people with TS and comorbid OCD and a control group. These authors found overall intact performance on a range of executive function and memory tests. But they found more errors in TS patients' performance of tasks requiring response flexibility, error detection and response inhibition, suggesting a hyperactive frontal–striatal thalamic frontal circuit.

There is, however, some consistent evidence, from neuropsychological studies in children with TS, of problems with motor skills and in particular visuomotor integration (Schultz et al., 1999). Here, though, the child populations studied frequently had comorbid ADHD. Several research workers have noted that apparent differences in perceptual-motor functioning of TD may be due to comorbidity of other disorders such as ADHD, as well as from the distracting interference of the tics at the time of testing (Channon et al., 1992; Randolph et al., 1993; Silverstein et al., 1995). Such neuropsychological tests have reported abnormalities in severe TS patients in skilled motor tasks like the Purdue pegboard and Groove tasks in children (Bornstein et al., 1991; Hagin et al., 1982), pre-adolescents (Bornstein, 1990) and adults (Bornstein, 1991a). There is also robust evidence of a higher level of overall motor activation in TD/TS. This activation takes the form of a higher cortical arousal, and higher behavioral arousal as shown in problems inhibiting automated motor actions (e.g., O'Connor et al., 2000, in press) and restless legs (Leckman & Cohen, 1999).

Rettew et al. (1991) compared 21 people with trichotillomania with 12 people with OCD, 17 people with other anxiety disorders and 16 controls on performance of the Money Road Map test and the Stylus Maze test. There was no difference in performance between pathological subgroups, but the trichotillomania group had more route errors and rule violations than the normals, while the OCD participants and normal participants differed only on the number of rule breaks. Enoch et al. (1995) reported visual field defects in OCD, TS and major affective disorder, but the field defects were unrelated to clinical severity and, in the authors' opinion, had no clinical significance. However, Clemenz et al. (1996) found no difference between the OCD group and controls in smooth pursuit eye movements of slowly moving targets.

Channon et al. (2003) note that evidence for impairment in executive functions is patchy, with little support for impairment in over-planning, rule finding or set shifting, but there may be implicit skill-learning impairment. In a study carefully controlling for comorbidity, Channon et al. (2003) examined abilities in inhibition and strategy generation, multi-tasking and rule following and set shifting and memory and learning in a group of 29 adult TS patients. The TS patients showed impairment in the ability to inhibit automated verbal responses. However, when there was comorbidity with ADHD, a wide range of executive functions were impaired. The study supported the lack of overall deficit in TS except for inhibitory aspects of executive function.

Channon et al. (2003) have also reported that adults with TS have a difficulty in controlling attentional resources, and in a real-life situation involving executive function, they have difficulties with problem solving and selecting relevant decisions. Channon et al. (2003) tried to move outside the constraints of abstract testing to look at problem solving in real-life social functioning. They found that although there was no absolute impairment in problem solving in patients with TS, they had problems generating socially appropriate solutions. The TS group also showed stronger emotional reactions to the problems, and Channon et al. (2003) conclude that factors such as emotion or knowledge structures could explain executive function deficit.

▶ EMOTIONAL REGULATION

Indeed, problems in autonomic regulation in tics may lead to impaired modulation of neuronal activity, and produce performance problems (Peterson et al., 1998). The precise mechanism underlying autonomic regulation is unclear but such regulation might influence catecholamine and DA levels (Tulen et al., 1998). Clients with a comorbid TD showed larger electrodermal responses than those without TD to novel stimuli, which might reflect greater autonomic sensitivity. Behavioral and autonomic regulation could contribute to changes in DA activity associated both with TD and TS (Ernst et al., 1999).

▶ LEARNING MODEL

An alternative approach to tic development comes in the learning model initially proposed by Azrin and Nunn (1973) which views tics as learned responses or, more specifically, adapted startle reflexes. A traumatic event evokes a reflex which develops into a tic which is then maintained by self-reinforcing factors (see Figure 2.1). Likewise, according to Corbett (1976) and Commander et al. (1991), the tic is a form of startle reflex that is learned in response to an aversive event, although, according to these authors, the propensity to be startled and over-stimulated may be biochemically determined. Azrin and Nunn (1977) hypothesized that tics develop following some physical trauma because they relieve muscle tension resulting from the injury or in other ways protect from injury. Tics are then negatively reinforced by the tension reduction that follows the occurrence of the tic behavior (Evers & van de Wetering, 1994), or by other external factors such as social attention. Additional contingencies encourage the propagation of the tic. For example, since the person lacks awareness of the tic, he or she can never exert complete control over it. Also, the tic may occur as an adjunct to other self-reinforcing behavior on an intermittent schedule of reinforcement, which leads the tic to become an auto-reinforced overlearned habit, difficult to extinguish.

Evidence supporting the early developmental part of the learning model is patchy. Sachdev et al. (1997) found no evidence of abnormal audiogenic startle reflex in 15 TS patients compared to 15 controls using stimuli at 88 and 114 dB. More recently, however, Gironell et al. (2000) did report an exaggerated acoustic startle reflex in 10 TS patients compared to 10 controls presenting 110 dB signals in a start–react paradigm. There is evidence of tics developing subsequent to peripheral physical injuries, and Factor and Molho (1997) report two such cases. Tijssen et al. (1999) reported three late-onset startle-induced tics, two linked to physical trauma and one linked to emotional stress. Some tics can be traced to learned gestures (e.g., scratching developing after a bout of acne, blinking after an eye operation, a head tic beginning due to the long hair worn during adolescence). This information, clinically useful though it may be in helping the person to increase awareness of the form of the tic, proves nothing about the learned nature of the tic because such

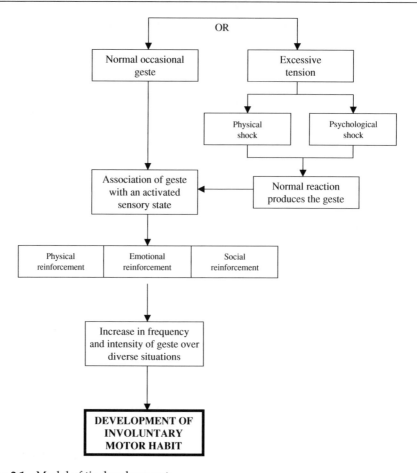

Figure 2.1   Model of tic development
Source: From Azrin and Nunn (1973). Habit reversal: A method of eliminating nervous habits and tics. *Behaviour Research and Therapy,* **11**, 619–628.

a situation may simply have been the occasion for the tic developing. In TS, in particular, tics can wax and wane, and be adopted on the basis of suggestion as an echo phenomenon (Seligman, 1991). There is also some evidence that tics may respond to hypnotic suggestion (Walters et al., 1988).

The claim that tics result from trauma or injury has some support, but not every tic develops subsequent to startle or injury, and the injury hypothesis does not account for tic substitution where a tic in one part of the body may substitute for or replace a tic in a distant part. Also, the precise reinforcer for the tic habit is unclear within the learning model (Turpin, 1983). Does the person engage in the tic habit to stimulate the self, or to rid the self of unpleasant sensations? In other words, is the tic reinforced by positive (stimulation) or negative (discomfort avoidance) reinforcement?

Evers and van de Wetering (1994) have put forward another model suggesting that the tic habit is most likely reinforced through tension release. They argue that among motor disorders, tics are unique in being preceded by a sensory urge, and they suggest a stimulus–response relationship between the urge, the subsequent tension and the ensuing tic to relieve tension (see Figure 2.4 on p. 36). However, any relief is short lived. Physiologically, the tic takes the form of a series of tense–relax muscle cycles in an already tense muscle where, however, the relax phase does not reduce tension to zero, but effectively returns it to an already elevated baseline. The long-term result of ticcing is hence maintained or increased muscle tension. The tense–release cycle could be seen to function in a way similar to rituals and other neutralizations in obsessional and habit disorders, which subjectively comfort while augmenting or maintaining the problem in the long run.

However, the tense–release cycle maintenance model of tic behavior is contested by another model emphasizing heightened sensory awareness as the maintaining factor in TS/TD (Fahn, 1993). This model proposes that tics represent a reaction to a heightened sensitivity towards sensory signals or, alternatively, an intolerance of such sensations. This heightened awareness model principally challenges the assumed involuntary nature of ticcing (implicit in the tension–release model). Is the tic, as Hollander (1993) suggested, a sign of lack of control over motor inhibition? Or is it the sensory, premonitory urge or sensation which is involuntary and leads to the tic action? Bliss (1980) also suggested that it is the premonitory urge to tic that is compelling, not the action. The tic action then constitutes an automatic response to the premonitory urge. If the tic is an automatic response to cope with the hypersensitivity, then the preferred treatment strategy for tic management would be exposure and habituation to the premonitory sensory urge as an alternative to reversing the motor tic habit through habit reversal (Bullen & Hemsley, 1983; Hoogduin et al., 1997).

But this latter treatment approach begs the question: What exactly is the premonitory sensation or urge? Its nature seems at the same time sensorial and attentional, and it is difficult phenomenologically to distinguish the two aspects (see Figure 2.2). The sensation is usually considered a sensory tic, indicating tension in the surrounding area. It is not clear if this sensation serves as a warning, a precipitator or is in fact part of the tic, because the sensation can persist even when treatment eliminates the actual tic movement. One possible interpretation of premonitory

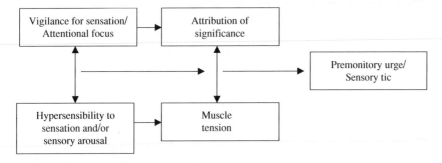

Figure 2.2   Possible inputs to the sensory tics and premonitory urges
Source: From O'Connor (2002). A cognitive-behavioral/psychophysiological model of tic disorders. *Behaviour Research and Therapy,* **40,** 1113–11142.

sensory tics is that they represent the subjective experience of neural dysfunction below the threshold for motor or vocal tic production (Chee & Sachdev, 1997). Kane (1994) has suggested that premonitory urges represent a heightened attention to physical sensations. He suggests that a particularly heightened sensitivity of the person with tics to somatic sensation produces an attentional focus that provokes the tic. If heightened awareness or attentional hypersensitivity to a particular tension becomes a preoccupation, and the attempt to suppress such a preoccupation provokes a tic, then this tic-producing process resembles the thought suppression analog of obsessional thought patterns, where the attempt to suppress an intrusive thought results in its resurgence (Purdon, 1999). Although the premonitory urge clearly correlates with tic frequency, it can arise independently, can persist when the tic behavior is eliminated, and can be modified independently by distraction and habituation (O'Connor, 2001). The premonitory urge may have similarities to the craving to smoke, which although seemingly inciting the smoking behavior actually varies independently of smoking and has a cognitive component (Tiffany, 1990). In the case of cigarette craving, the decision to smoke or the anticipation of smoking can produce the craving (O'Connor & Langlois, 1998). Possibly, then, the premonitory urge may be a product rather than a cause of attentional focus and may constitute an anticipation of ticcing subsequently reinforced by the ensuing tic behavior rather than an independent sensory precursor (see Figure 2.2).

▶ PSYCHOLOGICAL TREATMENTS

A number of diverse therapies have been undertaken over the years with Gilles de la Tourette syndrome (Azrin & Nunn, 1973; Cohen et al., 1988; Comings, 1990; Robertson, 2000). These have included hypnosis, psychoanalytic therapy and behavioral therapy, and cognitive-behavior therapy. In addition, there is family counseling and support.

Hypnosis has been used in case reports to change the location of tics to a more convenient body site. Family counseling and support has formed the basis for several interventions. Essentially, such therapy addresses coping difficulties due to TS behavior and offers parents and close others support in management strategies and environmental contingencies. The ethos of support groups for TS is actively promoted by TS foundations and frequently entails a consumer animating a meeting of fellow consumers, relatives or friends in sharing and discussing everyday problems. The support groups are distinct from educational groups and therapy and the little evaluation so far carried out suggests that they are highly valued by consumers (Grondin & O'Connor, 2001).

Psychoanalysis, once in vogue in the fifties, is now declining in popularity. The psychoanalytic view of tics is as diverted aggressive or erotic discharges, due to suppressed aggression or hostility. The therapy consists in gaining insight into the repression. However, there is no evidence to support this assertion and to the author's knowledge no empirically documented case exists where psychoanalysis has led to remission of tics. There is, however, some evidence reported by Peterson and Cohen (1998) and Robertson (2000) that non-directive psychotherapy may aid low self-esteem, learning difficulty, depression and other aversive emotional consequences of TS.

Other humanistic types of psychotherapy may help the person to understand his or her experience and alleviate internal distress (Lussier & Flessas, 2001). Peterson and Cohen (1998) recommend a flexible approach in psychotherapy permitting the targeting of whatever problem seems predominant in the TS family or educational setting.

► BEHAVIORAL APPROACHES

Behavioral approaches have taken several forms, namely: aversive negative reinforcement, positive reinforcement, counter-conditioning, and contingency management (Anderson et al., 2002; Clarke et al., 2001; Roane et al., 2002). The approach depends on whether the tic is conceptualized as a classically conditioned reflex, or as part of an operantly conditioned response. One early approach based on the assumption that tics are learned habits is extensive negative practice. In this technique, the tic is repeated voluntarily as quickly and with as much effort as possible over a fixed period of between 5 and 30 minutes, including several short rest periods to deal with fatigue (Peterson & Azrin, 1992, 1993). This approach, which has also been used in smoking cessation, aims to produce, on the one hand, a reactive inhibition which renders the act aversive and, on the other hand, to take practice of the act outside the usual contingencies.

Negative practice clearly has a short-term effect in reducing the targeted tic by around 58% drop in frequency. However, the effect is usually not maintained for longer than a few days. The exercise is very demanding and frustrating, and, furthermore, it is not clear whether it creates further tension and, hence, the need for tic substitution.

In the past, under the impression that the tic is an over-learned, rather than a non-voluntary response, other approaches have employed various forms of punishment to eliminate the tic response. One favoured approach is "time out" where the person is excluded from a place or activity in order to calm the tic. If the tics do diminish due to time out, they rapidly return when the period is over, and there is no generalization of any learning process to other tics. In effect, punishment strategies are not a recommended strategy to deal with tics since they are not efficient in the long term, and may negatively affect self-esteem, increase tension and lead to more attempts to camouflage or hide the tic.

Different types of positive reinforcement have, however, showed more success. In particular, it is widely recommended that patients with TS receive positive feedback and encouragement for abilities other than the tics. This permits establishment of a distinction between the person and the problem. It also relieves the pressure on the person to not always feel under scrutiny and judgment. It may also increase awareness that the person is not always ticcing.

Another technique that gives positive feedback is relaxation itself. The most popular form of relaxation is progressive muscle relaxation, where the person alternatively learns tense–release exercises for each major muscle group in the body (Jacobson, 1938). In addition, these exercises can be combined with respiration and visual imagery (Azrin & Peterson, 1988a; Lussier & Flessas, 2001). The exercises by themselves can be effective in reducing tics for short periods of time. However, they need to be adapted to make them interesting for children. If learned, they can be particularly useful in reducing tension when the tic occurs. However, it also must be appreciated that learning relaxation takes time with the need to pass through different stages in acquisition of the skill. Bergin et al. (1998) conducted a controlled trial randomly allocating 23 TS clients (mean age 11.8 years) to either a relaxation condition or a minimal therapy condition. The sample was stratified according to tic severity and ADHD comorbidity. Relaxation involved awareness training, breathing, postural relaxation, applied relaxation, biofeedback, while minimal therapy had the same number of visits but included awareness training, exposure to tapes about coping with tics, daily monitoring and positive thinking. At six weeks, there was a greater improvement in the relaxation group than in the minimal group but this advantage disappeared at three-month follow-up. Although relaxation by itself may not be an optional treatment for tics, it can be combined with other CBT approaches. Prominent among other approaches is awareness training.

Awareness training is one of the earliest approaches to changing habits, and follows the rationale of functional analysis that in order to modify behavior, knowledge of its form and contingencies is essential, in particular, in the case of tics when the person may not be aware at all. Rendering the person more aware of tics is likely to be an important element in control. Awareness techniques include: self-observation and record-keeping using a diary, a counter, mirror or video. Slowing down the tic voluntarily, or with the help of another person mimicking the tic, and speak aloud procedures permit recording each component of the tic. Somatic focus can be important to focus on the sensations and tensions preceding the tic. Studies have shown that awareness by itself can be effective on light tics or routine habits, and can reduce them by 75 to 100% (Azrin & Peterson, 1988a, 1989; Clarke et al., 2001; Cohen et al., 1988; Hadley, 1984; Sallee & Spratt, 1998).

▶ Habit Reversal

The learning model has produced the most compelling behavioral treatment for tics to date: habit reversal (HR). A great many behavioral treatment techniques have shown some success with tic management, including relaxation, hypnotism, muscle feedback, awareness training, negative self-practice, response prevention and massed practice (see Azrin & Peterson, 1988a), but the most impressive results have been reported by Azrin and coworkers using HR. Using this method, Azrin and Peterson (1988a, 1989, 1990), Peterson and Azrin (1992, 1993) and Peterson et al. (1994) report a reduction in tic frequency in the home environment of up to 99% in several studies involving TD, HD and TS. The HR package involves multiple stages, including relaxation, awareness, contingency training for positive reinforcement of non-ticcing and training in a competitive antagonistic response

Multimodal model

Awareness training

- Self-observation and diary monitoring of frequency and severity of tic movements.
- Identification of circumstance ssurrounding tic occurrence.
- Focus on sensations preceding tic onset.
- Inconvenience review of impairments induced by tics.

Relaxation training

- Practice in tension–release in muscle groups.
- Combine with respiration and mental imagery.

Training in an incompatible response (antagonist action)

- Implementing action antagonist to tic contraction to normalize tic action.
- Choose and model socially convenient antagonist action.
- Practice of incompatible response in contingent and non-contingent moments.

Contingency management

- Importance of social support and positive reinforcement.

Generalization of training

- Practice control in all situations. Apply to other tics.

Figure 2.3   Five principal stages of habit reversal
Source: From Azrin and Nunn (1973). Habit reversal: A method of eliminating nervous habits and tics. *Behaviour Research and Therapy,* **11**, 619–628.

(see Figure 2.3). This latter technique involves tensing the muscle antithetical and incompatible with the tic-implicated muscle. Awareness training and competing response training seem to be the crucial elements of the program (Miltenberger et al., 1985).

▶ The Incompatible Response

The aim of the competing incompatible response is to render the tic onset impossible because muscles antagonist to tic are contracted and hence impede its occurrence. Learning the antagonistic response involves finding an action that is socially acceptable and not visually prominent which permits willful contracting of opposing muscle groups. The response is maintained for several minutes and is practiced in and out of the tic-eliciting situation. Examples of appropriate actions to counteract tic actions are detailed by Carr (1995).

Although in some cases the incompatible response is a simple antagonist muscle action (neck contraction to impede a head tic), in other cases the response is a qualitatively different action which simply impedes the tic by being functionally non-equivalent. For example, slow breathing for a vocal tic or slow blinking for an eye tic.

The competing response (CR) theoretically installs an alternative response or habit to counter the tic movement and hence eliminate it. But there are alternative accounts of the CR. For example, the CR may function as a *geste antagonistic* whereby a random movement or reaction in a different part of the body by itself modifies the tic or habit. The CR might function as a movement distraction. Equally the CR may function as a punishment for habit onset (Turpin, 1983). It may function as a negative or positive reinforcer or as a social reinforcer, or as automatic reinforcer, or by some as yet to be identified means. Alternatively, the CR may be effective as a class of schedule or adjunctive behavior occurring as a side-effect of other time-based reinforcement schedules. In other words, the tics/habits may simply be performed when the person has no time limit and they can easily be replaced by the CR (Woods & Miltenberger, 1995). Although HR shows good response in isolated cases and seems to be equally effective in TD, TS and HD, its psychosocial impact and generalization are not clear. Unfortunately, Azrin and coworkers do not give sufficient information on the psychiatric comorbidity of their sample to permit adequate sample comparisons. Also, it is clear that the latter's criteria of success is limited to tic prevention and does not measure the impact on other behavioral or psychosocial factors. Studies of HR continue to show useful gains in clinical practice (Wilhelm et al., 2001), and O'Connor and coworkers (O'Connor et al., 1997a, 1997b, 2001b) reported a successful outcome of the HR package compared to the waitlist in the treatment of TD. Wilhelm et al. (2003) randomly assigned 32 TS clients to 14 sessions of either training or supportive psychotherapy. The HR training involved: awareness, relaxation, competing response, training contingency management and inconvenience review. The supportive psychotherapy involved mainly sharing experiences, feelings and expressing life issues. At 14 sessions, the HR condition had reduced to 19.81 on the Yale Global Tic Severity Scale (YGTSS) compared to 26.88 for the psychotherapy group, but this difference was no longer significant at 10-month follow-up due to relapse in the HR group. Clearly, more studies aimed at elaborating the theoretical basis of HR, standardizing application and establishing generalizability of findings across tic subtypes would be helpful.

▶ ABBREVIATED VERSIONS OF HABIT REVERSAL

HR has been the most rigorously investigated behavioral treatment, and which, in general, has shown considerable success. Several case studies, with TD, HR, TS, and in children and adults, have reported between 75 and 100% success in reducing tic frequency, maintained at two-year follow-up. The approach has also been validated in a school setting (Clarke et al., 2001). There is also evidence that the technique improves self-esteem since it accords a means of control (Woods & Miltenberger, 2001).

However, several problems remain with these studies: the majority are with small numbers of participants (1–12) of whom clinical data is often incomplete. The sole measure of outcome seems to be tic frequency and differences in this measure between clinic and home environment have been noted. There is no uniform treatment period. Some incompatible responses risk becoming substitutes for the tic. It is unclear what component of the HR therapy is responsible, and if this is the incompatible response, how this functions. Finally, several researchers have not supported the necessity of making the incompatible response functionally antagonist to the tic (e.g. Verdellen et al., 2004). Evers and van de Wetering (1994) have noted that it is not necessary to deal with one tic at a time, as recommended by Azrin and Nunn (1973).

Miltenberger et al. (1998) have noted that many authors consider HR to be a lengthy procedure and have attempted to develop shorter versions using less components. Allen (1998) employed awareness training and incompatible response training only to control rage attacks in a 14-year-old boy whose anger diminished after four to five months. Peterson and Azrin (1992) reported that a short version involving either HR, awareness training or relaxation reduced tics by proportions of 55%, 44% and 32% respectively, in four adults and two children. Wright and Miltenberger (1987) established that awareness training alone was sufficient to reduce a head tic with a six-year history. However, Miltenberger et al. (1985) implemented a brief program of awareness and incompatible response to treat diverse motor tics.

Douglas Woods and his team (Woods et al., 1996a, 1996b, 2003; Woods & Miltenberger, 2001), at the University of Wisconsin, have pursued numerous researches to determine the active component of HR in children. They have settled on a program of three major components: awareness training through self-rating diaries; incompatible response; and positive reinforcement and social support.

Woods et al. (2003) have developed a modified version of HR for treating vocal tics. This consisted of a three-session format comprising awareness training, competing response training and social support training. The competing response was diaphragmatic breathing. The vocal tics had reduced to zero at three-month follow-up according to parent ratings, while motor tics were not substantially affected. Interestingly, Woods et al. (1996b), in a sequential application of awareness training, competing response and social skills, showed that awareness training by itself is not enough to reduce tics, but there was wide variation of treatment lock-in at different stages for different clients. Clarke et al. (2001) used a two-component package consisting of HR and video self-modeling of the competing response. The HR consisted of two-week daily training maintaining the competing response for 1–3 minutes. Jones et al. (1997) applied an abbreviated HR on an adolescent self-biting tic. The therapy included relaxation and a competing response of chewing gum to prevent moving the lips over the mouth and not to bite the cheek. The number of sessions was not clear but at follow-up the tic was eliminated. Studies often use both contingent and non-contingent practice of the competing response which colors the function of this response. Is it simply developing another tic?

Verdellen et al. (2004) note that competing responses do not need to be antagonistic to reduce tic urge. They suggest exposure to the urge together with tic resistance is more effective with TS than HR.

▶ OTHER TENSION PREVENTION AND EXPOSURE TECHNIQUES

Other behavioral programs have paid more attention to the stimuli provoking tics, whether these be in stress or sensory states (Evers & van de Wetering, 1994), and suggested restructuring stimulus or environment, or learning a more appropriate socially acceptable response (Figure 2.4). Evers and van de Wetering (1994) hypothesized that tics were a way of reducing tension, which was itself a reaction to aversive sensory stimulus, and they reported two cases where implementation of alternative methods of tension reduction, such as making small movements when practiced over a six-week period, produced a significant decrease in tic frequency, with elimination of the tic in one case and maintained at three-month follow-up. An alternative treatment approach, as noted previously, is exposure to the premonitory urge during response prevention of the tic. This treatment approach is similar to the exposure and response prevention treatment model in other problems where exposure to the anxiety-provoking object, thought or sensation induces habituation and reduces the need to neutralize the sensation (i.e., to tic). Hoogduin et al. (1997) based their method of intervention on an exposure and response prevention approach which viewed tics as voluntary responses to neutralize unpleasant sensations. They reported significant decrease (68–75%) in tics in four cases after people with severe TS were exposed for 10 two-hour sessions.

In a subsequent, larger, controlled cross-over study, 45 people diagnosed with TS were randomly allocated to either HR or exposure treatment. Both treatments lasted for 10 sessions plus home practice. In the HR, participants learned to apply a competing response and hold it for one minute to counteract the tic. In the exposure, the participants focused on the sensory location of the tics and provoked the urge to tic, but resisted every desire to tic for a two-hour period. Exposure treated all tics, while in HR, tics were addressed one at a time. Both treatments were equivalent and there were less tics post-treatment but both showed low effect sizes. There

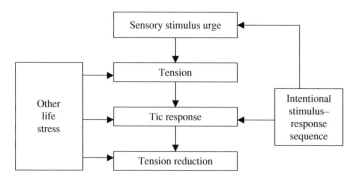

Figure 2.4   Sensory response model
Source: From Evers and van de Wetering (1994). A treatment model for motor tics based on a specific tension-reduction technique. *Journal of Behavior Therapy and Experimental Psychiatry*, **25**, 255–260.
Note: In this model, therapy consists of changing tic response for other tension-reduction movements to reduce sensory urge and replace tension with relaxation.

seemed a slight benefit if exposure followed HR. The authors conclude that both treatments may address the same processes of habituation or may increase feelings of mastery and control.

▶ CONCLUSIONS

The etiology of tic TD remains a mystery. Despite evidence of impairment in some aspects of executive functioning and visuomotor performance, in particular, performance inhibition, it remains unclear at what level this deficit is located. Is it impaired strategy or hard wired loss of function? Most neurobiological models see a principal role for the basal ganglia and frontal lobe circuit, but consistent evidence for structural abnormality is lacking. Nor can TS or TD be consistently characterized according to involvement of neurochemical systems such as DA since the effect of neuroleptic medications is far from universally effective. Neuropsychological findings suggest problems, particularly in TS, with visuomotor integration. When we break down the components of visuomotor performance (see Figure 31, p. 40), however, it seems that executive functions are largely intact, but that inhibitory functions are impaired. Selectivity and choice among alternatives are not optimal and there are problems allocating attentional resources, particularly in complex controlled tasks and where continuous action monitoring is required. Initial sensory information processes seem either intact or more active than normal. However, preparation and enactment of the later stages of response and accurate evaluation of feedback for response resolution seem suboptimal and may be linked to difficulties in dual task performance and the division of attention. On the behavioral front, a number of theories have been proposed to explain the appearance of tics via early learning experiences, but none has proved systematically supported. Occasionally, a tic can be traced to a traumatic event, but this does not explain the ease with which tics are substituted in TS. Tic onset cannot be accounted for by a conditioned stimulus–response sequence and may be mediated by other intra-organismic factors. The success of behavioral management strategies such as HR does, however, raise hopes that behavioral control over tics is possible. Unfortunately, it is unclear as yet which components are effective and how indeed the key element of the competing response operates within operant conditioning theory. Does the competing response work as a punishment, a distraction or a counter-conditioning of a contingency reinforcement, or does it simply improve feelings of self-control? It may not even be necessary to implement the competing response as an antagonist action to the tic and that any competing movement will serve the purpose if it reduces tension. If so, this challenges the functional role of the competing response as a contingency management device. Douglas Woods and collaborators have been active in trying to isolate habit reversal components and have, in fact, developed an abbreviated version that is composed of two or three components and seems to be as equally effective as the original multicomponent package.

Despite the success of current HR, such behavioral approaches are grounded more in behavioral theory than in the phenomenology of tic onset. The etiological model that tics are learned responses currently lacks support in other than isolated cases. Although learning principles apply to maintenance of the tic, the onset and course of tics cannot be adequately accounted for by a conditioning model. On the other hand, the environmental contingencies operating and the situational profile of the tic onset discount a purely neurobiological origin. In between brain and behavior is the motor psychology and psychophysiology of action concerned with the dynamic everyday enactment of voluntary and involuntary action. An empirically based model of TD may more likely emerge from understanding the process of ticcing rather than trying to fit ticcing into what we already know of brain function or behavioral theory. In the next chapter, we explore how this understanding may help to complement other approaches by bridging the gap between neurobiology and behavior.

Chapter 3

MOTOR PROCESSING IN TIC DISORDERS

▶ MOTOR PROCESSING

Although the work of some researchers (e.g., Channon et al., 2003) has tried to make sense of impairment on standard tasks of executive function by relating tasks more to the everyday performance of people with TS or TD, the significance of such performance is still not clear, nor do we know the level at which these apparent impairments operate. Looking to central brain structure for explanations in terms of, for example, basal ganglia disorder may be premature until we know the behavioral process involved and are able to separate strategy from deficit. In order to get information on process, we can turn to the psychology and psychophysiology of action, and in particular look in detail at the brain and its behavior as the person plans and executes actions that might relate to tic onset.

▶ PSYCHOLOGY OF ACTION

The first point to appreciate in a motor-processing perspective is the complete integration of mind and body, motor and sensory aspects at every stage of performance. The notion of stages of action is very important since different processes operate at different stages of performance. The planning stage of action is almost entirely cognitive. In comparison, the final point is guided entirely by automated motor feedback. The initial decisions to act can influence the whole progress of the act, and an instructional set can modify performance. When we say "instructional set", this also applies to all sorts of implicit expectations of the participant about his or her performance. For example, the person may simply believe the task has to be completed in a particularly fast or effortful manner and this will influence outcome. The effect of motivation on task performance as well as anxiety about performance is well documented. Pre-existing beliefs can affect self-regulatory factors and strategies adopted in the acquisition and execution of complex skills (Caudill et al., 1983). Coordination and accuracy of movement depend on self-efficacy. Anxiety generally leads patients to anticipate negative consequences, or be so concerned with the task that they monitor themselves performing the task rather than complete the task. People who perform tasks with higher confidence in their ability to perform

Cognitive-Behavioral Management of Tic Disorders by K. O'Connor.
Copyright © 2005 John Wiley & Sons, Ltd.

show a higher level of skill acquisition, particularly in complex tasks (e.g., Jourden et al., 1991).

After the planning stage, there is the preparation and execution stage of the task. Preparation can be broken down into a general orienting preparation where appropriate resources and energy are mobilized and a later specific goal-directed preparation where the fine-tuned motor program leads to accurate and satisfactory enactment of the task (Meyer et al., 1988). Various factors influence efficient preparation. The first is the undivided nature of the task. If the task has two potential goals, as in a complex reaction time, then the preparation may be slower and less efficient, compared to a simple reaction time (Friedman et al., 1988). Distraction by other competing stimuli or task demand can also impede optimal performance (Abernethy, 1988), as can the degree of state arousal (Fisk & Rogers, 1988). Finally, as we shall see later, physiological aspects at the time of performance, autonomic signals, muscle tension and respiration can also influence preparation in addition to trait factors such as anxiety and personality (Eysenck & Thompson, 1966).

At the general preparation stage as well as the next selective preparation stage, feedforward and feedback in equal measure modulate and guide performance (Karoly, 1993). Feedforward involves a delicate balancing act between activation or inhibition of psychological and behavioral factors. A sudden change in anticipation or intention will guide or redirect the movement. Conversely, feedback involves a delicate balance between efferent and afferent inputs, whereby emotional, proprioceptive, somatosensory, kinesiological, visuomotor systems give the feedback on the accuracy of the position of action. In the absence of visual feedback, somesthetic feedback is more likely (Grover & Craske, 1992) and this feedback may mislead positional sense (Hollins & Goble, 1988). Of particular importance here is the potential conflict between "feeling" and "knowing". In some tasks, we need to rely on feedback from "feeling" almost exclusively in order to be sure of success (Turvey et al., 1978), but in other tasks, it is important to be influenced more by "knowing" information such as provided by visual input. Inevitably, as the term implies, in visuomotor performance (Figure 3.1), there is likely to be some rivalry and even conflict between these two systems during performance;

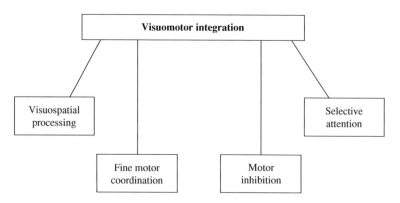

Figure 3.1   Neuropsychological features affected in Tourette's syndrome

for example, guiding a stylus requires both accurate grip strength and accurate perception.

Another important distinction in motor preparation is between skilled and un-skilled performance (Jaegers et al., 1989). Paradoxically, skilled performers are more likely to make errors at the precision end of the task than are debutants. One of the reasons is the different emphasis on automated and controlled components of the tasks at distinct stages of enactment. Debutants' performance is likely to be via controlled action throughout all early and middle stages of the performance process due to unfamiliarity, while skilled performers are likely to put early stages under automatic control, which can lead to problems in advance planning (Garcia-Colera & Semjen, 1988) and in articulating components when needed, and carries a danger of collapsing stages too quickly together and jumping over them to antic-ipate a further stage (Keele, 1968; Savelsbergh & Whiting, 1988). Blindly following a chain of automated actions can lead to erroneous performance, particularly feed-back connection, while feedforward errors are more likely to result from controlled actions. This point leads on to a key distinction in motor performance: distinguish-ing automated and controlled action (Shiffrin & Schneider, 1977). Controlled action requires conscious effort, while automated action requires less thought and per-mits quicker response. Conceptually, automated and controlled functions serve distinct purposes, but in practice they are found together in most actions. Indeed, at a certain point we must let go of reflection and control on the action in order to engage in execution. This "letting go" has been termed the "point of no return" (Osman et al., 1990a). Generally speaking, the "point of no return" occurs very late in the execution phase, mostly one can reverse or stop a motor program, par-ticularly a complex one, very late in the enactment process by countermanding. However, since programming and execution are independent processes, this may not be the case in automated movements – that is to say, movements with little or no complex programming, and where the point of no return is initiated early in the response process (van Donkelaar & Franks, 1991). In the stage model, cer-tain stages of the same movement are related, while others are independent. For example, early stages of preparation tend to lead on to one another but the later execution stage may be independent of these earlier stages, and this is particularly so where the execution stage is initiated early at the expense of prolonged prepa-ration in an automated task. Once a point of no return is reached, it is extremely difficult to inhibit according to a race model (Osman et al., 1990a). A race model is where control races after automated execution in case of the need for inhibition, such as, for example, in a countermanding paradigm, where an executed response must be stopped as soon as possible. In summary, then, it is difficult to classify any overall action as voluntary or non-voluntary, since in the stages of enactment of any action, different stages may involve automated and controlled functions. Hence, the behavioral act is a cognitive-motor, voluntary–non-voluntary entity.

As Dietrich (2004) notes, skilled flow of action is a question of balance between implicit (automated) and explicit (controlled) systems. Implicit programs are task-specific and less accessible to other systems and also less versatile. Explicit knowledge gives more flexibility and more self-reference and reflection, and in-creases computational complexity. Paradoxically, the skill level of a task is directly related to the number of distinct response patterns and their degree of automaticity. Optimal performance involves real-time sensorimotor integration and maximal implicitness of task execution. The effortlessness of a flow experience requires an autotelic merging of action and awareness with no metacognitive thoughts of failure or distraction.

► TICS AS BEHAVIORAL ACTS

One of the most important intellectual movements in motor psychology over the last 20 years has been the move away from trying to understand movement in terms of associated reflexology, to seeing all movement including reflexes inside a behavioral act. In the act model, telic action necessarily controls both motor and sensory components. As Weimer (1977) puts it: "The mind is intrinsically a motor system and everything mental is a product of constructive motor skills."

Although most of us are used to thinking of our sensory and motor apparatus as distinct, in practice this is not the case and the sensorimotor distinction, like the mind–body split, springs from Cartesian dualism. In fact, as several researchers have shown, there is thought–action coupling in all aspects of everyday life. We are constantly going back and forth between thinking and acting, and in the same way that sensory factors guide movement, so motor factors gate sensory input and both are subservient to an over-riding servocontrol monitoring of action reflected by the operation of the gamma efference system. Viewing the stages of movement as an "act" rather than a chain of reflexes and associated contractions explains well the fluid and continuous nature of movement flow. Indeed, the process of learning a skill seems parsimoniously accounted for by an "act" model where overall intention guides the connection of subcomponents. Deciding what to do and how to do it are distinct but interwoven processes.

Another important development largely due to motor theorists such as Bernstein (1967), Kelso (1994), and Kugler and Turvey (1990) is the view that information during action is processed in a dynamic way. In other words, the way we move generates information to the motor system. The information serving motor regulation is not static but is constantly adapting, developing in consequence of new movement positions. This notion of an ecology of action realigns old ideas of stimulus–response compatibility into notions of environmental affordance, particularly positionability or positional compatibility of an object with an action and posture. Indeed, the well-known Simon effect of reaction to stimulus compatibility, where response preference is given to signals physically compatible with responses, may be mediated by positional affordance together with intention (Michaels, 1988).

These dynamic notions of motor representation challenge older ideas of innate programs and fixed motor schemas, or stored prototype examples, since motor task similarity in the absence of environmental context does not guarantee transferability of skills (Chambertin & Magill, 1992). Labile intersensory interactions may produce motor illusions. The kinesthetic illusions produced by vibration, illusions or phantom limb position may be a result of discordance-driven dynamic adjustment when visual and kinesthetic signals are in conflict. In particular, reliance on the pro-prioception may lead peripheral cues on position to conflict with central feedback (Jones, 1988). The reciprocal interplay between periphery and central command has been further illustrated in the work of Brunia et al. (1982) investigating the interaction between posture, preparation and monosynaptic reflexes. Basically, this work has shown that amplitude of the spinal reflex depends crucially on activation of background factors and even the activation of irrelevant muscle groups. On the other hand, people themselves also show characteristic invariant action profiles in their activation of everyday motor patterns. For example, the tangential velocity profile of a goal-directed arm movement has a characteristic individual profile invariant across tasks, indeed, even transferable across tasks (Baker et al., 1988; Kahn et al., 1988). Personal style of movement therefore interacts with task demand to produce idiosyncratic ecological adaptation of movement. The aim of the movement is to maintain a flow of action through all the stages, and clearly one role of the feedback mechanisms serving motor regulation is to compensate for external interruption in flow. For example, the characteristic profile of an arm movement can be disturbed by the need for irregular step-like tracking movements and intermittent arrests of movement which then produce damped oscillations in the system. In this case, overall adjustment and recalibration of the movement will involve both proprioception and reafference.

Meyer and coworkers (Meyer et al., 1988) have also pointed to the utility of considering movement in terms of a first submovement, followed by a corrective second submovement. If the first submovement fails to reach target due to neural noise, corrective submovements seek to re-establish movement position. The subcomponent acts also on itself. So the corrective action may itself need further correction. For example, oscillations are likely to come into play to correct stepwise movements or when there are several intentional stops (Beuter et al., 1989), and these oscillations may need to be corrected by further muscle contractions.

Paradoxically, studies of the physical biology of movement emphasize not a purely neurobiological but a cognitive psychophysiological view and, in particular, that all types of action take place against an intentional act (Kugler & Turvey, 1990). What appears at first sight to be reflexive and automated is, in fact, set up by a wider intentional act and cannot be viewed outside of this act. Also, acts are continually evolving and, by definition, any persisting action is itself maintained by generated patterns of movement change deemed appropriate to the living system and its surround relation. There is a form of coalition or cooperation of organization within movement, what Kugler and Turvey (1990) term the "self-assembly of movement". It is only by constantly recruiting its own assembly that a system can be stable (Kugler & Turvey, 1990, p. 255): so an act is a relation. It is enacted only by reciprocal arrangement of a wide range of muscle groups. Kimura et al. (2002) have noted how pretension levels of a muscle affect speed of response and degree of preparation. In order to reach the arm out, the rest of the body has to be aligned to support such a reach. A rapid button press requires priming of the muscle but also anchoring of the feet in a forward poise. The monosynaptic Hoffman spinal reflex depends on posture for its intensity. Therefore, the nature of a non-voluntary tic reflex could likewise depend on the surround telic activity pattern.

▶ HUMAN ECOLOGY OF ACTION

We have noted that, physiologically, a tic is a contraction of an already tense muscle. Tics can or cannot be preceded by premonitory urges, and the most likely explanation of a premonitory urge is detection and attribution of a creeping tension. Simple tics seem non-sensical and reflex-like in that they are distant from volitional control and telic action and apparently pointless. They are not preceded by intention, as are, say, compulsive rituals, and seem, in fact, to form the opposite impulsive end of an impulsive–compulsive dimension. However, they do fulfill a function which is sensory release, and this release is more a conscious aim in complex tics where a person may adjust his or her body to "feel just right". Simple tics also release muscle tension. So muscle tension is present prior to a tic, since tics like all reflexes require tension to operate. But what is the nature of this tension? Is it ultimately a form of activity? How is it set up? Is it set up by some kind of telic action? When we look into background factors producing the tic, rather like looking beneath the tip of an iceberg, we find that a cognitive psychophysiological approach helps us to understand the human ecology of tics.

In the medical notion of tic as movement disorder, focus is on the central brain structures controlling movement, and whose functioning is clearly impaired in neurological problems. However, if we take an ecological viewpoint, tics as movements take place against a coordinated assembly of other muscle activity. The whole body as an action system is involved in the tic production. This action must have as its overall goal a telic aim even if subcomponents are automated. Our overall acts are driven by intention, possess meaning and are responded to and evaluated by others as such. The person is never outside an intentional goal-directed action, even if the intention is to do nothing. The action has physiological support from autonomic and central nervous systems, and our physiology supports and responds to the psychological qualities of movement. A planned goal-oriented action will evoke a different response than a vague hesitant action even if the same motor structures are in use. Furthermore, our actions are constantly modified by feedback, and feedforward from sensory, proprioceptive and visual perception, which respond to our overall intention.

▶ MOTOR PSYCHOPHYSIOLOGY

Any action is a constant interplay between inhibition and excitation which determines sensory gating of input. What we take in from the environment depends on our action and posture. Hence, in action there is always thought–action coupling. This interplay interacts with the stage of movement. Thinking while in the preparatory stage of movement is distinct from thoughts during execution, and requires activation of different cortical areas to a different degree. Electrocortical indices are good markers of dysfunction in preparation and the presence of a preparation potential distinguishes preparation from execution. Interestingly, such a potential may not develop optimally in TD (see Chapter 4).

A motor-processing approach also makes it more evident that strategy differences can play a greater role in unwanted movement and responses and in visuomotor performance. For example, activation for a response can be impeded by inhibition, but also by chronic preparation, particularly when the preparation is in a non-relevant muscle. Preparation can be impeded by distraction but less so when the preparation nears execution. Metacognition can also affect preparation since it controls investment in action and confidence in outcome. Such metacognitive control can often over-ride otherwise disabling cognitive factors. For example, although general dual task performance diminishes speed of preparation, paradoxically, performing two acts at once can aid performance if the nature of the separate tasks complements the overall intention. For example, an automatic tapping or rhymic movement can screen distraction and aid more complex attentional performance (O'Connor, 1989).

Also underlying this notion that movement always forms part of an act is the idea that all action, both voluntary and non-voluntary, serves a function within the act. A reflex is automated not because it escapes voluntary control or is a side-effect of deficient control, but because it helps issues of capacity and defence. Faster movements can energize a system and boost reafference better than slower movements, so reflex-like action may give an idiosyncratic but effective and unique type of motivating feedback that is not available from controlled action.

We can thus draw several conclusions from an ecological approach to action. Movement can be divided into several subcomponents. It can be abrupt, ramp-like discontinuous or it can flow smoothly and continuously. It can be controlled or automatic, it can be reflex-like and beyond the point of no return or it can be changed at will. Movement requires different stages which serve distinct functions, planning, preparation, feedback correction and execution, that occur in sequence, and each ingredient is related to the whole action which constitutes a reciprocal assembly of both cognitive and behavioral components in the service of a goal-directed telic activity.

Moving from knowledge of the mechanics of movement, we can infer how muscle tension is produced in the interaction of muscle and brain processes. Muscle contraction itself depends on a number of parameters. It is a function of innervational condition, and muscle length, and the velocity with which length changes over time. The length of a muscle is, in turn, a function of the angle of articulation, and the tension can be modified by momentum and load. A muscle movement is never isolated and responds as part of an overall program, hence sustained tension is a combination of central input and external load. Also sustained rhythmic movements risk developing an oscillatory movement if its flow is disturbed since where the action is indecisive, intentional tremor can arise. It is important to note that during a period of sustained contraction, reactive inhibition develops which can also lead to oscillatory movement. This movement impedes or dampens action and can be effectively corrected by reafference through a fast relax–contract cycle.

Any component of this sequence, whether abrupt and automatic or controlled, serves a function in the action cycle. There is no such thing as a non-functional movement within an act, although the goal of an activity may be overall maladaptive. So tics, although involuntary actions, form a part of a larger telic behavioral activity. Locally, the activity is reflected in a functional distribution of tension in selected muscle groups according to their potential use within an act. The function of a tic lies precisely in its nature as an automated action enacted beyond the point of no return. The nature of this action allows it to provide feedback on muscle state and primarily affect "feeling" feedback from proprioceptive factors and so contribute to the sensory or effort regulation of action.

We could consider that the tic, as a fast, automated, contract–relax sequence, serves several functions. It may serve to correct tension level where this chronic preparation risks becoming oscillatory due to sustained inhibition of movement. It may serve to stimulate reafference and goal-directedness of an action temporally arrested. It may serve to withhold a late preparation from the point of no return by recalibrating its position to an early stage of preparation but within the same goal angle. The precise function of the tic seems to be to release temporarily chronic tension or motor activation. This chronic motor activation itself seems built up via the telic action pattern. In other words, for some reason the overall pattern leads to conflict or impediment in the normal stages of action. Since the tension and hence tic is localized in a specific muscle, we may tentatively infer that the stage of processing affected is between specific preparation and execution. This hypothesis would predict that tic onset occurs during preparation or early stages of movement initiation and not during later execution stages. The motor literature suggests several candidates for producing conflict, including a conflict between competing goals and an inappropriate attempt to jump ahead of current stage of action. The problem may also lie with inappropriate feedback in guiding action. In particular, there may be a failure in the self-correcting metacognitive subcomponent monitoring movement.

The tension-producing tics may then arise through conflict resulting from an overall style of planning motor action. So, to understand tics we need to look at the more precise parameters affecting coordination and planning of movement, and this approach places tics in a less isolated and more holistic light. It is interesting to note that one of the most famous laws of movement, Fitts' law, was devised using a visuomotor task, in this case, stylus tapping. The original Fitts' law that duration and accuracy of targeted action bears a logarithmic relation has since been modified to accommodate a more linear relation when there are time constraints. Hence, the desire to complete a task both quickly and accurately under time constraints could lead to conflict.

Table 3.1 shows the principal stages of action, together with the different levels of function plus regulatory function, and different modalities of function at each stage of action.

Table 3.2 lists potential planning strategies which may influence visuomotor performance impeding flow from preparation to execution. Clearly, modalities of function may interact and over-ride each other at any stage of action. For example, change in goal will modify preparation stages. However, the table illustrates the predominant modalities likely to operate at each stage in an optimal uncorrected action.

Table 3.1 Stages of motor action

Control function	Action function	Energy function	Regulatory function
1. Goal setting	Choosing type and parameters of action required	General level of activation	Self-efficacy, self-awareness, self-monitoring
2. Planning the standard of performance	Preliminary orienting, preparation, balance of auto-mated/controlled action	Mobilization of relevant resources	Intentional feedforward
3. Specifying sub-components, subgroups of action	Specific preparation, initiation of movement	Specific muscle, sensorimotor activation plus support physiology	Visuomotor feedback
4. Correcting feedback mismatch	Point of no return, execution/enactment of action	Inhibition of irrelevant activities/activation	Proprioceptive/sensorimotor feedback
5. Evaluation of outcome for further action	Resolution of action	Reafference and readaptation of resources for further actions	Environmental, social, emotional feedback

The literature on motor processing and psychophysiology of TS suggests that problems are mostly at stages 2 and 3, in other words, between the later stage of preparation and initiation of movement in particular enacting and guiding responses efficiently to goal. The present hypothesis is that this problem is more strategy than deficit. People with tics and TS may over-prepare for actions, or prepare inappropriate muscles. They may end up preparing for two incompatible tasks instead of one. They may, in addition, jump ahead prematurely to the later stages of

Table 3.2 Potential planning strategies producing motor conflict

- Planning two conflicting goals at the same time
- Investing too much effort in a task, mobilizing too many resources
- Activating irrelevant muscles
- Preparing to do two competing tasks at once
- Trying to jump ahead to the end of a task or positioned prematurely
- Relying on the feel of an action rather than on visual or positional feedback as performance criterion
- Using automated mode to complete an action when controlled mode would be better for correcting error
- Arriving at the point of no return too quickly and needing to adjust action automatically
- Difficulty managing competing sources of feedback on the same action (e.g., somesthetic versus kinesological)

preparation and hence end up relying on inappropriate sources of feedback for current stage of action while ignoring more relevant feedback. The result seems to be a rupture in the flow and normal progression of final degrees of preparation past the point of no return to enactment. The action may become blocked prior to enactment and the tic occurs as a form of recalibration of muscle tension in order to maintain specific preparation.

In the following sections, we examine evidence to see if the characteristics of TD fit a cognitive–psychophysiological model of tic development which follows the ecological action model of movement. In particular, what is the evidence that tics result from sustained motor contraction resulting from conflicting or maladapted goal-directed actions? In the first section, we look at the evidence for the association of muscle tension with tic onset.

▶ CHRONIC MUSCLE TENSION

Is there a relationship between tic onset and muscle tension? The tic-implicated muscle is frequently a muscle implicated in a task where the action–frustration cycle is most notable and recurrent. Electromyographic (EMG) recordings of tic-affected muscles show that these muscles are rarely associated with zero tension and have a greater difficulty compared to non-affected muscles achieving different degrees of tension rather just an all or nothing state of tension (O'Connor et al., 1995). People suffering from tics also subjectively report chronic tension. Hoogduin et al. (1997) reported high overall muscle tension as a consistent feeling in all patients when identifying premonitory urges.

So how would such muscular tension be built up prior to tic onset? Behaviorally speaking, tension may be a product of inappropriate over-investment in action, or disproportionate anticipatory activation of the muscle at a premature stage in motor execution. On rare occasions, the tic may be traceable to a learned action, particularly in TD, or an accelerated series of actions learned in reaction to stress or other related situations.

Examples of exaggerated reactions in TS:

- A person who from birth felt that he had to add voluntary use of the cheek muscles to the involuntary blink reflex of the eyelids.
- A person who, when his eyes shut, thought he must use his cheek muscles to open them, otherwise they wouldn't open.
- A person who thought every time he placed an object, he needed to grunt to place it correctly.
- A person who, when paying attention, has to occupy leg muscles, moving them up and down in order to concentrate.

However, use of redundant muscles in carrying out a task is likely to lead to: (1) difficulties in inhibition; (2) difficulties in flexibility of action; (3) difficulties with complex performance; and (4) habit of relying on somatosensory feedback. In a recent electrophysiological study (O'Connor et al., in press) looking at electrocortical preparation and movement execution potentials, participants with TD showed no consistent relationship between preparation and execution stages of action, suggesting that preparation stages were not modulated efficiently, possibly due to a high level of activation. Anticipation and preparation can themselves induce muscle activation through the influence of the gamma-efferent system, and clients report that anticipation of a tic and focus on the tic muscle can by itself produce the tic (Kane, 1994). Even purely intellectual recall of a past tic can reactivate it (Peterson et al., 1999, p. 257). High tension generally would be maintained by over-preparation, which would not permit the muscle to profit from a normal relaxation cycle. The tic cycle is a series of tense–release contractions whose goal is to release tension temporarily or alleviate an aversive sensation, but which effectively maintains tension. The tense–release cycle keeps the muscle in a chronic state of preparation to act, and this chronic state in turn simulates a state of readiness (O'Connor, 1989). Consequently, progressive muscle relaxation as a therapeutic strategy seems beneficial and forms an important component of HR treatment. The tic is like the tip of an iceberg with a more general high level of background tension below the surface and, as we discuss later, it is necessary in treatment to reduce the tension and activation level overall as part of behavioral restructuring as well as addressing the tic in isolation in order to avoid tic substitution. A behavioral analogue of a high-risk tic situation of over-preparation is scripted in Table 3.3. So the notion that a tic serves to release chronic contraction in the tic-affected muscle seems to be upheld. The tense–release cycle, however, serves to maintain chronic preparation in the muscle. In other words, the preparation stage for whatever reason does not pass to the execution stage. This may be due to a conflict of goals or premature preparation. A clue to the reason for the chronic preparation and the need to sustain it comes from accompanying emotions.

Table 3.3 Analog of a high-risk situation inducing frustration–action motor tense–release cycle

General plan
You are preparing an action with a specific set of muscles in order to carry out a complex task with several unknowns (a skilled action, making a speech). You wish to get the task over with as soon as possible and feel you should always be further ahead in your performance. Just as you are about to execute the action, you decide to hold the action but stay attentive and ready to restart it again. In order to keep your prepared position, you quickly relax and retense the muscle or repeatedly pronounce the first syllable of the speech between sharp breaths.

Result
Chronic over-preparation accompanied by frustration–action, followed by a repetitive tense–release cycle in task-related muscle groups.

Specific example
Over-tense the arm, shoulder, hand and neck muscles in a forward position in preparation to catch a ball. Ask a confederate to feint throwing the ball to you randomly nine times out of 10 in unpredictable sequence over a period of several minutes, so that you do not know on which of the 10 throws the ball will really be thrown. You must thus react "as if" it will be thrown on each feint throw and then, if it is not, hold your position in preparation for the next throw. You will naturally tense and relax after each feint throw to readjust preparation.

► **THE ROLE OF FRUSTRATION IN TIC ONSET**

The tic occurrence is often accompanied by feelings of frustration or dissatisfaction. O'Connor et al. (1994) looked at situations likely to evoke tics and found that these were not necessarily related to anxiety but rather to thoughts or events of frustration. In particular, low-risk tic perceptions of "feeling free to act" or "being myself" were opposed to high-risk feelings of constraint, obligation and being judged by others.

Tic occurrence has a situation–activity profile. In other words, the tic is more likely to appear in some situations or activities rather than others, or is more likely to be worse during some situations or activities than others. The high-risk situations or activities may, objectively speaking, be very idiosyncratic. One person tics when reading, another when out walking. Despite the personalized nature of high-risk situations or activities, appraisals of such activities tend to be more uniform. During such situations or activities, the person feels dissatisfied, bored, frustrated, dissatisfied and under pressure. A more recent study (Brisebois et al., 2001; O'Connor et al., 2003) confirmed that tic onset is predominantly associated with dissatisfying and tension-producing activities.

Tics always occur in situations that represent to the person sources of dissatisfaction or frustration. Being late for an appointment, for example, by itself may not be enough to evoke a tic, but being, in addition, late and caught in the traffic and anticipating a stressful interview may cumulatively elicit the tic. The tense–release muscle cycle then seems to be linked with an emotional frustration–action cycle (Figure 3.2). So the chronic preparation is associated with feeling of constraint, but is the constraint generally self-imposed style or is it task-related?

► **TIC ONSET AND MUSCLE USE: THE FRUSTRATION–ACTION/TENSE–RELEASE CYCLE**

Tic onset occurs against a general background of tension. But why does the tic onset occur in one group of muscles and not others? In our clients, muscle implication in the tic seems ultimately linked to muscle usage. Although in TS tics can move around the body, this fact would still support the usage model as long as the tic occurs in muscles linked to a frustration–action cycle. Tics occur in otherwise voluntary muscles linked either by usage or expression to a high-risk tic activity. For example: a masseuse develops a twitch in her most forceful dominant hand when she is trying to rush a massage; a trombone player develops a tic in his lips, mouth and tongue during a hasty rehearsal; and, more symbolically, another person grimaces and makes a sound like "tsk tsk" with her mouth when anticipating problems. The sound and movement resemble an expression of negative self-judgment and frustration.

The tic then usually occurs in muscles linked either by symbolic or physical association with use, or preparation for use, in a high-risk tic onset situation. The

Background intentions introducing conflict into planning action

↓

Examples: I must be quick and accurate
I must watch everything I do
I must always be ahead of myself
I must do more than one task at the same time

Conflict between implicit/explicit–automated/controlled motor programming

↓

Examples: Automated program activated as expense of controlled program
Stage of program jumped over too quickly
Two competing programs activated at the same time

Excessive preparation for action

↓

Examples: Chronic tension in muscles linked to use
Motor restlessness
Tension in irrelevant muscles

Reliance on inappropriate feedback for regulating action

↓

Examples: Attention to somesthetic cues rather than visuomotor or kinesthetic cues
Feeling of frustration as motor program ready to execute action
but controlled monitoring seeks to correct action

Self-correction of motor preparation within intentional plan

↓

Examples: Difficulty countermanding executive action through controlled processing
Muscle constantly corrected through proprioceptive reafference at the point of no return
Increased reliance on "feeling" of action as sign of accomplishment, or completeness

Tic onset

↓

Automated tense–release tic cycle in muscles tied to use

Figure 3.2 Frustration–action cycle

tic-affected muscle might be implicated in an expression of emotion or action adapted for use in the high-risk situation or activity. For example, a client with an eye tic, whose style of action involves always speaking forcefully and over-involving face and cheek muscles in speech, feels that he must fixate his addressee in order to not miss information in an encounter. He considers quick blinking an

Table 3.4   Cognitive influences relevant to feedforward planning

Beliefs about tic disorder	"I'll never control my tics" "My tics make me appear mad"
Expectations about tic onset	"If I feel a tension, it means I'm bound to tic" "If I try to hold in my tic, I'll need to let it out eventually or I'll explode"
Evaluations of high-risk tic activities which produce tension	"This meeting will make me frustrated and upset" "This activity, which I feel obliged to do, is boring and unsatisfying"
Anticipation of ticcing	"I'm afraid if I tic in this situation, people will laugh at me" "What if I started ticcing now, that would be terrible"
Metacognitive influences on ticcing	"Just thinking about ticcing makes me feel like ticcing" "I focus on my tic to be vigilant to prevent it, but this provokes the tic"
Social cognitions and ticcing	"If people see me tic, I'll lose their respect" "Nobody would invite me to a party if they knew I would tic"
Planning strategies for coping with tics	"I'll rush through this job and hope I don't tic" "If I keep my body tense, I might impede the tic"

asset to help "use" in interpersonal encounters. So the tic action may serve part of a more general behavioral purpose and be linked to cognitive, emotional, as well as to physical goals. Obviously, a defensive or startle reaction (as proposed by the learning model) would count as one example of such use, but such a reaction is only one category of use. Mckinlay and Dixon (2001) suggest tic muscles may become incidentally associated with goal-directed actions.

At first sight, it might appear that this link with muscle use applies selectively to certain complex tics, but not to more simple tics. But the ecological model would hold that all tics serve a function. Of course, tension may be present in muscles irrelevant to the task, as long as they are activated by the task demand. In all cases, the tic would be activated by sustained chronic preparation in the service of an identifiable activity. The frustration–action cycle is also maintained by coping reactions to the tic, which may try to disguise it or hold it in and so increase tension level. We have discussed the emotional or feel factors associated with action. There are also consistent cognitive factors influencing feedforward planning strategies (see Table 3.4)?

▶ PERFECTIONIST STYLES OF ACTION

People with TD, TS and, to a lesser extent, HD seem to score higher than controls on subscales of the Frost Multidimensional Perfectionist Scale (MPS) related to personal standards and organization. However, people with TD do *not* necessarily score high overall on measures of perfectionism or obsessionality (O'Connor et al., 2001a). The cognitive aspect of this perfectionism manifests itself in beliefs about the importance of being efficient, of doing as much as possible, and not wasting time, or appearing to do so. These perfectionist beliefs are accompanied by a premeditated style of action involving a tendency to attempt too much at once, premature abandonment of tasks, unwillingness to relax, pace action appropriately, invest more effort than necessary, be in advance of self and foresee the unforeseeable (see Chapter 4).

The behavioral aspects of this style of planning action first came to notice in the clinic when clients could not find time to do the homework exercises because they already had too much to do. It would be tempting to connect this planning style with ADHD in terms of impulsivity, distraction, hyperactivity or even with "type A" behavior. This over-active style clearly bears a "family resemblance" both to hyperactivity and possibly type A behavior. As Leckman and Cohen (1999, p. 71) note, there are few studies assessing hyperactivity in adults. Hicks et al. (1990) have previously reported increased type A behavior in people with HD. However, the term "over-activity" is preferred here since it avoids assumptions of a link to childhood hyperactivity and grounds the description in the precise behavioral observation in the adult of over-investment in planning action. The style of planning here is clearly premeditated and aimed at achieving a perfectionist goal. Although the style of action may be idiosyncratic and situation-specific to the person, the perfectionist appraisals are uniform and persistent and represent a stable belief in the over-active style as the most efficient way of acting. The person with TD may report rigid black and white beliefs such as: "Either I do everything at once or I'm lazy." Or there may be unspoken rules and assumptions which make the person feel that he or she must act in this way, e.g., "Not feeling well is not a good enough excuse to change a scheduled appointment/activity." "People will not tolerate me if I'm a little late." There may also be deep core assumptions fuelling over-activity such as: "I could be inadequate and if I don't act as quickly as possible, everyone will know I can't perform." Such a perfectionist style of action becomes self-perpetuating.

Typically, the over-active person will have several tasks planned at the same period time (e.g., go to the mall, return library book, visit a friend, go to the bank, etc.). The result, apart from always being in a rush, is that the person feels stretched and strained and constantly in conflict between what he or she is doing and what he or she feels should be done. Frequently this conflict adds in an unnecessary stress to current tasks and sabotages feelings of accomplishment. The offshoot is that the person is dissatisfied, frustrated, irritable, feels trapped and makes a poor personal judgment. The second dimension, over-investment, relates to doing more than is necessary, and expending more effort than necessary on an intellectual, emotional and physical level. On a physical level, the person may invest irrelevant tension in another part of the body or in the same muscle group, for example, blinking with cheek or forehead muscles in addition to eyelid muscles, or respond to an isolated task with a block movement (lift up a pen with the complete arm, not just the fingers). The tic action itself is often visible precisely due to the implication of non-pertinent muscles. This extra physical effort can be normalized with practice but there may also be a tendency to over-invest intellectually and emotionally in the reaction to, and anticipation of, an event. Even if the person is immobile during the tic, thoughts can create unnecessary frustration and an over-investment in negative anticipation and preparation (O'Connor et al., 1994).

► HEIGHTENED SENSORIMOTOR AWARENESS

The hypersensibility of people with TS/TD has been noted by several authors in visual, auditory and tactile modalities (e.g., Bliss, 1980; Kane, 1994). Such sensitivity can lead directly to the development of tic-like responses in coping. For example, as noted, eye blinks may originate as defensive responses to light. Subjectively, people with TS/TD report increased sensory discomfort, tingling or itches, sometimes resulting directly in scratching, rubbing or moving (e.g., Leckman & Cohen, 1999, p. 27). The hypersensibility in people with TS can also take the form of irritation with hair, sweat, skin texture or an over-reaction to light, sound, or touch, smell or taste. As noted earlier, the premonitory urge prior to ticcing could itself be a result of such hypersensitivity, and there is some experimental evidence of sensory excitability and augmented sensory-evoked potentials in people with TS/TD (Johannes et al., 2001; van Woerkom et al., 1994). However, there is a potentially cognitive aspect to this sensory element, albeit relatively under-explored (see Figure 2.2, p. 29). Increased attentional focus might augment hypersensibility to sensations, and the possible attributions of negative significance to the sensations may further increase their importance in a similar way to the cognitive distortions and appraisal assumptions in other psychiatric disorders (e.g., panic, somatoform disorders) (Salkovskis & Clark, 1993). In addition, enhanced self-attention and self-awareness may result from increased self-focus. A fairly consistent finding with TS/TD groups is the sensitivity of such clients to the judgment of others (Leckman & Cohen, 1999, p. 149). People with TD are over-concerned with self-image, that others will pass judgment (including on appearance of the tic), and detect subtle deficits in reaction and style, leaving them dissatisfied with themselves. In a recent study, items of self-image distinguishing TD groups from controls were mainly concerned with feelings of being ill, at ease with others, and dissatisfied with self-image (O'Connor et al., 2001b). Although such self-focus and sensitivity could, of course, result from the experience of ticcing through conditioned evaluation and subsequent generalization, the person's awareness of the tic and its social effect is sometimes limited and the self-focus can be present even in situations at low risk for ticcing.

So there could be a reciprocal influence between the cognitive/emotive and behavioral/psychophysiological manifestations of ticcing. A perfectionist concern with personal standards could lead to a heightened self-attention, sensory awareness and a self-focus on appearance. Likewise, a heightened hypersensorial state could lead to heightened agitation and an over-concern to regulate personal actions and appearance. Both positions independently would, in any case, ultimately enhance sensory stimulation and feed sensorimotor activation. A high level of motor activation has been documented in clients with TS/TD (see previous section). There is evidence of motor neuron excitability, enhanced motor preparation, difficulty inhibiting responses or modulating arousal when initiating complex responses. Enhanced motor activation would, in turn, affect neurochemical regulation which could, in turn, produce increased motor restlessness, and further encourage motor activity and impulsivity. Cath et al. (2001b), in a study examining serotonin activity in people with TD and OCD, have suggested that low serotonin syndrome and 5-HT hypo-functionality is associated with impulsivity. The complex relation between, say, serotonin and DA may not, in this case, be pathology-specific. Hence, differences in neurochemical levels may be less a state function and more a long-term compensation/adaptation mechanism in response to chronic dysregulation of activity and arousal.

This reciprocal path between neurochemical and sensorimotor activation leads at the same time to both greater stimulation and the need for more such movement and stimulation. This, in turn, would feed sensorimotor activity and result in a difficulty to remain calm. Motor activation would also be sustained directly by continued beliefs about the need to be always on the move. All these influences could produce a ceiling level of motor activation or "motor excess" (Tryon, 1993).

▶ DYSREGULATION OF MOTOR ACTIVATION CYCLE AND SENSORY FEEDBACK MECHANISMS

This ceiling effect due to chronic over-activation could plausibly lead to problems in short-term arousal regulation. But this arousal regulation could also be disrupted by distraction from the perfectionist desire to be always ahead of oneself. The latter tendency could lead to less attentional focus on performance in the here and now, with thoughts focused more on the next task or on future or other events. Anecdotally, clients with tics frequently complain of being "in the moon" and not being entirely focused on the here and now. Sample quotes: "I'm always ahead of myself; I'm doing one task and already I'm daydreaming about what I must do next and so on"; "I'm rarely reacting in the here and now, to the present"; "I find it difficult to not think on ahead. There always needs to be something going on in the back of my head." There may be difficulty in optimally adapting arousal/activation level to task demand. Because of the emphasis on feeding sensorimotor stimulation, feedback signals indicating when tasks are satisfactorily done, or the appropriate state for a task, may be trumped by information from proprioceptive feedback, rather than adjusted in accordance with complex integration of current visuospatial information. This reliance on intensity of muscle tension and effort may resemble the proprioceptive focus typical of somatoform disorder (Scholz et al., 2001).

An over-active trying-to-do-too-much-at-once and over-investing-too-much-effort style of action could well impair efficient regulation of arousal and attention. Difficulties in regulating attention/arousal would result in, and, in turn, be reinforced by, restlessness. Such difficulties in regulating arousal and attention could explain the specific problems of people with TD/TS in initiating and carrying through complex tasks (which require controlled allocation of resources). Problems in initiating complex tasks could lead to a level of frustration associated both with the consequences and with the anticipation of complex task performance, particularly those tests requiring open-loop planning (i.e., controlled rather than automated regulation). This frustration might also impair the ability and/or desire of people with TD/TS to plan actions on the basis of visuospatial cues and so integrate these into movement planning. Problems in visuomotor integration (noted earlier) could thus result from an over-reliance on sensory and proprioceptive "feel" to know when the action is accomplished or when enough effort has been invested. The frustration and impatience would then lead to enhanced tension as the muscles are continually over-readied for action (frustration–action cycle) and kept in a state of over-preparation relying on somesthetic and proprioceptive (rather than visual) information on accomplishment.

▶   A COGNITIVE-BEHAVIORAL/MOTOR-PSYCHOPHYSIOLOGICAL MODEL OF TIC DISORDER

The current cognitive–psychophysiological (CP) model, while building on previous behavioral research into the development, maintenance and modification of learned habits, integrates a motor-psychophysiology approach with CBT and so proposes that cognitive factors play a much larger role both in the emergence and maintenance of tic behavior. The development and modification of tic behavior are best understood in terms of a reciprocal interaction between psychological and physiological factors in the course of motor action.

A key distinguishing factor of the CP model of tic onset is precisely the reciprocity in everyday practice between cognitive/emotive and behavioral/physiological factors. In accordance with a stage model of motor activity, each successive stage, working back from tic onset, represents the cognitive-behavioral background from which factors at the preceding stage emerge. There is a cognitive style concerning the right way to organize and plan activities, on the one hand, coupled with a heightened self-attention and sensory focus which monitors action and also functions at the psychophysiological level (Figure 3.3). The starting point from the cognitive side is a perfectionist style of planning action. The perfectionism relates most closely to the personal organization and the personal standards subscales of the MPS (Frost et al., 1990). On the behavioral/physiological side, there is heightened sensory focus, hypersensitivity and heightened self-awareness. All elements of the model are already established attributes of TS/TD. The model, as elaborated in the following sections, offers an account of how the reciprocity between elements of sensorimotor activation influences tic onset.

▶   CLINICAL IMPLICATIONS

The CP model would suggest that, in addition to functional analysis, topography of the tic itself should be studied in detail to give information not only on function but on usage. If the model of multidetermined sensorimotor activation and chronic muscle tension production is correct, then the evaluation should also seek

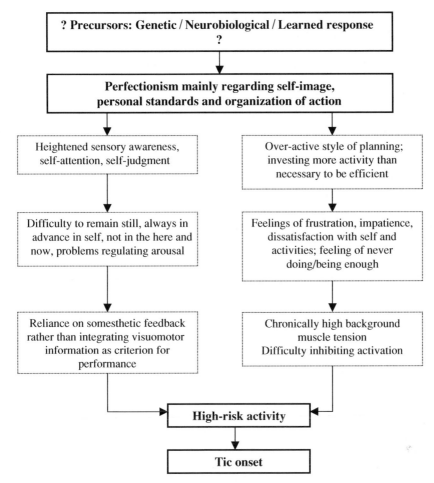

Figure 3.3 Cognitive Psychophysiological Model
Source: From O'Connor (2002). A cognitive-behavioral/psychological model of tic disorders. *Behaviour Research and Therapy*, **40**, 1113–1142.

out a profile of high-risk activity/situations and associated cognitive appraisals and coping strategies defining these high-risk activities. Psychophysiological evaluation would be a useful measure by which to objectively evaluate the level of central motor action and peripheral muscle tension during ticcing.

Treatment based on a CP model would thus necessarily focus on reduction of background motor activation by both cognitive and behavioral means. In the CP model, the local precursor of the tic onset is background tension. Reducing tension overall, however, requires addressing input from four separate sources: muscle tension itself, over-active style of action, effortful preparation in anticipation of the high-risk situation, and the maintaining coping behaviors. The premonitory urge is a combination of sensory awareness, over-prepared muscle tension, attentional focus and the subsequent attribution of inevitability of the tic onset which might feed the attentional focus. Such heightened sensory awareness could be targeted and attenuated by producing habituation through interoceptive exposure to sensations coupled with response prevention. The response prevention would lead to eventual extinction both of the attentional focus behavior maintaining hypersensitive awareness and of the attribution according significance to the premonitory urge, and to the subsequent imminence of the tic. Cognitive strategies would also be useful to challenge hyperattentiveness to self- and excessive self-consciousness and concern over self-image. However, in severe cases of tics where associated behavior is more self-destructive, the preoccupation with ticcing may take on a life of its own and create a separate, very short-term reinforcement schedule. A constant cycle of premonitory urge and frustration will produce – and, in turn, be maintained by – increasingly disinhibited tension/sensation-relieving tic behavior. Here, clearly, habituation to sensory state and increasing tolerance of frustration might be essential initial elements to a treatment program prior to cognitive restructuring (Hood et al., 2004). There is, indeed, some evidence that exposure to premonitory urge is more effective than HR in people with severe TS (Verdellen et al., 2002).

The onset of the tic itself is spurred on by the high level of background motor tension, but, in addition, there seems to be a low degree of flexibility in the tic-affected muscle. The tic-implicated muscle may be in an all-or-nothing state of tension (and never completely at zero tension level). Retraining the muscle to achieve more graded levels of tension may change its habitual use, and at the same time gives the person more flexibility and control over self-regulatory muscle use (O'Connor et al., 1995). In some tic actions, there is also the tendency to involve more muscles than necessary, for example, blinking with cheek muscles in addition to eyelid muscles. Such unnecessary over-investment of effort in response could be normalized through education.

Such education in muscle use involves normalization of muscle use, exclusion of non-relevant muscles, use of appropriate effort and developing the ability to discriminate and articulate, with the help of biofeedback, the parts of an overgeneral reaction (e.g., learning to blink with eyelid rather than cheek muscle). Another technique aimed at preventing tension is "prevention by relaxation", which involves monitoring the tic-affected muscle to keep it in a state of relaxation in order to prevent the tic. This technique can be learned and practiced as a form of habit reversal (O'Connor & Gareau, 1994, p. 66). Rather than containing or suppressing the tics, if the person focuses on relaxation of the tic-implicated muscle, then the tic is prevented. Such competing slow response development has been used as a treatment strategy by Miltenberger et al. (1998). However, the CP model predicts that prevention by relaxation is more likely to reduce muscle tension itself than another type of CR in the long run. The CR component, crucial to HR, is likely by itself to result in increasing tension as the muscle contracts antagonistically to the tic.

At the same time, coping strategies and appraisals maintaining muscle tension and stress – indeed, all effortful ways of disguising or holding in the tic – would ideally be extinguished and replaced by relaxation responses. Such coping strategies would include containment strategies which result in both enhanced vigilance to stress cues and preoccupation with the tic which, in turn, can amplify tension and sensory awareness. Thus, the preferred strategies to reduce tension involve: increasing muscle flexibility, decreasing behavioral activation, correcting the perfectionist beliefs tied to planning action, and the secondary appraisals and coping behaviors maintaining arousal, coupled with an education in economic muscle use.

▶ CONCLUSIONS

The CP model introduces the role of cognitive factors in tic onset. The current chapter has outlined the rationale for adapting a CP approach to tics, based on a motor model which views tics as a functional by-product of overall telic action style. Underlying perfectionist styles of action impairs attention/arousal and mood regulation in people with TD, TS or HD, and addressing such cognitive factors aids general muscle relaxation and prevents tension build-up in tic-affected muscles. Addressing cognitive appraisals about tics also aids habituation to hypersensitivity by shifting attentional attribution and self-focus. The CP approach predicts that all tics and habits in TD/TS/HD show a characteristic situation/activity profile associated with onset and that the muscles affected in tics can be linked by usage or habitual expression to a frustration–action cycle in high-risk tic-onset situations/ activities. The CP model also suggests that preventing a build-up of tension by addressing the excessive activation will be a more effective intervention strategy in the long run than attempting to reverse or resist the habit after it has arrived, and will be more likely to prevent tic substitution. Reducing the level of motor activation in people with TS or TD should also result in changes in experimental motor performance as measured, for example, in studies of motor preparation, visuomotor performance and response inhibition. The CP model should apply equally to people with TD or TS clients, although treatment might differentially target emotional and sensory or cognitive reinforcers of the tic behavior depending on tic severity.

Chapter 4

EMPIRICAL STUDIES TESTING THE COGNITIVE–PSYCHOPHYSIOLOGICAL MODEL

▶ OVERVIEW

The cognitive-behavioral/psychophysiological model makes various claims about the nature of tics. Firstly, that they need to be understood against the background of current telic activity. Secondly, that tics are the result of tension produced by a particular style of action which leads to conflict between stages of motor action. Thirdly, that this local style of action relates to a wider style of planning action which pervades the person's life and leads to an over-active tension-producing activity style. The model also suggests that this chronic activity style will be reflected in an abnormal psychophysiological sensorimotor activation present at both central and peripheral levels. Furthermore, the model suggests that this level of motor activity – as it is due to strategy, not deficit – would be modified by a program that directly addressed style of action in the therapy.

Some of these claims have found support, as detailed in the final sections of the previous chapter, from existing clinical and research literature. In this chapter, we describe empirical studies designed to directly operationalize some of the components of the model and experimentally validate the claims. The selection of studies presented here are not exhaustive but have been chosen to cover key points of the model.

▶ BEHAVIORAL ACTIVITY ASSOCIATED WITH TIC ONSET IN CHRONIC TIC AND HABIT DISORDERS

(Adapted from O'Connor et al., 2003)

▶ Background

The etiology of tics is unknown, but Azrin and Nunn (1973) view tics and habits as developing according to the laws of learning. In a clinical context, functional analysis is frequently employed to clarify the antecedents and consequences reinforcing tic behavior. Azrin and Nunn (1977) recognized that different strategies need to be applied in HR depending on different situations. However, few studies have systematically examined situational profiles associated with TD or HD.

A previous series of studies (O'Connor et al., 1993, 1994, 2001b) reported that clients with tics identified situations when the tic occurred and when it did not occur. High-risk situations could be either high or low arousal situations – for example, one client was most likely to tic when active at work, another when relaxing at home. However, the accompanying thoughts and feelings most frequently concerned impatience and frustration, being judged or not performing as desired. Furthermore, anticipation of a high-risk situation can by itself elicit the tic, suggesting a strong potential role of cognitions (and cognitive appraisal processes) in tic production.

▶ Aim

The aims of the present study were to examine activity profiles linked to tic onset and associated subjective appraisals of the activities in people suffering from chronic TD and HD, and to compare these profiles among different subgroups of TD and HD.

▶ Recruitment

Seventy-six people (out of 83 recruited) aged 18–62 (38 male and 38 female; mean age = 38.2, SD = 10.0; 70% with partners) diagnosed with either chronic TD, TS, or HD participated in the study. We distinguished two diagnostic categories (Table 4.1): *Habit disorders*, encompassing trichotillomania ($n = 15$), bruxism (with daytime component) ($n = 6$), scabiomania (scratching) ($n = 4$) and onycophagia (nail or finger biting) ($n = 15$); and *simple chronic tics*, comprising shoulder movement ($n = 5$), head motion ($n = 18$), eye blinking ($n = 15$), and TS ($n = 4$). Mean chronicity of problems was 24.6 years (SD = 11.0).

▶ Method

The participants completed with an evaluator a form ranking the three most frequent high-risk activities and the three most frequent low-risk activities linked to tic or habit onset. Appraisals associated with the low- and high-risk activities were established by asking the persons to evaluate how they thought any two high-risk activities were similar in a way not shared by low-risk activities (triadic sorting). The appraisals were ranked 1–7, corresponding to how they applied to each individual's low- and high-risk situation.

Table 4.1 Activity profiles associated with low- and high-risk tic and habit onset

Activity type	Example	Habit disorders		Simple tics	
		Low risk	High risk	Low risk	High risk
Study or intellectual activity	Attending class or lecture		Tricho nail biting	Head tics, eye blink tics	
Passive attendance	Watching TV, attending a hockey game		Nail biting	Eye blink tics	Shoulder tics
Relaxation	Relaxing in bed, meditating		Scratching	All tics	
Socialization	Talking in a group or at a party	All habit disorders, especially tricho		Eye blink tics, face tics	
Waiting	Awaiting test results, waiting in line		All habits	Head tics	Other tics
Manual work	Digging a ditch	All habits		Other tics	Shoulder tics

Source: From O'Connor et al. (2003). Behavioral activity associated with onset in chronic tic and habit disorders. *Behavior Research and Therapy,* **41**, 241–249.

► Classification of Activities

The individual reports on the low- and high-risk activities had enough characteristics in common to enable them to be regrouped into the 12 activity categories (study activity, intellectual work, grooming, manual work, passive attendance, eating, relaxing, leisure pursuits, socialization, sport activity, in transit, waiting for an appointment). The same categorization was used for both low- and high-risk activities. Each activity was allocated to one category. As a small proportion of the activities (8 out of 456) did not fit into any of these categories, they were not included in the analysis. The test–retest reliability of the categorization assessed at two points, two months apart, was 1.00. The initial category sorting was replicated by an independent rater. Inter-rater agreement tests conducted on a subset comprising 15 subjects yielded kappa values ranging from 0.60 ($p < 0.02$) to 1.00 ($p < 0.00$).

► Classification of Appraisals

The elicited appraisals related to the low- and high-risk activities were classified into eight constructs: active–inactive; calm–tense; satisfied–dissatisfied; interested – bored; in control–not in control; judged–not judged; energized–tired; and open–reserved. Again, a few entries (5 out of 311) did not belong in any construct category and were omitted. Inter-rater agreement was measured for all categories, again using 15 subjects; kappa values were between 0.53 ($p < 0.04$) and 1.00 ($p < 0.00$).

► Statistical Analysis

In order to compare differences in activity profiles and cognitive appraisals across types of TD and HD, chi-square analyses were conducted. A two-way chi-square compared the presence or absence of activity types or cognitive appraisals in low- and high-risk categories between the two TD/HD groups. Separate analyses were conducted for low- and high-risk activities. If the overall chi-square was significant, the adjusted residuals (non-parametric equivalent of z-scores) for the cell percentage of each subgroup were examined. An adjusted residual score greater than 1.96 for a given subgroup percentage indicated that the subgroup differed significantly from the overall group percentage.

► Results

High-risk Activities

- Study/active listening was a prominent high-risk activity for people suffering from trichotillomania (it was mentioned 60% of the time; adjusted residual = 2.2), and nail biting (64%; adjusted residual = 2.5), whereas it was notably absent from the high-risk activities recorded by people with head movements (11.8%; adjusted residual = −2.3) and eye blinking (13%; adjusted residual = −2.0).
- Passive listening was absent from the high-risk activities of those with shoulder tics significantly more often than for the other subgroups (0%; adjusted residual = −2.2).
- Relaxation was a high-risk activity for scratching (75%; adjusted residual = 3.5).
- Social occasions constituted a high-risk activity for eye blinking (73%; adjusted residual = 3.6) but were included significantly less often in the high-risk activities for trichotillomania (6.7%; adjusted residual = −2.5).

Low-risk Activities

- Social occasions were a low-risk activity for HD (53%; adjusted residual = 2.0).
- Passive listening was a common low-risk activity for eye blinking (67%; adjusted residual = 3.6) while it was ranked significantly more often as a low-risk activity for nail biting (7%; adjusted residual = −2.0).
- Eating was also a low-risk activity for scratching (100%; adjusted residual = 3.6).

Associated Appraisals of Activities

- The tense–calm construct seemed the most relevant to the manifestation of both TD/HD. A tense state was associated with onset of the disorder in 64 out of 76, or 84% of participants.
- A high-risk activity was most likely to be appraised as active by those with simple tics (30%; adjusted residual = 2.7), while appraisal of a high-risk activity as inactive was most likely in HD (56%; adjusted residual = 2.7).

- Appraisals of inactivity were disproportionately absent from the high-risk appraisals of those with eye blink tics (13%; adjusted residual $= -2.3$).
- Appraisal of a high-risk activity as tense was also characteristic of simple tics (93%; adjusted residual $= 2.1$) whereas appraisals of boredom were associated with high-risk situations in HD (44%; adjusted residual $= 3.4$).
- Appraisals of boredom were associated with high risk in trichotillomania (53%; adjusted residual $= 2.7$) and scratching (75%; adjusted residual $= 2.3$), but such appraisals were likely not to constitute a high-risk appraisal for people with a head movement tic (6%; adjusted residual $= -2.2$).
- Appraisal of an activity as inactive was associated with high risk in nail biting (64%; adjusted residual $= 2.1$).
- The appraisal of a high-risk activity as unsatisfying was cited by a large proportion of subjects with head tics (88%) and bruxism (67%), and was also mentioned by 48% of the other subjects.
- Finally, the energized–tired construct as a high-risk appraisal was cited most frequently in trichotillomania (73%), eye blinking (67%) and head movements (71%) but again was also cited by 52% of people in other subgroups.

▶ Discussion

This study demonstrated the existence of an idiosyncratic pattern of high- and low-risk activities for individuals with TD and HD. Moreover, there were also consistent differences in activity profiles between HD and simple tics.

HD (especially trichotillomania, scratching and nail biting) shared common activity profiles, which distinguished them from eye tics particularly. Trichotillomania was associated with intellectual activity. Shoulder tics were associated with manual activities and the onset of eye tics seemed to occur more in social occasions.

People with trichotillomania and nail biting seem to perceive themselves more as inactive when they experience the urge to perform the habit. Also, people with trichotillomania and scratching habits more often feel bored in situations in which they do their habit than do people with other tics/habits.

Conversely, people with tics tend to view themselves as active and tense when ticcing. There was some uniformity of the appraisals regardless of the type of activities, suggesting that despite diversity of activities, the activities themselves are similarly perceived and evaluated across TD and HD. The evaluations seem to reflect boredom, dissatisfaction and tenseness as high-risk state–situation products, regardless of situation or type and level of activity.

The importance of this activity profiling specific to different types of TD cannot be underestimated from a behavioral point of view. Classically, environmental contingencies form the operants for behavioral management, whereas internal states may be classically conditioned to form state-dependent reinforcers and hence maintainers of the problem behavior. Behavior is hence seen as a response to the environmental or state contingencies. Functional analysis forms the cornerstone of behavioral case management, and has always examined precursors and consequences to a behavior as a prelude to applying behavioral principles. Operants previously tied to tic onset include social attention, stress, family dynamics. Onset of HD has also been previously tied to states of depression and boredom. However, the findings from the specific activity profiles fit more within an ecological than a conditioning model, since the association is between location of the tic, the type of tic onset and the type of telic behavioral activity. In other words, tics are more likely to occur at certain sites under some but not other telic activities. Furthermore, tics tend to occur in the muscles most likely to be used in those encounters in either a functional or an expressive way. The analysis of activities was not only confined to high risk but include low risk, so permitting a more thorough appreciation of the functional distinctions between tics, since it tied tic onset in a particular group to use of the muscle during activity, and lack of tic onset in the same muscle to non-use of the muscle within activity.

The findings show that the tic is present when the affected muscle is tied to functional use in a situation (e.g. facial tics during socialization, but that it is absent in another activity. The claim that tics do not occur in a behavioral vacuum seems in part supported and, if so, supports the further claim that tics are associated with wider strategic behavioral plans. Tics could still be learned or copied or substituted, but only within a wider coordinated activity that is also learned or copied.

The next study explores this claim further by investigating the wider behavioral style of planning of people who suffer from tics. It has already been noted that clinical observation has shown this population to have problems with motor restlessness and higher sensorimotor activation. But what is the precise form of this high activation? How would such activation be directly related to tension and to ticcing?

► VALIDATION OF A STYLE OF PLANNING ACTION (STOP) AS A DISCRIMINATOR BETWEEN TIC DISORDER, OBSESSIVE-COMPULSIVE DISORDER AND GENERALIZED ANXIETY

(Adapted from O'Connor et al., 2001a)

► Background

TS and TD are characterized by tics which are non-voluntary repetitive movements that may occur singly or in series and be complex or simple in nature. Subjective report suggests that the role of tics may be tension reduction and there is some evidence that some people with TD may be chronically aroused and show greater startle reflex. Behavioral aspects of such high activation levels include the stressful way adults with tics and, to some degree, with HD tend to adopt tension-producing styles of action where they attempt to do too much and jump from one task to another. These clinical observations provided the basis for constructing a 30-item STOP questionnaire. The aim was to examine the reliability and validity of the STOP instrument and, in particular, to examine the extent to which the style of action was typical of TS and TD compared to other diagnostically close groups with obsessive-compulsive and generalized anxiety disorder, and whether response to the STOP items were trait factors or part of tic symptomatology by examining change in scores pre- and post-behavioral treatment.

▶ Aim

The aim was to assess internal structure, reliability, convergent validity, discriminant validity, clinical validity and predictive validity of the STOP questionnaire.

▶ Questionnaire Items: Content Validity

The STOP questionnaire was designed to systematically assess style of planning action in adults with TS, TD and HD. Thirty items with clinical face validity were chosen on the basis of clinical experience, clinician consensus and preliminary testing. The items were selected on the basis of consensus among experienced clinicians working in our team.

▶ Design

In order to anchor the range of responses, the items were presented in the form of a choice between two alternatives along a continuous line, with the over-active style item at one end of the dimension and its opposite style at the other end. The participants had then to place a vertical line at the point along the horizontal line corresponding to their habitual style (see Appendix 1e). Responses along the dimensional line were scored on a scale from -50 to $+50$ according to whether the response was on the side of the over-active items (0–50) or on the side of the line representing the non-over-active alternatives (0–+50). Scale items were balanced for right or left response bias.

▶ Method

The STOP questionnaire was administered to a sample of 259 people. The data of 241 were entered as complete: the sample included 87 controls (CON) selected from normal population and screened for psychopathology, 53 TS/TD, 45 HD, 42 OCD, including both obsessions with and without overt compulsions (ruminators), and 14 generalized anxiety disorder (GAD). All participants in the clinical groups were about to enter treatment protocols and were diagnosed according to DSM-IV criteria by a psychiatrist and a psychologist using a semistructured interview. There was no diagnostic overlap in the groups selected. In other words, the TS/TD and HD were screened for GAD and OCD and the OCD and GAD were screened for TD.

Table 4.2   Factor scores for clinical groups on STOP – two-factor solution

Factor 1: Over-preparation 3,4,5,6*,14*,15,16,17,26,27,28,29,30				Factor 2: Over-activity 1,2,8,10,11*,18*,19,21,22*,23*			
Group	(N)	Mean	Alpha	Group	(N)	Mean	Alpha
GAD	(14)	−16.77	0.85	GAD	(14)	−3.19	0.18
CON	(87)	10.50	0.81	CON	(87)	−0.12	0.46
TD	(53)	0.29	0.79	TD	(53)	−9.72	0.66
OCD	(36)	−6.85	0.79	OCD	(36)	−3.13	0.23

Note: *Indicates that item is reversed when scoring.

► Factor Analysis

Factor analysis (Table 4.2) with varimax rotation revealed three factors with eigenvalues greater than 2.0 and which accounted for 35% of the item variance. A two-factor solution was retained accounting for 28% of the item variance.

The first factor (18%) grouped together items representing over-preparation/over-investment in planning (e.g., planning for unforeseen events, complicating activities, investing more effort than necessary). The second factor (10%) related more directly to over-activity and the need to be always on the move and doing something, and inability to relax (e.g., unable to keep still, talking too quickly, trying to do too much).

► Test–retest reliability

Test–retest reliability was calculated on TS/TD + HD and CON samples through readministration of the STOP questionnaire 1–2 months later. Alpha reliability for the TD + HD sample ($n = 30$): Factor 1 (over-preparedness) = 0.94, Factor 2 (over-activity) = 0.91; alpha reliability for CON sample ($n = 28$): Factor 1 (over-preparedness) = 0.55, Factor 2 (over-activity) = 0.38.

► Convergent Validity

Convergent validity (Table 4.3) was assessed through correlations between standardized measures of anxiety (Speilberger: State–Trait Anxiety Inventory [STAI]), perfectionism (Frost et al.: Multidimensional Perfectionism Scale [MPC]), obsessions (Rachman & Hodgson: Maudsley Obsessive-Compulsive Inventory [MOCI]), self-esteem (Lawson et al.: Social Self-esteem Inventory [SSI]), depression (Beck Depression Inventory [BDI]), and were correlated with the two major STOP factor scores, in a subsample of participants (who completed all instruments) (number in brackets).

Table 4.3 Correlations between measures and subscales of STOP questionnaire

	Factor 1 **Over-preparedness** subscale correlated with a number of anxiety measures				Factor 2 **Over-activity** subscale correlated only with two perfectionist subscales		
	(N)	Pearson r	Sig.		(N)	Pearson r	Sig.
STAI state anxiety	(89)	−0.29	$p < 0.005$	Personal standards	(96)	−0.35	$p < 0.000$
STAI trait anxiety	(89)	−0.59	$p < 0.000$	Personal organization	(97)	−0.24	$p < 0.02$
MPI subscales:							
• Concern over mistakes	(98)	−0.30	$p < 0.003$				
• Doubts about actions	(99)	−0.52	$p < 0.000$				
• Parental criticism	(99)	−0.19	$p < 0.049$				
MOCI total	(93)	0.44	$p < 0.000$				
MOCI subscales:							
• Checking	(97)	0.38	$p < 0.000$				
• Washing	(94)	0.20	$p < 0.045$				
• Slowness	(96)	0.34	$p < 0.001$				
• Doubt	(98)	0.29	$p < 0.003$				
SSI self-esteem	(96)	0.35	$p < 0.000$				

▶ Discriminant Validity

Discriminant function analysis was computed to compare TS/TD + HD, GAD and OCD groups. There was a significant difference between TS/TD + HD, GAD, OCD and CON groups on both STOP subscales. Over-preparedness: Wilks lambda = 0.91, F ratio equivalent = 10.50, $p < 0.000$; over-activity: Wilks lambda = 0.85, F ratio equivalent = 9.18, $p < 0.000$. The best discrimination was found between TS/TD + HD grouped together compared to GAD and OCD on highest loading items from the two subscales. This discriminant analysis correctly classified: 71.4% of GAD, 72.4% of TS/TD + HD and 80.6% of OCD, for an overall correct classification of 74.3%. Discriminant analysis comparing TS/HD and CON and GAD correctly classified: 35.7% of GAD, 78.2% of CON and 73.5% of TS/TD + HD responses, with 72.9% of cases correctly classified. However, there were only 14 GAD cases.

▶ Internal Consistency

The internal consistency (alpha coefficients) on each scale for each subgroup based on the two-factor solution are given in Table 4.2.

▶ Clinical Validity

The questionnaire was measured pre- and post-behavioral treatment with waitlist control where aspects of both over-preparedness and over-activity were targeted in treatment. The STOP was administered to 74 participants pre- and post-treatment and 24 pre- and post-waitlist. Degree of control over tic or habit was monitored pre- and post-treatment and/or waitlist and at two-month and two-year follow-up.

There were no systematic differences in STOP profiles between TS/TD and HD groups. Significant change on the STOP items after the return from the waitlist control were confined to item 2 (finding it difficult to relax) (t [−2.06], $p < 0.05$), and item 26 (obliged to play a role) (t [−2.34], $p < 0.03$). The changes in both cases were not in a beneficial direction (i.e., post-waitlist, the client groups found it more difficult to relax and more obliged to play a role).

There were significant pre- and post-treatment differences on the following STOP items: post-treatment, both TS/TD and HD clients found it easier to relax (item 2) (F [1, 72] = 12.44, $p < 0.001$); easier to keep still for 15 minutes at a time (item 8) (F [1, 72] = 10.34, $p < 0.002$); easier to complete a task under pressure (item 14) (F [1, 72] = 8.06, $p < 0.006$); unnecessary to always accomplish a task in haste (item 20) (F [1, 72] = 9.47, $p < 0.003$); more important to take time to make a decision than to decide rapidly (item 24) (F [1, 72] = 8.87, $p < 0.004$); preferable to quit or modify boring encounters than tolerate them impatiently (item 25) (F [1, 72] = 10.35, $p < 0.002$). The clients' scores on the STOP questionnaire tended to revert to a less over-active and less over-prepared profile post-treatment.

Factor 1: Over-preparation (examples of high loading items)
   Loading (0.55)
6.   Do you have the impression that you prepare too much for a task and make more effort than necessary?

   ....|..
   Always   Never

   Loading (0.71)
17.   You anticipate the arrival of an unusual or unknown event. Do you:

   ....|..
   Become immediately tense   Adapt to it easily

   Loading (0.66)
26.   Do you feel obligated to play a role rather than be yourself?

   ....|..
   Always   Never

   Loading (0.73)
27.   Do you have a tendency to complicate situations that seem simple to others?

   ....|..
   Always   Never

   Loading (0.61)
29.   During planning for tasks, do you sometimes anticipate unforeseen events that make it more difficult to plan?

   ....|..
   Always   Never

Factor 2: Over-activity (examples of high loading items)
   Loading (0.37)
1.   You have five different tasks to do at home. Would you tend to:

   ....|..
   Begin them all at   Start with the one you
   the same time   consider a priority

   Loading (0.44)
2.   You decide to rest during one hour and to do nothing. Do you find that:

   ....|..
   Very difficult   Very easy

   Loading (0.58)
8.   If you were asked to not move during 15 minutes, would you find this:

   ....|..
   Impossible   Easily realizable

   Loading (0.57)
10.   In a general way, do you speak:

   ....|..
   Quicker than   Slower than
   most people   most people

   Loading (−0.61)
11.   When you plan your schedule for the day, do you:

   ....|..
   Have a realistic conception   Overload yourself
   of what you can achieve   with jobs to do

   Figure 4.1   STOP items (Style of planning questionnarie)

▶ Multiple Regression

Multiple stepwise regression was carried out with degree of control over tic or habit reported at follow-up as the dependent variable and change pre- and post-treatment in style of planning action, STOP anxiety, depression, self-esteem, perfectionism as independent measures. There was a minimal multicolinearity among independent variables and tolerances were good. Change in overall STOP score post-treatment predicted degree of control at two-month follow-up (F [2, 57] $= 6.73$, $p < 0.002$). Changes in selected STOP items ($n = 52$) (items 1, $p < 0.003$; 16, $p < 0.001$; 20, $p < 0.004$; 24, $p < 0.001$) were revealed as highly significant predictors of degree of control over tic at two-year follow-up.

▶ Discussion

People with TD and HD do share a similar profile of STOP which distinguishes them significantly from controls and GAD and OCD. Although the overall variance accounted for by the two-factor solution (35%) was slightly low, other psychometric properties were satisfactory. The test–retest coefficients for the controls were low, but this might be explained by the generally low scores of this group on the high loading STOP items, and hence the lack of consistent over-active styles in controls. The style of planning seems to consist of two subscales which have good consistency and reliability within the tic group. The tic group, however, seems particularly high on the over-activity scale, although the profile on both scales seems important to a satisfactory group discrimination. STOP items are sensitive to clinical change and show predictive validity, so suggesting that style of planning is an index of successful tic or habit management and is therefore modifiable. The discriminative validity of the STOP suggests its potential utility as an aid to diagnosis.

Clinically speaking, people with chronic TD and TS and, to a lesser extent, HD typically do show an over-active style of planning action involving: attempting to accomplish too much; performing several tasks at once; and placing unrealistic expectations on performance (O'Connor et al., 1994). Such a style of action would concord with psychophysiological and experimental evidence of problems in the central organization and preparation of action. Indeed, some of these STOP characteristics resemble the distractibility, impulsivity and hyperactivity of ADHD, which is known to have a significant comorbidity in children with TS. But, on the other hand, this over-active style of planning in adults is linked clinically with convictions about the correct way to organize activity and with perfectionism as measured on MPS (Frost et al., 1990) of personal organization and standards (O'Connor et al., 1997b, 2001a). Other research has suggested a higher prevalence of type A behavior (Hicks et al., 1990). So the over-active style of planning may be driven more by perfectionist ideas than impulsiveness, but so far there has been no systematic evaluation of hyperactivity in adults or in adults with tics or habits. The current STOP scale possesses satisfactory psychometric properties and is being administered in a larger-scale study of hyperactivity in adults.

One of the main functions of both tic and habit cycles may be to release tension, and muscle tension is usually elevated in TD and HD groups. Consequently, relaxation is frequently integrated into habit management programs as an effective treatment strategy. The over-active style of planning might contribute to tension and so may be addressed as part of relaxation. The strong link of this STOP subscale with subscales of perfectionism suggests, however, that cognitive restructuring of activity may also be a beneficial treatment strategy. The change pre- and post-treatment in STOP items suggests this style of action can be modified. Furthermore, change in style of action seemed a good predictor of outcome at follow-up.

The GAD and OCD groups also scored high on the over-preparation scale, with the tic group showing wide variability. The clinical observations were tied specifically to physical over-preparation. We had noted that people with tics often involve redundant muscles in actions – blinking using the cheek muscles, moving in block actions to perform a fine motor task, or simply investing more muscle effort in a task. However, in the questionnaire, we decided to explore this in the wider behavioral perspective of emotional and behavioral over-preparation. One of the features of anxiety disorders is that there is an increasing emotional and cognitive preparation prior to anxiogenic events, which has the effect of increasing activation. A key distinction between controls and social phobics is the amount of preparation prior to speaking (Roy et al., 2002). Clearly, the questionnaire responses reflected more extra-emotional and behavioral effort, and not specifically physical over-preparation.

In the over-activity dimension, however, which was a fairly monolithic construct, TD + HD showed highest scores and supported the claim of a hyperactivity characteristic of TD. However, the study is in the process of replication adding items more relevant to physical over-preparation and more related to physical over-activity to the STOP questionnaire.

Tics arise against background activity and also if this activity is undertaken within a particularly over-active style of planning; in addition, this over-activity seems related to perfectionism which indicates a cognitive and possibly strategic purpose to the hyperactivity. In the next section, we review our psychophysiological studies of TD designed to examine cortical and autonomic and behavioral indices of activation during performance of simple and complex tasks, and so connect planning and motor action through motor psychophysiology.

▶ Muscle Control in Chronic Tic Disorder

Some tics are markedly asymmetrical, for example, shoulder, neck, face and sometimes eye tics can occur only on one side. In our clinical treatment of these problems, we have frequently noted that the person experiencing a tic has difficulty in contracting the affected muscle or muscles slowly. In the case of a unilateral tic, the person is less able to modulate the level of contraction on the tic-affected side than on the contralateral non-affected side between completely contracted and completely relaxed. The tic-affected muscle, when contracted to any degree, immediately jumps to a full contraction. No level of tension other than a full contraction can be sustained and the muscle appears to have reflex-like qualities.

In a systematic study of 18 patients with asymmetrical tics, this lack of flexibility in the tic-affected muscle was confirmed (O'Connor et al., 1995), by recording muscle activity, pre and post, a series of discrimination exercises designed to train graded contraction in tic-affected muscles. Prior to treatment, neither muscle was able to relax to zero. The tic-affected muscle was clearly less controllable than the non-affected muscle and subjects had more difficulty learning to discriminate and control contraction level. But increasing control over the contraction did increase the degree of control over the tic in the majority of subjects.

All subjects achieved the discrimination criterion of identifying unaided degrees of muscle contraction, but, subsequently, we have refined this criteria as the ability to smoothly and continuously increase and decrease muscle activity level between 0 and full-scale contraction. A visually displayed computer graphic gave feedback as an indication of the continuity of contraction. Our clinical experience has suggested that it is important to achieve isolation of the muscle or muscle group from surrounding groups affected during the discrimination exercise. Successful control over muscle contraction was followed in six cases by a clinically significant decrease (>40% of initial value). The lack of change in the measures at a neutral site and in heart rate suggested that changes in the tic-affected muscles were not due to general state changes in arousal or habituation.

The findings provide some psychophysiological evidence for Corbett's (1976) proposal that the muscles implicated in simple tics exhibit a reflex-like quality in that they are under less voluntary control than non-affected sites, and that modifying the "reflexive" nature of the muscle does have some immediate effect on tic frequency. Replacing the tic with a soft response over a period of several weeks has been reported in the literature as a form of competing response which, when practised contingently with the tic, can reverse the tic habit when it occurs (Azrin & Peterson, 1989). But in our case the exercises were non-contingent and simply involved increasing control of the muscle contraction with the aid of biofeedback. The study, though preliminary, suggested that increasing control over tic-affected muscles may be an important factor in augmenting control over the tic. The next study looked specifically at preparation and execution stages of action while monitoring electrophysiological measures of cortical activation.

► BRAIN–BEHAVIOR RELATIONS DURING MOTOR PROCESSING IN CHRONIC TIC AND HABIT DISORDERS

(Adapted from O'Connor et al., in press)

► Background

In accordance with the stage model, motor processing begins with a planning stage, involving a generalized motor program. A preparation stage "tunes" the response, and an execution stage with decreasing degrees of freedom accompanied by error correction, if necessary, terminates in an action end point (Schmidt, 1988). The preparation stage does not necessarily overlap with the execution stage (Leuthold and Jentzsch, 2002). Motor action itself can be decomposed into different stages, each associated respectively with distinct cortical event-related potentials (ERP) components. For instance, ERP components such as readiness potential (RP) and movement associated potential (MAP) are thought to reflect respectively processes of response preparation (Brunia, 1980; Brunia & Damen, 1988; Kornhuber & Deecke, 1977), and response execution (Rektor et al., 2001). RP typically shows a slow negative going deflection prior to movement and maximal at the pre-central motor cortex. RP precedes voluntary movement and is largest when preparation for movement involves planned effort (Kornhuber, 1978). RP seems higher during activation of selective complex responses, particularly during performance of sequential complex finger movements (Cui et al., 2000a, 2000b). It is nearly or entirely absent during reflex actions (Obeso et al., 1981), although tics themselves may sometimes appear semivoluntary with accompanying RP (Duggal & Haque Nizamie, 2002; Karp et al., 1996). Movement itself produces a potential maximal over the vertex called MAP. MAP represents a composite index of pre-central cortex motor activation while generating the pyramidal tract volley following response and may also be a function of reafferent and proprioceptive feedback to cortical areas from subcortical structures (Brunia & Vuister, 1979; Brunia et al., 1982; Rektor et al., 1998). RP shows higher amplitude in the sensorimotor areas, whereas MAP is localized more posteriorly. Hence RP and MAP measures appear as independent processes, but their electrocortical topography is sensitive to type of planned motor execution (O'Connor, 1980). In particular, the parameters of movement may vary depending on whether the intended action is controlled or automated. All movements involve some degree of controlled and automated components, but these components may be differentially emphasized depending on task demand and complexity of the act required. The key influence on whether controlled or automated planning has priority seems to be related to the complexity of movement (Osman et al., 1990b). There is evidence that separate cortical systems are linked to automated timing (motor and pre-motor circuits) and cognitively controlled tasks (pre-frontal and parietal circuits) (Lewis & Miall, 2003). Thus, anticipation of the nature of the act, its complexity and consequences becomes of paramount importance in determining the preparation and enactment of controlled acts.

Chronically high levels of activation may predispose the tic person to perform automated ballistic actions as a way of trying to regulate proprioceptive (sensory) feedback on state. Under conditions of stress, the person with a tic may find it more difficult to initiate a controlled action and stop an automated action. This hypothesis was partially supported in previous studies examining automated and controlled performance during countermanding STOP and GO paradigms (O'Connor et al., 1999, 2000). These studies reported that whereas the control group showed faster reaction time (RT) for automated than for controlled response conditions, the TD group showed no condition effects (37). Furthermore, O'Connor et al. (2000) reported no differences between TD, HD and control groups in GO reaction time (GO RT) but a difference in the ability to inhibit an automated response (STOP RT) as reflected in a slower STOP RT to automated than controlled responses in the TD group. The control group (CON) showed a practice effect over time in both STOP and GO RT, whereas the patient groups showed no practice effect in either STOP or GO RT over two trial blocks. The results were interpreted as showing that in TD there is a difficulty in modulating motor activation level in accordance with task demand and that such patients have a tendency to be chronically over-aroused.

The aim of the current report was to examine the electrocortical chronometry of motor processing in clinical groups affected with either TD or HD compared to a non-psychiatric CON group, as recorded before (RP) and during (MAP) the generation of controlled and automated RT. In accordance with our previous RT results and with brain-imaging studies, we hypothesized that the TD and HD groups would show a heightened cortical arousal compared to the CON group and consequently (a) the TD and HD groups would show no systematic difference in RP or MAP peak latency or amplitude between automated and controlled performance, and (b) the TD and HD groups would show no practice effect for either the RP or MAP amplitude or RT across two consecutive trial blocks due to chronic activation. We also predicted that the correlation between RP latency and MAP latency, and between RP latency and RT, would be lower in TD compared to the CON group, where suboptimal modulation of response planning in TD would presumably produce a more variable relationship between preparation and the processes involved in response execution.

► Materials and Methods

Participants

Participants entering a behavioral management program for tics were recruited pre-treatment. Scalp recording electrodes were placed over frontal left and right central and parietal areas. Eighteen TD, 24 HD, and 24 controls (CON) originally participated in our study. After elimination due to movement artefact or technical problems, 44 participants remained (14 CON, 17 HD and 13 TD). The TD group comprised 8F, 5M (all right-handed [assessed by the Edinburgh Handedness Questionnaire] [39], age 39.54 [11.4]). Six had eye tics, 4 head tics, 2 vocal tics, and 1 shoulder tic. The HD group comprised 12F, 5M (15 right-handed, age 38.3 [10.3]). Seven had trichotillomania, 8 onychophagia and 2 had bruxism. Mean chronicity of the problem in the TD group was 26.4 [11.2] and for the HD group 22.3 [9.2]. The non-psychiatric control group comprised 9F, 5M (13 right-handed, age 36.4 [9.5]). Those diagnosed with chronic TD scored between 2.5 and 12.0 on the global calculation of the Tourette's Syndrome Global Scale (TSGS) (Harcherik et al., 1984), which is in the mild–moderate range. Typically, apart from the presence of tics causing distress and at least some disruption of activities, social and other functioning was not significantly impaired with the exception of some degree of motor restlessness.

The Traffic Light Task

The traffic light paradigm (O'Connor & Lapierre, 1994) was a fixed 4-second foreperiod reaction time task. The 4-second warning period permitted adequate preparation for controlled and automated responses. The inter-stimulus interval (ISI) was constant at 4 seconds and the inter-trial interval (ITI) varied randomly between 5 and 15 seconds. The longer foreperiod permitted adequate distinction between early sensory components and ensured that RP was unconfounded by orienting processes (Cui et al., 2000a, 2000b). The paradigm allowed us to compare cortical events during the time to initiate an automated and controlled response. Two sets of three lights appeared side by side on a computer screen in the form of traffic lights. One set signaled an automated, and the other a controlled, response sequence. Each trial began with one of the two yellow READY lights signaling that, in 4 seconds, the green GO light would appear and the participant would have to make either a controlled or an automated response. The *automated response* was three taps on a lever with the two fingers of the dominant hand (– – –). The *controlled response* was three taps of Morse code "dash-dot-dash" (–·–) on another lever but using the same two fingers of the dominant hand. After a period of acclimatization of 20 trials, all participants received two replications of 52 trials, with a short rest period between replications.

▶ Results

There was a significant group by condition interaction ($F[2,41] = 4.01$, $p < 0.03$). A subsequent ANOVA, comparing TD and CON groups, revealed that the interaction was mainly due to the difference between TD and CON, which produced a significant group by condition interaction ($F[1,25] = 7.31$, $p < 0.02$). However, the ANOVA comparing HD and CON groups showed no significant interaction ($F[1,29] = 0.358$, $p = 0.55$), whereas the CON group showed higher MAP amplitude under automated compared to controlled response conditions across both blocks. These group differences in MAP amplitude were reflected more significantly in the discrepancy between RP and MAP amplitude across groups. This difference measure (RP minus MP peak amplitude) showed a significant group by condition effect ($F[2,41] = 5.11$, $p < 0.01$) over all electrode sites during the controlled condition, especially in the first block of trials. The Scheffé post hoc test revealed that the TD group showed the largest difference and the CON group the least difference.

Relationships between Behavioral (RT) and Electrophysiological (RP–MAP) Measures

There was regression between RP peak latency and RT. The CON group showed a linear relationship between RP latency and RT under automated and controlled conditions in all electrode sites (Table 4.4). The HD and TD groups showed no linear relationship between RP latency and RT under any performance conditions. This latter finding was not confounded by heterogeneity of variance across groups and represented a genuine difference in association between response time and preparation processes in the clinical groups.

In sum, the TD group showed no correlation between electrocortical and behavioral processes engaged in motor preparation and those reflecting execution of the motor responses. In the CON group, these two stages were highly associated. The HD group fell midway between the TD and CON groups.

▶ Discussion

Results revealed that the CON group was better able than the clinical groups to modulate RP and MAP peak amplitude in accordance with practice and task demand. The CON group showed larger MAP amplitude in the automated

Table 4.4   Linear regression coefficients between latency of readiness potentials and reaction time measures under automated and controlled conditions

ERP measures	Type of reaction time	Electrode placement	Control		Habit disorder		Chronic tic disorder	
			R^r	p	R^r	p	R^r	p
Readiness potential	Automated condition	Frontal	**0.55**	0.00	0.02	0.60	0.04	0.51
		Left central	**0.52**	0.00	0.01	0.70	0.01	0.70
		Right central	**0.42**	0.01	0.00	0.91	0.03	0.60
		Partial	**0.54**	0.00	0.02	0.59	0.02	0.62
	Controlled condition	Frontal	0.14	0.19	0.02	0.56	0.11	0.26
		Left central	**0.64**	0.00	0.01	0.67	0.07	0.37
		Right central	**0.35**	0.03	0.01	0.66	0.01	0.80
		Parietal	**0.37**	0.02	0.01	0.69	0.00	0.98

Source: From O'Conner et al. (in press). Brain–behavior relations during motor processing in chronic tic and habit disorder. *Cognitive and Behavioral Neurology.*
Note: Data in **bold** characters are significant at 0.05.

condition, so indicating that execution of the response was more readily achieved under automated processing. In contrast, neither clinical group showed a systematic distinction in either preparatory or motor associated responses between controlled and automated responses.

The lack of a systematic condition or practice effects in TD and HD groups could suggest high cortical activation. Alternatively, the difficulty in TD may be to inhibit non-relevant activation so impeding selective efficient preparation for the corresponding response execution, particularly under complex task demand.

The linear regression results between RT and RP peak latency revealed a strong linear association in the CON group, indicating a temporal synchrony between central motor decisions and response times. This synchrony was absent in both the HD and TD groups where there was no association between RP peak latency and RT under any conditions.

The participants in the current study were diagnosed with TD rather than TS. However, the restricted range of scores on the TSGS in our TD group was largely due to the absence of impairment in social and other functioning in everyday life. Motor tic frequency covered the complete range [1–5] of the scale. Since tics are the defining characteristic of both TS and TD, it seems reasonable to speculate that the current results would generalize to a more severe TS group.

The current differences in cortical indices of preparation support the hypothesis that difficulties in planning actions optimally are characteristic of chronic TD.

► **Summary of Psychophysiological Investigations**

The psychophysiological findings then support the claim that people with TD have higher activation levels at both cortical and motor level. The findings support other studies that have shown that the problems with TD lie more with inhibition than with activation. Furthermore, the activation levels are chronic and people with tics seem unable to ever completely relax tension. Cognitively speaking, the event-related potential studies indicate no problem in planning as such, or in executing, but a lack of consistent relationship between planning and response. We speculate that over-activation at a cortical level may produce this discrepancy by impeding normal flow. But the particular motor strategy that induces conflict is unclear, and awaits further investigation. More light might be shed on this problem by studying the relation between ERPs recorded at all stages of planning. In particular, it would be interesting to study the relationship between attentional and motor components of ERPs to see which is predominantly affected in TD and if there is a covariation.

The experimental psychophysiological findings so far reviewed have empirically supported claims of the model to the extent of tying tic to background activity, background activity to general style of planning and a cognitive perfectionism, and TD to chronic tension and over-activation and also to discontinuity between planning and execution.

The next study reports the evaluation of a therapy directly addressing issues in the planning of action, and introducing a cognitive-motor component into the habit reversal package aimed at modifying planning and preparation for action both in and out of high-risk tic situations.

▶ A COGNITIVE-BEHAVIORAL PROGRAM FOR THE MANAGEMENT OF CHRONIC TIC DISORDERS

(Adapted from O'Connor et al., 2001b)

▶ Background

The most compelling behavioral treatment for managing the tics in TD or TS seems to be HR (Azrin & Nunn, 1973). This package involves multiple stages, including relaxation, awareness, contingency training for positive reinforcement of not ticcing and the crucial element of practice of a competitive antagonistic response. HR has also been found effective for HD such as nail biting, hair pulling and oral habits, again with small-scale uncontrolled studies, variable treatment and follow-up periods (Peterson et al., 1994). Although HR has shown startling success in individual selected cases and in small-scale controlled studies, there have been no large-scale randomized-controlled studies of the efficacy of HR.

In a previous study of six cases who did not respond to HR treatment (O'Connor et al., 1999), five showed substantial improvement (80–100%) following a cognitive intervention targeting style of action. Tic clients reported that challenging the beliefs and assumptions underlying the client's general style of action, increased the likelihood of applying the tic control strategy to new and diverse situations, possibly since the client gained more opportunity to understand the way in which anticipation influences preparation, and tension levels. At the beginning of cognitive therapy, many tic clients were skeptical of how thoughts can affect what they perceived as a physical problem. However, in our experience, after reading the relevant sections of the manual (O'Connor & Gareau, 1994), the clients were struck by how many of the list of styles of action "clicked" as applying to them. Subsequently, the exercises aimed at modifying planning reaffirmed the link between the action styles and tension. Only one client relapsed in the group of six who benefited from the style of action intervention, and all six clients, themselves, reported that changing their style of action was a key factor in improving their tension regulation.

The model that served as a heuristic guide to clinical practice was as follows: perfectionism regarding self-image, personal standards and personal organization creates unrealistic expectations of performance which lead to a counterproductive style of action (e.g., attempting too much). Subsequently, frustration at not performing as desired produces heightened tension, part of which involves over-preparing muscles for the anticipated task (associated with the frustration). This tension, which can be relieved short term by repetitive tense–release cycles, provokes the tic habit. In support of this last claim, muscle tension values decreased in tic-affected sites post-treatment, though higher tension pre-treatment may only be present in high-risk tic situations and not when the person is at rest (O'Connor et al., 1995, 1997b).

The present waitlist control study evaluates the efficacy of a manualized cognitive-behavioral treatment program based on the HR package with an additional cognitive component addressing style of action, and administered under standardized conditions to a large sample of both HD and TD recruited from the general population.

Incompatible competing responses took three forms: prevention by relaxation (localized relaxation to counteract onset of the tic in the high-risk situations, see Table 4.5, p. 83); normalization (a more normal response substituted for the tic or habit by pacing the tic response, e.g., correcting excessive blinking through training in the use of correct muscles and rhythm); and behaviorally antagonist response in accordance with HR recommendations (Carr, 1995). The *cognitive* aspect of restructuring action aimed at introducing flexibility into judgments and anticipations about intended action, both in high-risk and other situations. Perfectionist beliefs about personal organization were specifically addressed including: developing realistic expectations about performance; investing appropriate effort in performance; accepting realistic feedback on performance ability; and avoiding strategies that create tension and frustration.

Relapse prevention and generalization strategies (e.g., Marlatt & Gordon, 1985) included: foreseeing stressful states and excitable events likely to occur in the future; adopting a rational approach to any future relapse; and not catastrophizing any recurrence of the problem.

▶ Participants

Participants were recruited from announcements in the local and metropolitan jour-
nals. A psychiatric interview assessed participants according to DSM criteria and
on personal history and severity of tic symptoms. Baseline clinical and questionnaire data were available on a maximum of 105 (54 TS/TD, 51 HD) participants.
At the end of pre–post waitlist/treatment, questionnaire data was available on
a maximum of 90 participants, although missing values reduced this number on
some items. These 90 broke down into 47 chronic TD and 43 other HD. The sites
of the simple tics broke down further according to principal tic-causing distress as:
eye, 15; head/shoulders/neck, 19; face, 6; hands, 2; abdomen, 2; legs, 1; vocal tics
(including respiration-related tics), 2. The type of HD included: trichotillomania,
13; onychophagia, 12; scabiomania (scratching/skin pulling), 6; bruxism, 4; complex finger/hand routines, 3; other body movements, 5. Thirteen participants met
criteria for Tourette's syndrome.

▶ Waitlist

Thirty-eight people were randomly allocated to the waitlist and this included
22 TS/TD and 16 HD. The intention-to-treat waitlist period was designed to control for the initial effect of volunteering, the passage of time and the spontaneous
variations in tic severity (tics may wax and wane over time). The treatment or waitlist period lasted 14–16 weeks. After retest, those on the waitlist then received the
cognitive-behavioural treatment package and follow-up procedures.

▶ Questionnaire Measures

Questionnaire measures to assess psychosocial function and psychopathology
included: the Social Self-esteem Inventory (SSI) (Lawson et al., 1979); the Life Experience Survey (LES) (Sarason et al., 1978); the Speilberger State–Trait Anxiety
Inventory (STAI) (Speilberger et al., 1970); the Beck Depressive Inventory (BDI)
(Beck, 1970); the General Health Questionnaire (GHQ) – 12-item version (Goldberg, 1972); the Maudsley Obsessional–Compulsive Inventory (MOCI) (Rachman
& Hodgson, 1980); the Eysenck Personality Inventory (EPI) (Eysenck & Eysenck,
1980). This style of planning action was measured by a 30-item Style of Planning (STOP) questionnaire measuring personal organization, the need to be over-
prepared, always on the move, and accomplishing as much as possible. The Multidimensional Perfectionism Scale (MPS) (Frost et al., 1990) was also administered.

▶ Clinical Measures

The clinical measures included a *daily tic diary* which recorded frequency (total
number per period), intensity (weak 1, strong 5) and degree of control over the

tic (none 0, complete 100) on a daily basis in a specially prepared booklet. The participants were trained in the use of the booklet and a unit of tic (tics) or habit was defined at the beginning of the evaluation.

A separate *situational grid* identified the high- and low-risk situations for tic occurrence and also measured the probability of the tic occurring in each high- and low-risk situation. *Videos* were recorded for all participants pre- and post-treatment/waitlist for 10 minutes in a conversation with the therapist about the tic problem and for 10 minutes during re-creation of a high-risk situation likely to provoke the tic. An external rating of a *close other* was obtained (when possible) on the change in frequency, intensity and other relevant aspects of behavior.

▶ Cognitive-behavioral Program

The entire treatment package was administered for a standard period of 12 weekly sessions with a further one-month home practice and then full post-treatment evaluation. All stages of the program were administered to all participants who did not abandon.

In the information stage, the person was presented with the rationale of the program, definition of the problem habit, information on motor habits and inappropriate strategies of dealing with them (e.g., suppression).

The *awareness* stage comprised auto-observation, monitoring exercises, completing a situational profile, and identifying the cognitive factors (e.g., anticipations/expectations) associated with the high-risk tic situations.

The next stage involved relaxation and muscle discrimination exercises aimed at: (1) demonstrating, with the aid of biofeedback, how behavioral strategies induce a change in motor and autonomic arousal; (2) increasing knowledge of different tension levels; (3) learning standard applied relaxation techniques (Bernstein & Borkovec, 1973; Ost, 1987).

The final *cognitive-behavioral restructuring* stage aimed to modify anticipations and evaluations linked to high-risk situations; challenge beliefs about planning and organization of action; and rehearse incompatible cognitive-behavioral responses to prevent tic onset (Table 4.5).

▶ Changes Following Treatment

Clinical Outcome

Seventy-one (88%) of the completers (with diaries) showed a significant decrease in both tic/habit frequency and intensity post-treatment on diary, clinical and video measures. Fifty-two (65%) reported control between 75 and 100% over the tic/habit post-treatment, 16 (20%) reported between 50 and 75% control, and 12 (15%)

reported less than 50% control. At two-month follow-up, there was no relapse. Eleven TD and 16 HD had completely eliminated the tic/habit at two-month follow-up, and, of these, three TD and six HD reported some degree of relapse at two-year follow-up. Conversely, four TD and three HD who had not eliminated post-treatment reported complete elimination at two-year follow-up. Two-year follow-up was conducted by a structured telephone interview with a total of 56 participants who had successfully completed the program. At two-year follow-up, 43 (77%) of those contacted had maintained or improved their control, and 29 (52%) still reported 75–100% control.

▶ Participant Evaluations

Of the 90% of participants who reported practicing the *awareness exercises*, 39% found them very useful; 96% used the *auto-observations* (daily diary), and 70% found this very useful; 91% practiced the *physiological* and *relaxation* exercises and 68% found them useful; 96% used *cognitive and behavioral restructuring* of whom 66% reported finding it very useful; 98% reported changing *style of action* at least somewhat, of whom 65% reported finding it very useful; finally, 91% reported that interaction with the *therapist* was very useful. There were no differences between the TD and HD groups in the type and use of strategies or in the strategies used or found helpful.

▶ Questionnaire Measures Pre- and Post-treatment

There was a significant decrease post-treatment in both state and trait on the STAI (state: $F [1,78] = 8.21$, $p < 0.005$; trait: $F [1,77] = 11.09$, $p < 0.001$) score and on the BDI ($F [1,75] = 31.83$, $p < 0.001$). On the MPS, there was a significant decrease in the subscale: concern over mistakes ($F [1,77] = 6.84$, $p < 0.01$), but no change on other subscales. There was a significant decrease in the GHQ ($F [1,77] = 32.40$, $p < 0.001$). The SSI showed an overall significant increase post-treatment ($F [1,77] = 14.05$, $p < 0.01$). There were no equivalent significant changes in the waitlist group (Figure 4.2).

▶ Conclusion

The active cognitive-behavioral treatment program was more effective than a waitlist condition and was equally effective for TD, HD and TS. Completion of the program also produced beneficial effects on mood and psychosocial functioning. The lack of substantial differences in change parameters between TD and HD groups suggests these two disorders respond identically to the same cognitive-behavioral approach. The idiosyncratic situational profile found in every case of TD, TS and HD in the present study underscores the importance of functional analysis in the treatment of both disorders. The presence of cognitive appraisals

Degree of control over tic

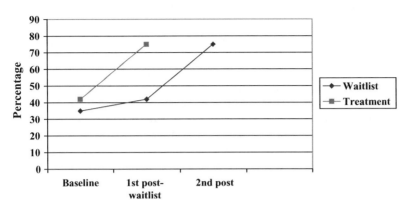

Figure 4.2   Change in tic frequency pre- and post-waitlist and post-CBT treatment

Table 4.5   Competing responses antagonistic to tension build-up

Hand movements	Keep hands in contact with surface or object or a part of the body (e.g., thighs) which can give feedback on position and state of tension. Alternatively, place hands in a location or position antagonistic to tension in the pocket or lightly gripping an object
Arm movements	Keep arms hanging close to the body when not in use and be aware of unnecessarily tensing forearms and raising to "half-most", bent tense at the elbow. Place forearms resting across each other at waste level
Shoulder movements	Keep shoulders down below neck level. Be aware of shoulders rising unnecessarily during manual actions. Monitor for small "adjustment" movements which may alter position and create tension. If sitting, place shoulder blades against seat back to give feedback on position and state
Neck	Be aware of habitual postures involving neck torsion or tendencies to place neck at an angle when writing or attending or holding neck in when speaking
Head	Head should follow gaze direction and face object of attention. Be aware of holding head in fixed position to avoid full focus
Eye blinks	Focus on slow blinking at rate 3–5 per second. Be aware of any over-fixation of gaze when attending to someone/something. Shift gaze every 5–10 seconds to a reduced tension. Be aware of implication of other facial muscles besides eye muscles and eye lids when blinking or looking
Vocal tics	Slow diaphragmatic breathing. Relax throat and neck muscles. Extend outbreaths
Legs	Keep feet sole-down on the floor, legs apart. Be aware of sitting or standing on toes, or of pressing thighs together

Source: Inspired by Carr (1995). Competing responses for the treatment of Tourette's syndrome and tic disorders. *Behavioural Research and Therapy,* **33** (4), 455–456.

associated with tic situations and their modification post-treatment points also to the potential clinical utility of targeting cognitions. If cognitive factors play a defining role in the phenomenology of TD and HD and contribute substantially to the chance of successful maintenance of habit change, then the addition of a more time-consuming cognitive approach to the already successful HR as the behavioral treatment of choice seems justified. The over-active STOP, which was identified and addressed as part of treatment, also emerged as an important predictor of relapse at follow-up. Modifying a tension-producing mode of action might be expected to help to reduce build-up of muscle tension. Our results strongly suggest that a cognitive-behavioral approach to treating tics and habit disorders should be considered either as an alternative to, or in conjunction with, medication. One problem in trying to isolate active components in the treatment is that all components seem to be active, but for different people at different times. Hence, the contributions have to be assessed statistically and quantitatively.

The modification of style of action did seem to contribute to successful outcome. It also predicted relapse at two-year follow-up. Furthermore, key aspects of style of action changed post-treatment, suggesting that the program was successful in addressing cognitive and behavioral aspects. Although we were unable to record physiological measures post-treatment, motor performance measures were completed pre- and post-treatment and waitlist. The next section briefly reports these findings, since visuomotor ability is frequently associated with tics and TS, and any changes here might be important to reference to the debate on strategy versus deficit.

▶ DOES BEHAVIOR THERAPY MODIFY VISUO-MOTOR PERFORMANCE IN CHRONIC TIC DISORDER?

(Adapted from O'Connor et al., 2001c)

▶ Background

TS and TD have been associated with basal ganglia function and some clinical studies have reported abnormal movement parameters (Hollander et al., 1990) and difficulties inhibiting movements (Channon et al., 1992). However, studies of executive function have failed to show consistent poorer performance in either TD or TS (Bornstein, 1991b). But no studies to date have examined a range of purely motor tasks, covering different types of motor function.

The aim of the present study was to compare motor performance involved in aiming movements, hand coordination and fine control of steadiness in a group of TD, with a group of HD, and a non-pathological control group. In addition, the client groups were tested pre- and post-successful completion of a behavioral management program.

► Recruitment

One hundred and five tic- and habit-disordered participants (54 TD [of whom 13 were TS], 51 HD) were recruited at baseline from participants in a behavioral management program. Thirty-four controls were volunteers, matched on age and level of education to the client groups. Controls were screened on a battery of psychopathological questionnaires.

Thirty-six of the client group were randomly allocated to a waitlist control condition for three months. The rest received a three-month behavioral treatment package. All participants were retested at three months and two months, then at two-year follow-up. The behavioral program was based on Azrin and Nunn's (1973) and Azrin and Peterson's (1989) "habit-reversal" technique with an additional component addressing style of action. Exercises aimed at style of planning action and at improving motor control and efficiency were combined with relaxation techniques to aid control over tic or habit. Clinical outcome measures included a self-report diary recording tic habit, video situational ratings and close other ratings.

► Hypotheses

The hypotheses were: (1) the TS/TD group would show poorer performance on all motor measures than the HD group or controls – the controls showing best performance; (2) the TS/TD subjects who successfully completed a behavioral program to improve control over tics would show improved motor performance at three-month retest.

► Performance Tests

The performance tests included the Wisconsin card sorting test (WCST) (Heaton et al., 1993), the Purdue pegboard test (Lafayette Instrument Company), the groove steadiness test and the hole type steadiness test (see Table 4.6).

The WCST was scored according to the manual direction instructions. Scores included total number of categories sorted, number of trials administered, correct responses, errors, perseverative and non-perseverative errors and percentage conceptual level responses and learning to learn (conceptual efficiency across categories). Together these subscores yield a total score.

There were no differences between the TS/TD and HD groups in any of the WCST scores and all scores fell within the 16% or greater percentile range of the age-matched norms of WCST published in Heaton et al. (1993). So, there was no evidence of abnormal WCST performance in the TS/TD or HD groups in our sample.

Table 4.6 Purdue pegboard, groove test, hole steadiness test for each group

	Baseline		Waitlist		Post-treatment	
	Tic disorder ($n = 54$) (sd_{n-1})	Habit disorder ($n = 51$) (sd_{-1})	Tic disorder ($n = 22$) (sd_{n-1})	Habit disorder ($n = 14$) (sd_{n-1})	Tic disorder ($n = 43$) (sd_{n-1})	Habit disorder ($n = 37$) (sd_{n-1})
Groove test						
Dominant hand	21.57 (1.43)	21.34 (1.75)	21.42 (1.37)	21.34 (1.52)	21.67 (1.18)	21.52 (1.36)
Non-dominant hand	20.05 (2.0)	20.59 (1.56)	20.48 (1.75)	20.73 (1.68)	21.05 (1.49)	20.64 (1.62)
Hole test		($n = 47$)				
Dominant hand	64.16 (10.03)	62.50 (9.63)	65.94 (5.91)	60.29 (11.32)	63.81 (8.53)	64.15 (8.39)
Non-dominant hand	60.79 (10.21)	60.06 (10.37)	59.75 (8.60)	56.77 (11.66)	61.05 (9.01)	62.08 (8.29)
Purdue pegboard						
Dominant hand	45.75 (4.04)	46.30 (4.90)	47.82 (4.44)	47.79 (7.85)	46.84 (4.59)	47.66 (4.99)
Non-dominant hand	43.93 (3.69)	45.00 (4.91)	44.27 (4.80)	44.64 (6.08)	45.51 (3.38)	46.51 (3.48)

Source: Adapted from O'Connor et al. (2001c). Does behavior therapy modify motor performance in chronic tic disorder? Presented at *World Congress of Behavioral and Cognitive Therapy*. Vancouver, Canada (July).

Purdue Pegboard

This test has been validated as a measure of sensorimotor–motor performance efficiency in both normal and clinical populations, and is scored as the total number of small pegs, placed in a series of aligned holes by dominant/non-dominant hands separately and both at the same time. There was no significant difference between the TS/TD and HD groups in total pegs placed by the dominant hand, the non-dominant hand or by both hands simultaneously. All scores were in the top 10 percentile of the norms given by Lafayette and co-authors in the instruction manual.

There was, however, a significant difference in performance between client groups and the control subjects in the number of pegs placed by dominant, non-dominant and both hands simultaneously (dominant $F[2,134] = 5.28$, $p < 0.006$; non-dominant $F[2,134] = 3.11$, $p < 0.047$; together $F[2,123] = 7.74$, $p < 0.0007$; total $F[2,133] = 8.90$, $p < 0.0002$). The controls performed better than the client group and placed a greater number of pegs.

Groove Test

The groove test was scored as the distance in centimeters (max. 25 cm) traveled along the groove until the probe touched the side. The score was averaged over 10 trials. There were no differences between the TS/TD or HD groups in mean distance or between client and control groups.

The Hole Type Steadiness Test

The performance was measured as the total time for which the person was able to maintain the probe steady for 10 seconds within the nine successive holes of the test, each hole having an increasingly small diameter. Total time possible was 90 seconds (10×9) for each of three successive replications. The score was the total mean time over three replications for dominant and non-dominant hands, the time averaged over all trials for both hands, and the number of contacts between the probe and the side of the hole.

Again there was no difference between the TS/TD and HD groups in performance, but there was a significant difference between the control group and the client groups in performance for the dominant hand ($F[2,128] = 7.01$; $p < 0.001$), the non-dominant hand ($F[2,129] = 5.62$; $p < 0.005$) and a suggestive difference in overall mean score for both hands ($F[2,129] = 2.48$; $p < 0.08$). The client groups attempted more holes but the controls kept the probe steadier and made less contacts.

► **Pre- and Post-behavioral Treatment**

Scores on each of the motor performance tests were examined pre- and post-treatment and were compared with the scores from the waitlist group retested after an equivalent period of time without treatment.

In the groove test, there were no significant treatment effects for the dominant hand, or treatment by group interactions effects; but for the non-dominant hand, there was a suggestive effect over time (F [1, 75] = 3.70, p < 0.058) and a group by treatment effect (F [1, 75] = 3.57, p < 0.063) which indicated a significant improvement post-treatment for the TS/TD group and less improvement for the HD group.

The Purdue pegboard showed a significant improvement over treatment for the dominant hand performance (F [1, 76] = 6.52, p < 0.013) and non-dominant hand performance (F [1, 76] = 15.41, p < 0.0001). There were differences between the TS/TD and HD groups, and the tendency was for better performance post-treatment, but there was no improvement in the number of pegs placed by both hands simultaneously (F [1, 76] < 1).

▶ **Waitlist Group**

There was no significant improvement over time in the waitlist group for dominant or non-dominant performance of the groove test. There was, however, a significant improvement over time in performance of the dominant hand of the Purdue peg-board test (t [35] = −2.46; p < 0.02) and the diameter of the hole attempted on the hole test (t [35] = −2.39; p < 0.02) by the dominant hand. These changes in the waitlist group can be ascribed to practice effects, and again were not comparable to the more significant effects post-treatment.

▶ **Discussion**

There were differences between both the TS/TD and HD groups and the control group at baseline, indicating that both clinical groups showed poorer performance. There may be similarities in motor organization between these TS/TD and HD client groups.

There has been previous speculation that performance differences in the TS/TD group may be due to the presence of tics and their distracting effect, rather than basic organic deficit (Channon et al., 1992). Our results show that motor performance can be improved following successful tic management. Whether the improvement is due to the reduction in tics or the acquisition of improved strategies of motor control remains to be established.

▶ **CONCLUSIONS**

In this chapter, we have reviewed empirical evidence in support of the cognitive psychophysiological model. The research is a work in progress and we are currently extending and replicating the work to arrive at a surer understanding of the relationship between tics, motor activity, psychophysiological activation and cognitive and behavioral stages of planning and executing action.

These research findings, plus other developments in the literature, encouraged us to develop a program focusing on a cognitive-motor restructuring of action to regulate TD and modifying cognitive and behavioral aspects of action planning as the central platform for tic control.

Chapters 6 and 7 give a detailed account of the program with a client and therapist manual, plus four case studies illustrating the application.

Chapter 5

FUTURE DIRECTIONS

► **THE COGNITIVE-BEHAVIORAL/
PSYCHOPHYSIOLOGICAL CONCEPTUALIZATION
OF TIC DISORDERS**

The current model and program raise several questions for future research into tics and TS. In a cognitive psychophysiological model of TD, cognitive factors are accorded equal importance to behavioral factors as intervention strategies for regulating background motor activation. As noted in Table 3.4 of Chapter 3, cognitive factors play a larger role in tic onset than has been previously recognized, to the extent that we might suggest cognitive therapy as the first port of call for intervention strategies. Beliefs about the disorder would seem to be an important starting point. These beliefs determine expectations about tics and control over tics and subscribe often to self-fulfilling coping behavior, for example, by reacting to tics by tensing to contain the tic and so, in fact, making onset more likely.

Since clinical phenomenology (including psychological, behavioral, biographical and developmental aspects) is still the basis for the diagnosis of TS and TD, further refinement of cognitive and emotional and behavioral associations of tics should aid clinical precisions. As Pauls and collaborators (Pauls et al., 1995) noted, clarifying the phenotypic appearance of TS can only facilitate further genetic studies (p. 83) and indeed other types of research.

► **IMPLICATIONS FOR FUTURE RESEARCH**

As regards cognitive factors, TD seem to entail perfectionist thoughts but the perfectionism in tics seems more specific and related to personal standards and organization. Tics in TS/TD are often preceded by anticipations, even though the anticipations relate more to a situational appraisal than to a specific intrusive thought. The value of attending to cognitive factors is highlighted by the way that anticipations and appraisals may provoke the onset and maintenance of both disorders. Cognitive techniques such as distraction might alleviate the attentional focus producing the tics. Premonitory urges, even severe coprolalia-related ones, can be modified by distraction. In a vocal tic case treated recently by the author, distraction by thought or action was a useful strategy for breaking the link between the urge to make the noise and the onset of the vocal tic, and thereby demonstrating to the client the possibility of control. The debate on the role of cognition also raises the intriguing possibility that what is learned or acquired in both disorders is a cognitive structure which facilitates a type of planning and the accompanying emotional experience which provokes the tic or ritual. This overall cognitive psychophysiological style, rather than the specific movement it provokes, may prove to be a clearer marker of both TS and TD.

The specific link in our model between perfectionism and behavioral activation could have implications for the treatment of some aspects of hyperactivity. The restlessness of hyperactivity may be partly driven rather by perfectionist beliefs about personal organization. Interestingly, stimulants like MPH reportedly give subjective feelings of accomplishment and this may explain their paradoxical effect on hyperactivity. The effect may be produced not via motor pathways but by modifying the cognitive evaluations of action. The desire in the person with TS + hyperactivity to switch among many tasks may not reflect a loss of inhibition but rather a perfectionist need to do as much as possible. In the same way, other disinhibited behaviors in more severe TS, such as "forbidden touching" or other risky behaviors, may be a consequence of an over-prepared reaction aimed to control, not to abandon, behavior. In other words, knowing that a behavior is forbidden would lead the person without TS/TD to have confidence in his or her ability to refrain from doing it. In TS, however, the person immediately prepares actively not to do the action which, of course, paradoxically emphasizes the possibility that it could occur. This over-investment in restraining an activity maintains the importance of not doing it, and reinforces the thought of loss of control. This thought then leads to "tests" of control like half-extending and retracting the hand as though about to touch something forbidden. Such near-miss tests are intended to demonstrate control or rather disconfirm the idea that loss of control might occur. Such an over-investment in preventing an action was present in a TS patient whose phonic tic was to bark like a dog. Paradoxically, it was the thought that he might bark like a dog and the strong desire not to do so that led him to bark as a test of his self-control over barking. Throat-clearing urges in libraries, where noise is forbidden, are frequently preceded by preoccupations with controlling such urges; the over-investment and focus on the throat muscles in turn provoking the urge. This pattern of concern clearly resembles the obsessional person who constantly reminds himself not to forget, and who reacts to the thought of doing something "as if" it was equivalent to having done it.

Systematic application of *functional analysis* in TS and TD would generate data on environmental, behavioral, cognitive and affective associations. An activity profile is characteristic of tics, and such a profile could help to differentiate not only between tics and obsessions but between tics and neurological spasms. Also, a profile of activity associations linked to tic onset or intensity might provide insights into the role of learning in acquisition of tic disorders.

So far, studies employing parenting questionnaires have failed to reveal any consistent patterns of rearing styles in either TS/TD or OCD but a more refined focus

on *childhood experiences* and attachment in childhood other than a formal explo-
ration of parenting characteristics may reveal more vicarious learning experiences.
For example, the internalization of ambivalent messages may produce unrealistic
expectations about how to accomplish an action particularly at the pre-operational
stage of childhood. It may be the thought patterns of uncertainty or perfectionism
that are learned in childhood rather than the specific behavioral patterns. There is
the possibility of modelling if at least one parent suffers from tics. Perfectionism is,
in part, due to environmental factors (Frost et al., 1990), and we need to be clearer
on the functional analysis of tic onset to help us to determine if environmental
and interpersonal associations say whether tics are more likely to occur in interactions with parents. In particular, the current model would suggest that telic
action patterns, such as style of action and frustration action cycles, are behind
tic occurrence.

It seems crucial in future to employ *ecologically relevant experimental paradigms* to
factor in a psychological content as a mediator of apparent dysfunction. The regulation of emotion, thoughts and behavior can be the cause as well as the consequence
of neurochemical change, and a recursive psychoneurobiological model seems the
most appropriate to adopt when understanding the multidetermined nature of
tic disorders. Neuropsychological findings may be equivocal since such research
has, in the past, sought basic organic deficit, whereas the contextual aspects of
TD suggest functional and selective deficit. Behavioral or cognitive strategies, perfectionism or the style of planning can inhibit action and may produce apparent
neuropsychological impairment. Since these psychological variables can be targeted by psychological treatment, routine testing pre- and post-behavioral treatment could help to determine the generalizability of experimental effects such as
failures in selective inhibition. The creation of analog experimental paradigms with
the appropriate situational provocation or degree of emotionality could produce a
clinically credible high-risk activity in order to elicit corresponding physiological
changes, and tic-like behavior in people with and without the disorders.

► THE TS–OCD SPECTRUM

The notion of the OCD spectrum has been influential since Hollander (1993) proposed that the unifying factor for several impulsive and compulsive disorders was
a difficulty to inhibit or delay involuntary repetitive movement. However, from the
outset there were difficulties in specifying what exactly defined this continuum.
Initially, the continuum ranged from risk avoidance to risk seeking, but in a later
publication by Hollander and Benzaquen (1997), the spectrum was defined as a
continuum from overestimation of harm on the compulsive end to underestima-
tion of harm on the impulsive end (p. 99). The dimension was explicitly conceived
within a biological framework of hyperfrontality versus hypofrontality linked to
increased–decreased serotonergic sensitivity. In fact, where brain-imaging studies
do show differences in regional brain activity in OCD and TS, the picture is generally more complex and involving more cortical areas than can be subsumed under a

uniform frontal hypo–hyper functionality dimension (e.g., Busatto et al., 2000). Furthermore, the pattern of brain activity varies depending on symptom expression, state and task demand (Phillips et al., 2000), which suggests a reciprocal interaction between brain and behavior and the possible role of compensatory mechanisms producing cortical changes in both TS and OCD (Hugo et al., 1999; Peterson et al., 1999). One of the key emotional distinctions between tics and OCD compulsions is related to the emotional experience at the time of doing the tic or OCD ritual. In TS/TD, onset of and feedback from the tic is sensorially based. Although impulsive disorders give rise to pleasure (Hoogduin, 1986; Shapiro & Shapiro, 1986), tics seem triggered by psychasthenic feelings of sensory incompleteness or insufficiency (Leckman et al., 1994/1995). Cath et al. (1992b) view "felt emotion" as crucial to diagnosis. Summerfeldt et al. (1999) have suggested that sensory-based perfectionism may be at the root of feelings of incompleteness. Summerfeldt et al. (1999) distinguished between symmetry compulsions with and without superstitious obsessions.

A sensory-cognitive distinction between tic and OCD disorders is captured well in the distinct subtypes of "just rightness". The "just right" feeling accompanies ordering compulsions such as arranging books, or performing symmetrical movements, which seem to lack a rationale other than the need for everything to be "just right". Coles et al. (2003) have also suggested that the same actions may be performed on the basis of two distinct motivations: (1) something not being just right, and (2) the feared consequences.

People with tics do not appear to show the same cognitive sequence as in OCD. Tics are not preceded by an intentional thought and are not in general related to anxiety or anxious thoughts. Scores on the obsessional inventories are uniformly very low in TD except for ambivalent items concerning repetitive movements. People with TS/TD do not report concerns of responsibility, guilt about actions, need to control thoughts, which reflect standard appraisals in OCD, neither do they report doubt and low self-confidence, although they may have self-image concerns. Appraisals relate generally realistically to onset and consequences of the tic ("People will notice my tic and I'll be embarrassed"). The type of coping strategies used to contain or conceal tics are not equivalent to OCD-coping strategies (Wojcieszek & Lang, 1995).

The cognitive aspects of perfectionism are distinct in TD and involve beliefs about the importance of being efficient, of doing as much as possible, and not wasting time, or appearing to do so. Perfectionism in OCD more typically takes the form of doubts about actions, and concerns over mistakes (e.g., Frost et al., 2002; Rhéaume et al., 1995). Conversely, subscales of personal organization and personal standards do not relate to OCD (Rhéaume et al., 1995).

These distinctions in cognition between TS and OCD do not support the spectrum model. Furthermore, the spectrum model predicts an impulsive–compulsive dimension and would predict impulsive thoughts concerning short-term reward, stimulation or risky behavior to precede tics. In fact, there is very little evidence that TS or TD show high traits of impulsivity. They do not score more highly on trait

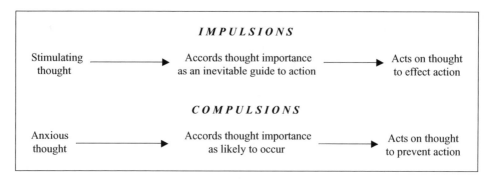

IMPULSIONS

Stimulating   ⟶   Accords thought importance   ⟶   Acts on thought
thought   as an inevitable guide to action   to effect action

COMPULSIONS

Anxious   ⟶   Accords thought importance   ⟶   Acts on thought
thought   as likely to occur   to prevent action

Figure 5.1   Impulsions and compulsions

measures of impulsivity, extraversion or other compulsive risk-taking behaviors like gambling or pyromania (Cath et al., 2001b, 2001d).

A key factor supporting the link between OCD and TS is the apparent high comorbidity between OCD and tics. Estimates of adults with TS and OCD vary between 28 and 63%, and OCD with tics around 17% (O'Connor, 2001). Distinctions between the two disorders, then, may be more apparent in a population with both OCD and tics. Cath et al. (2001d), in a series of studies differentiating between symptoms in OCD + tics and TS, noted that current instruments are probably not sensitive enough to discriminate complex tics from OCD compulsions. The authors developed their own interview schedule which discriminated repetitive action and thoughts from anxiety-related obsessional fears. Shapiro and Shapiro (1992, p. 157) noted this confusion and listed a series of complex movements that could count as tics. Both OCD and TS can report the same repetitive behaviors (Figure 5.1), depending on whether they are defined as impulsions or compulsions (distinguished according to the absence or presence of anxiety and goal-directedness). The only distinctions reported by Cath et al. (2001c) between OCD and TS on the basis of type of movement were rubbing and touching repetitions and echo phenomenon. The findings of Cath et al. (2001c, 2001d) also supported distinctions between a tic-related symmetry factor versus non-tic OCD-related washing factor. In this and other studies, TS with OCD is considered the most severe group in terms of symptomatology, and this may be because complex cognitive tics are confused with obsesssions.

▶ SEPARATING IMPULSE FROM COMPULSE: THE CASE OF COGNITIVE TICS

As noted in Chapter 1, Cath et al. (1992b) have introduced the notion of a "cognitive tic" as a means to clarify some of the confusion between intrusive mental impulses and obsessional ruminations. The distinguishing factor between "cognitive tics" and "ruminations", according to Cath et al. (1992b), is that the former are playful, often following simple urges with no rationale behind them, whereas ruminations are more purposeful. Therefore, counting a sequence of numbers for no reason would be classified as a "cognitive tic", whereas mentally repeating a scene of potential catastrophe would constitute an obsessional intrusion. However, in practice it is difficult to separate the two. Obsessions may come to resemble tics in their repetitive nonsensicalness when they become over-learned habits devoid of original cognitive motivation. In addition, a client may retrospectively ascribe an intentional motivation to a tic, and a purposeless movement may sometimes be given a sense by the person post-hoc (Cath et al., 1992a). A head movement may be interpreted by the person as meaning there was something to look at. A defining distinction between cognitive tics and obsessions is the presence of cognitive rituals accompanying mental obsessions. These are mental operations following the initial intrusion, such as wiping away or suppressing or substituting intrusive thoughts as a way of neutralizing their impact. Mental neutralization is equivalent to the overt neutralization of compulsive rituals. But the attempt to distinguish tics and rituals is further hampered by the sometimes limited insight and awareness of people with the problems. Hence, questionnaire approaches (e.g., Coles et al., 2003) to clarifying the distinctions and aiding differential diagnosis between complex tics and compulsions may be improved by assessing a wider behavioral context.

Further work clearly needs to be done on clarifying impulsive and compulsive thoughts and distinguishing mental tics from voluntary thoughts, worries and obsessional intrusions. Obsessive ruminations may be distinguishable from complex cognitive tics since the latter may be repeated in series, and may not develop as other intrusions do, nor be accompanied by the same level of awareness, and may, like other tics, show a situational or activity profile. In addition, like other tics, cognitive tics may not always reach the threshold of conscious awareness, but may need to be monitored in all their detail through awareness exercises. Also tics can be incorporated as part of obsessional behavior. A recent client at our clinic felt that the tics brought good luck and that otherwise something bad would happen later in the day. The superstitious thoughts were triggered by thoughts about events that would occur during the day, whereas the tics were provoked in situations of interpersonal frustrations. But the tics were sometimes voluntarily induced to assuage the conviction that otherwise bad luck would follow. Lang et al. (1993) also reported a case where tics were integrated into sign language, which blurred the division into voluntary and involuntary movement. A possible way of differentiating obsessions from mental or cognitive tics comes from evidence of a client's ability to substitute a cognitive tic for another type of tic. For example, a client who felt the urge to count numbers and letters on advertising hoardings by the roadside was able to interchange this mental routine with a leg tic. She felt the same immediate relief from doing either and could substitute one for the other depending on circumstance. The content of obsessional ruminations, by contrast, tends not to change although one neutralization strategy may substitute for another.

If some obsessions are mental tics, one might expect to find an activity profile associated with the cognitive tic in the same way that anticipations and beliefs associated with tic onset are revealed through functional analysis (Table 5.1). For example, in the case of the lady who mentally counted and rearranged the number of letters on roadside hoardings, the activity profile revealed a strong association between cognitive tic onset and travel activity which produced feelings of uncertainty and vulnerability.

Table 5.1 Examples of similar complex mental tics and obsessional compulsions

Sensorial compulsions	Obsessional compulsions
• Touching	• Intentional checking
• Repeating phrases	• Ritual repetition
• Mental games	• Aversive flashes/images
• Playful thoughts	• Disturbing ideas
• Running through mental scenes for fun	• Repeating events mentally to check for errors
• Copying what others do or say	• Stereotyped response due to OCD rules
• Saying or doing because it's stimulating or because it can't be inhibited	• Saying or doing to ward off bad luck

▶ ADAPTATION OF THE PROGRAM TO CHILDREN AND TO OTHER GROUPS WITH SPECIAL NEEDS

The studies reported here have almost exclusively focused on adult and adolescent tic sufferers. A major question hence remains concerning the applicability of the program to children. This is particularly pertinent, given that tics are at their peak in childhood. There have already been several reports adapting elements of the HR program to children. Relaxation can be induced in children with appropriate animation of the steps. Competing responses can be implemented in children with the help of child-friendly competing responses and appropriate social reinforcement.

It may be harder to discuss abstract cognitive constructs with children, but in terms of the motor model such constructs can be operationalized in terms of behavioral implications and physical attitudes. For example, the implications of feeling under pressure can be simply and concretely translated into "not getting the feeling that I am going to be told off by Mr . . . "

The components of the program can clearly be tailored according to need, but one major problem with trying to test out and isolate components is that no universal benefit seems to be drawn from any one component of the therapy. Some people start to benefit early from awareness, others only later. In the clinical study (see Chapter 4), although change in style of action components was predictive of outcome, subjective reports of benefit were distributed across all program components. Obviously, as noted earlier, if a person seems particularly affected by any one aspect of the problem, help can be focused on that problem. If the person is caught in the self-stimulation sensorimotor enforcement style to a self-destructive degree, then this aspect will need to be addressed in priority, by strategies to reduce importance and increase the tolerance given to the sensorimotor signals.

An issue with comparing children to adults is the difference in impact of the tic and associated comorbidities. It is rare, in fact, to find a child who does not have an associated behavioral disorder, whether this be hyperactivity, ADHD, obsession or rage syndrome. Most studies of children lack generalizability, precisely because the child population has significant comorbidity. The results may be further confounded by medication, and this is particularly relevant given the facility with which many clinicians prescribe neuroleptic medication to children.

Manifestations of hyperactivity and inattention frequently precede the appearance of tics in 40–50% of TS children, and ADHD is associated with 21–90% of TS children. On the other hand, other externalizing behaviors such as inattention, impulsivity, oppositional and antisocial behavior occur frequently in children with TS, as does OCD. Perhaps, most importantly, there is also an increased level of anxiety in children, not present in adults. Coffey et al. (2000) noted a 3.5 chance of anxiety being associated with severe tics in children. TS has also been reported to be more likely associated with depression, night terrors and sleep problems. Nearly a third of children suffering from TS also suffer learning difficulties and 60% of these children have difficulties at school. These difficulties are independent of intelligence and often represent the indirect effects of experiencing tics, which can disrupt performance and lead to low self-esteem and sense of rejection and isolation.

Another problem that is characteristic of children is aggressive behavior, in particular rage syndrome. Between 42 and 66% of children with TS experience aggressive episodes often set off by the frustration in trying to master their problem. Rage episodes are characterized by sudden uncontrollable explosions, often triggered by an apparently insignificant event. The child may attack objects or people and the intensity and absence of motivation distinguishes rage from anger, and parents often consider the rage the most unsettling symptom. Between 35 and 70% of children suffer rage syndrome compared to 8% of adults. It seems that as well as being related to severity of tics, the presence of anxiety and ADHD occurs in 92 and 95% of rage cases. If all three problems are present, the probability of rage is likely (Budman et al., 2000). Rage also seems to be linked to lower serotonin levels and stage factors such as lack of sleep, hunger and stress. After the rage has passed, the child is calm, often oblivious to what caused the rage.

Ways of dealing with rage and tics in children, apart from medication, have generally consisted of positive and negative reinforcement, punishment by time out, attempts to set limits, and muscle relaxation. The technique of self-modeling has also shown success.

Azrin and Peterson (1988a, 1988b) have shown a success rate of between 75 and 100% in reducing tic frequency in children through the use of HR techniques. The child observes and notes his tics on video. He or she then verbalizes the circumstances preceding tic onset, and practices relaxation, plus an incompatible response by auto-modeling. The child then practices the CR when the tic arrives and also receives home practice and non-contingent and relaxation training. The HR training has also been validated in a school setting.

An alternative transactional approach seeks to deal with tics and other underlying behaviors by resolving conflicts and reducing tensions and interpersonal aggressive styles in the family as a way of achieving calm (Greene, 2001). In such cases, protocols such as relaxation and incompatible responses need to be made concrete and identifiable to the child, and may take the form of a game (Berthiaume et al., 2004).

In the current program, the notion of thoughts evaluating the tic and leading to tension and ticcing may be difficult for the child's conceptual stage. But the exercise can easily work with whatever feelings the child expresses to distinguish high- and low-risk situations or activities. The behavioral restructuring can be achieved through role-play and games, and development of the children's version program is currently underway (Leclerc, 2004).

▶ APPLICATION OF THE PROGRAM TO OTHER TENSION PROBLEMS

The application to all types of HD is straightforward and has been successfully reported in a range of problems. Pélissier and O'Connor (2004) reported a case study of a lady with severe trichotillomania, where perfectionism was targeted successfully in treatment. In the clinical trial reported in Chapter 4, and in our subsequent clinical work, we have found the CP program equally effective in HD including bruxism, onychophagia, scabiomania, trichotillomania and tics. Stuttering may also be a form of HD where a similar style of action and associated beliefs about being efficient in verbal communication guide a style of speech which is continually ahead of itself.

Focal dystonias are a group which theoretically could be classified as a motor habit problem.

Dystonia is a syndrome of sustained muscle contractions, frequently causing twisting and repetitive movements, or abnormal postures (*Ad Hoc* Committee of the Dystonia Medical Research Foundation, 1984; see Fahn et al., 1987). A distinction is made between focal, segmental and generalized dystonia, depending on whether one part, two or more contiguous regions, or multiple parts of the body including the legs are affected by muscle spasms (Marsden et al., 1976). The site of the spasm in a focal dystonia may be the neck muscles (spasmodic torticollis), the orbicularis oculi muscles around the eyes (blepharospasm), the hand and forearm muscles during writing (writer's cramp), the muscles of the jaw, mouth and tongue (oro-mandibular dystonia), the laryngeal muscles involved in speech production (spasmodic dysphonia), or the pharyngeal muscles, resulting in difficulty with swallowing (spasmodic dysphagia). The exact prevalence and incidence of focal dystonias are unknown, although they are not uncommon disorders. The etiology of dystonia is uncertain. As with TD, the idiopathic dystonias are considered to be due to a functional biochemical abnormality in the basal ganglia, although the precise site or nature of this are at present unknown (Jahanshahi & Marsden, 1989; Yudofsky & Hales, 1992).

Features noted by Jahanshahi and Marsden (1989) as characteristic of the elec-
trophysiology of dystonias include: co-contraction of antagonist muscles, which
suggests an abnormality of reciprocal inhibition in dystonia; contraction to remote
muscles not engaged in the production of the voluntary movement; and paradoxic
contraction of passively shortened muscles, the so-called "Westphal phenomenon".

In spasmodic torticollis, involuntary contractions of the neck muscles result in abnormal head posture and/or involuntary head movement. The abnormal posture
can be rotation (torticollis) or tilt (laterocollis) to the left or right, forward flexion
(antecollis) or backward extension (retrocollis) of the head, or a combination. The
muscles most frequently involved are the sternocleidomastoids, the trapezius and
the splenius (Podivinsky, 1968). The ratio of male to female sufferers is roughly
equal (Patterson & Little, 1943). Onset is usually gradual, and typically occurs between 30 and 50 years of age (Patterson & Little, 1943). The severity of the abnormal
posture and of the involuntary movements of the head is affected by body position,
often being worse when upright and mobile and relieved when lying down. Like
people with tics, patients with torticollis use "trick" coping movements to keep the
head in the midline.

Sheehy and Marsden (1982) have suggested a distinction between simple and
dystonic writer's cramp. In the former, involuntary contractions of the hand and
forearm muscles occur when writing, other acts with the hand being performed
normally. In dystonic writer's cramp, muscle contractions in the hand occur not
only when writing but also during other manual acts such as handling everyday tools and objects. Simple writer's cramp may progress into the dystonic type.
Abnormal posture of the fingers, hands or wrists are evident when the person
attempts to write. People may often adapt to the problem by teaching themselves
to write with their other hand or to write in a special posture (Sheehy & Marsden,
1982). The hand may be bent at the wrist to grasp the pen. The onset of writer's
cramp is often between the ages of 20 and 50 years, and is most prevalent amongst
those who make their living through writing or use of their hands (for example, skilled muscians, artists or athletes). Sports dystonias such as dartitis and
snookeritis affect mainly skilled players. In skilled players there is far more reliance on forward planning (Abernathy et al., 1994), which, as noted in Chapter
3, may lead to conflict with current feedback. Other more modern occupational
cramps, very similar to writer's cramp, include masseur's cramp, where the sufferer often adopts similar coping strategies to writer's cramp. In one case seen by
the author, a clear motor conflict was produced by the desire to be further ahead
than possible with the massage plus an over-investment of effort. Computer con-
sole cramp can also be accompanied by posture cramps resembling repetitive strain
injury.

Biofeedback protocols for dystonia already exist, at least to an extent in muscle
training, implicate some aspects of the present program (Jahanshahi & Marsden,
1989). The major therapeutic aims in biofeedback for dystonias include training of:
recruitment of activity in non-functional or weak muscles; inhibition of undesired
excessive muscle activity; coordinated muscle activity (which may necessitate initial training as in [1] and [2] above), as, for example, in spasmodic torticollis, where

the two antagonist sternocleidomastoid muscles need to be trained to achieve muscular balance, and a midline posture of the head.

Research has shown that components of both relaxation and muscle feedback can have temporarily beneficial effects on muscle tension. Deepak and Behari (1999) looked at the use of specific muscle feedback for hand dystonia. The authors pointed to clinical evidence that there might be a coactivation of antagonist muscles and hyperactivity of muscles normally non-involved in activity. Interestingly, they note that attempts to write with the opposite hand usually lead to that hand also becoming dystonic. Relaxation and negative reinforcement show limited benefits. In the study, they trained people to use less effort when writing, using muscle feedback. People then practiced writing when relaxed 5–10 minutes per day over a two-month period. The muscle was sometimes difficult to locate for small hand movements. Nevertheless, there was a 90% improvement in pain ratings and writing fluency within sessions, but this was not carried over between sessions even if accompanied by relaxation and other skill training. However, other research has reported variable effects of biofeedback training on spasmodic torticollis (Leplow, 1990). Leplow notes a complex interaction in biofeedback training of 10 patients, between instructed control, biofeedback effects and cognitive processes, and suggests that attentional and cognitive aspects of pre-existing motor programs may need to be addressed for effective control over tension.

In conclusion, the focal dystonias as a group do show similarities to tics and habit disorders, in the way tension relates to overall motor action. The psychophysiological methods currently in use tend to alleviate the problems. These observations encourage further evaluation of the current CBT program in these disorders as an aid to treatment.

Chapter 6

THERAPIST MANUAL

▶ OVERVIEW OF THE PROGRAM

The 10 stages of the program are given in Figure 6.1. The 10 stages are cumulative and the person continues to practice all stages until the end of therapy. Appendices 1a–1h give assessment forms.

▶ Assessment Procedures

1. Assessment and diagnosis (see Table 6.1).
2. Detailed tic history/assessment (Appendix 1a).
3. Impact of tics on everyday life (Appendix 1b).
4. Tension Scale Questionnaire (Appendix 1c); Beliefs about Tics Questionnaire (Appendix 1d); Style of Planning (STOP) Questionnaire (Appendix 1e).
5. Motivation to participate (Appendix 1f); Inconvenience review (Appendix 1g); Coping strategies (Appendix 1h).
6. Tic quiz (Appendix 7).

▶ Ten-stage Program

1. Awareness: First stage/second stage/third stage: daily diary, situational monitoring, external rater, video assessment, tic quiz.
2. Discrimination protocol, biofeedback.
3. Relaxation exercises (stages 1–4).
4. Reduced sensorimotor activation, exposure, re-attribution.
5. Style of action planning (STOP) questionnaire, item analysis.
6. Cognitive restructuring, linking anticipation to belief, triple column technique.
7. Behavioral restructuring, integrating competing response, prevention by relaxation and normalization into new action script.
8. Cognitive-behavioral restructuring of high-risk activities.
9. Generalization over high-risk situations, post-treatment assessment.
10. Relapse prevention, home practice.

The anticipated length of treatment time is 14 sessions but the program may be completed in fewer sessions if the practice is sufficient; or, of course, it may

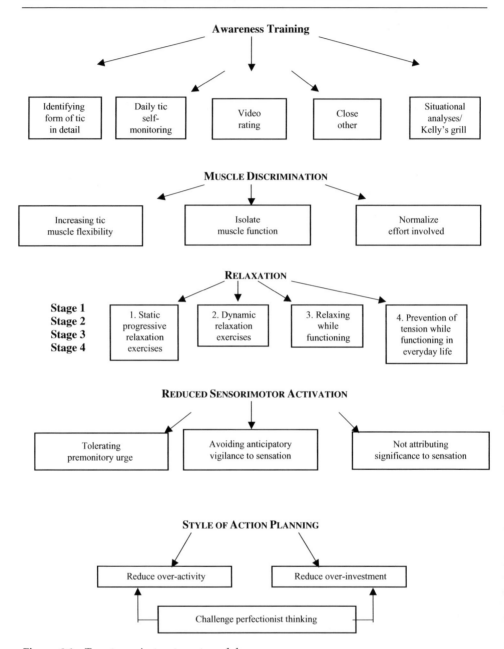

Figure 6.1   Ten stages in treatment model

take longer. Exercises should always be verified by the therapist with the help of forms where appropriate. At the end of the 14 weeks, there is a home-based practice period lasting four weeks where the clients implement procedures by themselves. It may be helpful to phone clients on a weekly basis at home to ensure compliance and deal with trouble shooting. Progress can be assessed

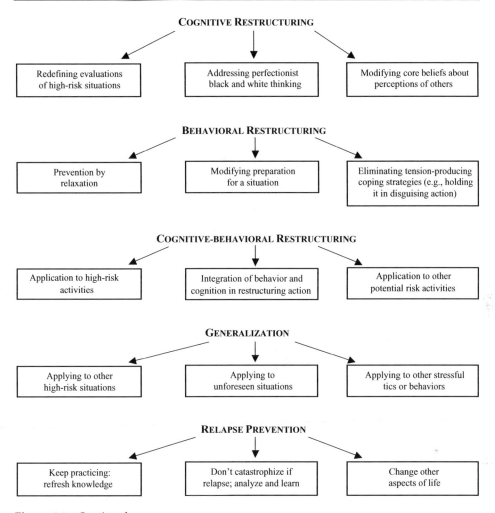

COGNITIVE RESTRUCTURING

| Redefining evaluations of high-risk situations | Addressing perfectionist black and white thinking | Modifying core beliefs about perceptions of others |

BEHAVIORAL RESTRUCTURING

| Prevention by relaxation | Modifying preparation for a situation | Eliminating tension-producing coping strategies (e.g., holding it in disguising action) |

COGNITIVE-BEHAVIORAL RESTRUCTURING

| Application to high-risk activities | Integration of behavior and cognition in restructuring action | Application to other potential risk activities |

GENERALIZATION

| Applying to other high-risk situations | Applying to unforeseen situations | Applying to other stressful tics or behaviors |

RELAPSE PREVENTION

| Keep practicing: refresh knowledge | Don't catastrophize if relapse; analyze and learn | Change other aspects of life |

Figure 6.1 *Continued*

post-treatment on daily diary measures and other questionnaires given in the appendices.

At the end of therapy, relapse prevention forms a crucial last step and clients are encouraged to continue to apply exercises to any remaining tics and habits, but not to expect some spontaneous remission without effort.

► ASSESSMENT PROCEDURES

The first part of the therapist manual discusses the principal aims of each stage, the second part discusses session by session procedures, and the third part covers main trouble-shooting issues.

Table 6.1 Evaluation instruments for assessing Gilles de la Tourette and related disorders

	Test	Authors	% of studies (n = 45)	Comments
1	Clinical interview with the DSM-III or IV criteria	Diagnostic interview for child and adolescents revised, child and parent version (DICA) – Reich (2000); Welner et al. (1987) Diagnostic interview for children (DISC) – Piacentini et al. (1993) Global assessment of functioning – American Psychiatric Association (1994) Structured clinical interview for DSM-III-R(SCID) Schedule for affective disorders and schizophrenia for school-age children present and lifetime version and epidemiologic version (K-SADS-E) – Kaufman et al. (1997) and Orvaschel and Puig-Antich (1987)	61.2%	Semistructured clinician-rated interview.
2	Yale Global Tic Severity Scale (YGTSS)	Leckman et al. (1989)	38%	This instrument classifies five dimensions of symptoms (number, frequency, intensity, complexity and disruptiveness) on a six-factor scale (0 = none to 5 = severe). It's a questionnaire for the teacher and/or parents. The psychometric properties are: validity: 0.74–0.85; video or observation counting, 0.49–0.62.
3	Direct observation or functional analysis		27%	
4	Tourette's Syndrome Global Scale (TSGS)	Harcherik et al. (1984)	16%	The TSGS has two major domains which contribute equally to the global score. The first domain is ratings of motor and phonic tics, and the second domain is an overall social functioning score. Each type of category is rated on a two-factor scale: frequency and disruptiveness of tics.

5	Motor tic, obsessions-compulsions, vocal tic evaluation survey (MOVES)	Gaffney et al. (1994)	0.4%	A self-report scale for the symptoms of Tourette's syndrome was designed to be quickly and easily completed by children, adolescents or adults. The MOVES generates scores on five subscales: motortics, vocal tics, obsessions, compulsions, associated symptoms. The MOVES subscales correlated significantly ($p = 0.6$–0.8) with independent examiner-rated scales, including YGTSS, Shapiro Tourette's Clinical Rating Scale, and two scales for OCD.
6	Schedule for Tourette's and other behavioral syndromes	Pauls & Hurst (1996)	0.4%	Clinical rating scale.
7	Behavior rating inventory of executive function (BRIEF)	Gioia et al. (2000); *see also* Mahone et al. (2002)	0.2%	The dynamic, multidimensional nature of executive function has been challenging to operationalize and assess in a clinical setting. This questionnaire, to be filled by parents and teacher, allows an assessment of the executive function but without a diagnostic evaluation of TS or ADHD.
8	Best estimate diagnostic procedure	Leckman et al. (1982)	0.2%	
9	Movement disorders checklist	Brasic (2001)	0.2%	
10	National hospital interview schedule for Gilles de la Tourette's syndrome	Robertson & Eapen (1996)	0.2%	

continues

Table 6.1 Continued

	Test	Authors	% of studies (n = 45)	Comments
11	The tic symptom self-report (TSSR)		0.2%	
12	Tourette's syndrome diagnostic confidence index (DCI)	Robertson et al. (1999)	0.2%	The DCI is a useful, practical instrument for use in the clinic or research practice allowing an assessment of lifetime likelihood of TS. Further work is needed to test the DCI's psychometric properties. Its correlation with other instruments and associations with psychopathology provide support for its being a lifelong measure of TS. This instrument uses life history information to contribute to a measurement of the likelihood of TS and it is a continuous rather than categorical measure of the likelihood of the disorder.
13	Yale schedule for Tourette's syndrome and other behavioral syndromes (YSTSOBS)	Pauls et al. (1991) Jagger et al. (1982)	0.2%	Clinician- or patient-rated schedule of tics, obsessions, compulsions and premonitions.
14	Shapiro Tourette's disorder severity scale (TS-Sev)	Shapiro et al. (1988)	0.2%	This allows an assessment of tic severity on a six-point scale (very mild to very severe) with a reliability of 0.82–0.92 and a validity of 0.50–0.72. It serves as a clinical instrument use to determine the level of disruption of tics.
15	Tourette's disorder scales (TODS)	Shytle et al. (2003)		

► Diagnostic Instruments

There is no standard semistructured interview (equivalent of the Anxiety Disorders Schedule [ADIS]) but individual researchers have developed their own interview protocols (e.g., Leiden protocol [Cath et al., 2001d; Robertson, 2001). The standard measure for clinical assessment of TD is the Yale Global Tic Severity Scale (Leckman et al., 1989). This scale records frequency, intensity, complexity and anatomical site of motor, sensory, phonic tics, and also interference in other areas of life. There are also other clinician-rated scales such as the Tourette's Syndrome Global Scale which scores degree of tic severity and assesses disruption due to tic multidimensionally (Harcherik et al., 1984). There have been attempts to adapt the Yale–Brown Obsessive Compulsive Scale (Y–BOCS) for use with tics and habits on the assumption that all form part of the same OCD spectrum (Stanley et al., 1993), but the Y–BOCS is generally likely to underscore the presence of tics and habits.

► Diagnostic Boundaries

Estimates of comorbidity of TS with ADHD in children vary between 20 and 90% depending on diagnostic criteria (Robertson & Eapen, 1992) as compared to 2–11% in non-TS populations (Costello & Angold, 1988). Comings and Comings (1984) and Shapiro and Shapiro (1986) both felt that ADHD was an integral part of TS. In adults with TD, as noted later, there also seems to be a particular style of action similar to hyperactivity, but with a clear cognitive component.

However, the two key diagnostic boundaries for TS/TD in adults are OCD and HD. Some researchers consider that all these disorders are part of the same OCD spectrum. The comorbidity of a TD with OCD in adults varies across studies from 25 to 63% and about 17% of adult OCD have tics (Holzer et al., 1994).

► Measuring Tic Behavior

There seem to be four preferred types of tic assessment: video rating, self-monitoring, clinician assessment or external observer assessment.

- *Video assessment* There do exist standard video-rating procedures (e.g., the Rush method [Goetz et al., 1987]). One obvious problem biasing video assessment is that tics are frequently suppressed, so simply videoing a person may not be a reliable way of identifying the presence of tics, *unless* a tic-provoking situation is constructed in collaboration with the person. For example, in a recent study in our laboratory, expert raters showed a poor hit rate in distinguishing tic- from non-tic-disordered clients during a standard videod psychiatric interview, but with nonetheless a good inter-rater agreement (O'Connor et al., 1998). But tic detection improves substantially during the video of a high-risk situation (see Video protocol, p. 110).

- *Self-monitoring* The status of the tic or habit and associated emotions can be monitored in a daily tic diary which records frequency, intensity of urge to tic and degree of control (resistance) over the tic on a daily basis in a specially prepared booklet (Appendices 4–6; printed prototypes are available in Appendix 6). Participants must be trained in the use of the booklet and a unit of tic (tics) or habit defined at the beginning of the evaluation.

  The way the person appraises both the tic occurrence, appearance, and the long-term effects of suffering from TD have not been systematically studied. It is possible that an appraisal-assumption instrument such as the OBQ-87 (Obsessive Beliefs Questionnaire [Obsessive Compulsive Cognitions Working Group, 1997]) could be adapted for this purpose (Anholt et al., 2002). Alternatively, O'Connor et al. (1993, 1994) have suggested modifying the Kelly's repertory grid to permit assessment of constructs defining reactions to high- and low-risk situations and to self as tic disordered (Blowers & O'Connor, 1996) (see Awareness 3, p. 110).

- *Clinician or external observer assessment* The clinician or observer rates the tic occurrence without the person's knowledge. This is useful for overall improvement ratings. Unfortunately, identification of tics will be limited unless the contextual nature and suppression of tics is taken into account.

Each of these four measures of tic behaviors has a different type of bias, but agreement between all four assessment measures on outcome gives some convergent validity to a finding of a clinically significant change, or not, on the triangulation principle adopted in other types of clinical methodology (Kay et al., 1993).

An important initial concern is motivation, since frequently the clients may not be seeking aid on their own initiative, or they may have many reservations about the utility of the tic program. Motivation is measured by the motivation questionnaire, beliefs about tics, and the tic quiz. There may be an identification with the tic as a part of their eccentricity, or there may be secondary gain due to dynamics of the home environment. The inconvenience review can be completed to aid or establish motivation. The clients need to understand that therapy is collaborative, adopts a learning model and requires consistent practice of exercises in and out of the sessions over the 12–14 weeks of therapy. If the clients lack motivation, they may benefit from motivational interviewing techniques.

Further information on a client's tic after taking the history involves completing the following forms given in Appendix 1: (1) the impact questionnaire to measure the impact of the tic in everyday life; (2) subjective tension level; (3) beliefs about tics; (4) the STOP questionnaire to identify style of planning.

► TEN-STAGE PROGRAM

► Stage 1: Awareness

Awareness 1

The first four weeks of the program are devoted to awareness learning. Preceding the first session and after diagnostic evaluation, the person can complete and read the first part of the tic manual giving information on habits, plus the overview and goals of treatment, and tic quiz and motivation scale, plus STOP, and impact questionnaire. The program targets one tic at a time, hence the need to identify a dominant tic as a target for treatment (see Appendices 2a and 2b).

All aspects of the tic need to be described from its onset as a premonitory urge right through to the coping strategies used. Identification of the tic is important since it constitutes the unit for the whole of the treatment. In a person with one predominant tic, this poses no problem, but for someone with multiple tics, it may be difficult to target just one tic. The solution effectively is to follow several criteria: (1) which is the most preoccupying? (2) which causes most distress? (3) which occurs frequently? and (4) which is most accessible to treatment? Normally, when treating a series of behavioral problems, the ideal is to start from the easiest and most controllable and progress up the hierarchy, but here this is not desirable, since client motivation is likely to be highest for the most troublesome tic.

In this first session, the therapist will also reply to questions the person has about the nature of the program, particularly about the learning model, since the person, if aid has been sought before, will almost certainly have encountered a more neurochemical model of tic management. The person's attitude, as perhaps revealed by motivational questionnaires and beliefs about tics, is important. The tic quiz can also provide a chance to discuss facts about tics. If the person is unmotivated or completely closed to the idea of behavioral control, it will be necessary to reconsider participation. On the other hand, as long as the person is a little open to try the exercises, this is fine.

At this stage, the rationale for awareness training is repeated with the emphasis on the important therapeutic effect for the person. Frequently, people look upon completing diaries and forms as a chore. The aim is to view the awareness exercises as a voyage of self-discovery. The person should read the tic diary manual.

Criteria for the first stage of awareness are that the person (1) is motivated to undertake program and exercises, (2) understands the model, (3) agrees to keep a diary, (4) understands the importance of awareness, (5) agrees to complete awareness exercises including diary keeping for two days and (6) agrees to read the relevant initials sections of the manual.

Awareness 2: Diary Keeping

It is important to get feedback on the first two-day monitoring stage. The person now progresses to daily monitoring with a fixed time period (minimum two hours, maximum all day). The time period depends on the severity of the tic and the monitoring ability. The results of the awareness sessions are linked to further education about situational profiling and further diary keeping. The idea of a situation or activity profile of tics and the implications for control can be explored. The person typically may have noticed that the tic intensity varies over time. Self-monitoring may have temporarily increased the tic frequency because the person is focused on it. Or if the tic is mild, it may have decreased in frequency. A tic unit must be finalized at this point which will remain constant throughout treatment. Hence, the focus of description will be on this unit. The therapist may need to model the tic to help the person to identify its form, and may require the person to describe the tic out loud. It will be useful to discuss the possibility with the person's permission of involving a close other in monitoring, and reinforcement and contingency management throughout the program.

The person will have read the overview of the program and understand the self-reinforcing nature of the tic, and tension-producing coping responses can be addressed. Outstanding answers to the tic quiz can be discussed. Criteria for this stage: (1) the client understands the daily diary exercises, and the tic unit is identified; (2) any questions about the model are satisfactorily answered; (3) if plausible, a close other can be nominated (external collaborator); (4) high- and low-risk activities can be identified, using Appendices 2d and 2e.

A close other can be implicated as co-therapist with the client's permission. The role of the close other is to understand the program and model, and to receive education on the nature of tics. The close other will act as an external evaluator, will rate the person's tic at the beginning and end of the program, and may act in certain roles to aid awareness. The close other will encourage the person in practice of the exercises, provide formal and informal contingency training and reward schedules, refrain from negative comments while the person is ticcing and act as a helpful source of feedback throughout the program. If necessary, separate or joint sessions can be scheduled with the close other to discuss progress on problems. The criteria for this final stage of awareness are: the person should be aware of all steps in the occurrence of the tic including the person's reaction and coping response; the person should be settled into diary keeping for one tic unit; the issue of close other involvement should be resolved and close other contacted and informed; high- and low-risk activities identified and the principle of Kelly's grid explained by the therapist (see Appendix 2j).

Awareness 3: Tic Profiling

At this stage, the diary is examined in detail to separate out activities of high and low risk of tic onset. Normally, there will be several of these activities, so choosing three should not be difficult. The evaluations of the situation allow us to see the activities that are most related to the occurrence or non-occurrence of the tic. Kelly's grid eliciting evaluations of low- and high-risk situations can be completed partly with the therapist and also at home. If possible, it is a good idea to make a video. We usually make a video of a low-risk and high-risk situation for 10 minutes each and a suitability situation or activity can be scripted with the person. The occurrence of the tic can then be viewed and scored by a hand-held counter.

Video Protocol

❑ Choose a low- and high-risk situation/activity from the self-monitoring form or Kelly's grid.
❑ The situation/activity preferably repeats on a regular daily basis.
❑ The high-risk scene should be scripted with the person. This might be easy and consist of the person waiting, reading or simply sitting during the video. Ideally,

a real-life experience will form the basis for the script – e.g., "I was asked to wait in the office while the boss went and found the problem dossier. I felt myself becoming more and more apprehensive just wondering what he would say. I tried to concentrate on reading the report but I became fidgety, etc."

❑ The low-risk situation should be filmed first of all since this will probably be found more relaxing and encourage acclimatization.

❑ If a high-risk situation/activity cannot be practically scripted, the person can use his or her imagination to live the scene.

❑ After filming the sequence for 10 minutes, the scene where tics are present is viewed together with the client.

If a video is not available, there are two options: (1) A close trusted other observes the person and then describes or notes the tic or imitates the tic. (2) A person can observe the tic in the mirror. This is appropriate for a facial tic. For other tics, the person can imitate the tic to match feeling the tic and visioning it.

► Stage 2: Discrimination Protocol

The clinical rationale for the discrimination exercise is also given in the client manual, which the client should read. The therapist can repeat the rationale to make sure it is understood, covering the following points:

(a) Tic-affected muscles tend to be less flexible and less able to contract gradually from one tension level to another. They tend to jump from all to nothing.

(b) This gradation of tension can be learned through practice, but, like all practice, it takes time and consistency.

(c) The exercises consist of slowly contracting and relaxing muscles by degrees (25%, 50%, 75%).

(d) If using a biofeedback machine, the machine helps to give feedback on this exercise and helps to identify the different grades of tension. The bar or other graphic feedback display goes up and down along with the degree of contraction and so gives feedback on the state of the muscle. But the idea is eventually to internalize and identify the sensation associated with the tension, to enable practice at home, away from the machine.

(e) The laboratory session will give some experience of controlling the tension level and start off the exercise, but to gain maximum effect, it must be practiced daily at home at least twice per day – or more if necessary. Watching the muscle in a mirror or light placing of the hand on the muscle will help to give feedback at the beginning.

(f) The goal of the exercise is to be able to change the level of tension reasonably smoothly between 0, 25%, 50%, 75% and full tension. The more the practice, the smoother the contraction becomes and the more there is control.

(g) This discrimination exercise is not a relaxation exercise. The relaxation is a complementary exercise aimed to relax tension. The discrimination exercises are devised to educate about muscle tension and give more control over the tic reflex-like action.

(h)   Another aspect to gaining control over the tic is isolating the action of contraction and relaxation of the muscle to the muscle group and not involving
other irrelevant muscle groups. This isolation is also important since people
with tics also over-prepare muscle actions, put in too much effort and move
using irrelevant muscle groups.

(i)   Normalizing the tic action involves not only control of its tension level but
using just the amount of effort required and not more.

(j)   Ask: Do you understand the rationale? Do you have any questions? Are you
ready to start? If no, repeat appropriate information.

If using a biofeedback machine:

1.   Ask the person to locate the muscle mass. Mark on a muscle anatomy chart
the exact location of the muscle mass and keep a copy in the files. Generally,
three surface electrode tabs should be placed as far as possible in the middle of
the muscle for maximum sensitivity (between one-third and two-thirds of the
distance between the point of origin of the muscle and the point of insertion).

2.   Follow procedures recommended by the recording device manufacturer for
application of electrodes or seek technical assistance from an electrophysiological technician. Wash and cleanse the skin. Attach electrode tabs onto the tic-
affected muscle or nearest related muscle group, and to an unaffected muscle
group. Ideally, the unaffected group will be symmetrically opposite the affected
group, i.e., opposite cheek, arm, leg, etc. Where this is not possible, the electrodes should be placed on the nearest accessible voluntary muscle group. Most
recording devices have a ground electrode which can be placed on a neutral site.

3.   Open the computer and create the personal file. Check that the muscle groups
are registering as expected and produce a recording on the computer monitor
by asking the person to contract and relax relevant muscles. Ensure that the
bar or other visual display on the computer responds to contraction and is
scaled to accommodate the full amplitude of the muscle feedback machine.

Discrimination Procedure

1.   The instructions and aim of the exercises are given to the person again, and
the person is asked to repeat the rationale. The rationale is that tic muscles lack
flexibility and tend to be in an all-or-nothing state. Hence, flexibility can be
learnt by slowly training the muscle in different degrees of contraction. This
exercise to be done slowly is a way of increasing control.

2.   The entire discrimination session is recorded, starting with the baseline. A five
(5) minutes baseline recording records activity in a normal resting state with as
little movement as possible. The person should ideally be sitting comfortably
in a chair with feet down, head upright and arms rested on the chair arms. "I'd
just like you to sit normally in a normal position and keep as still as possible
for 5 minutes." The experimenter keeps contact with the person to a minimum
during recording.

3.   The difference in flexibility between the non-affected and the affected site is
demonstrated by asking the person to increase tension slowly in the non-
affected site, and pass through four stages from 0 to 25%, 50%, 75% to full
tension level and then slowly decrease through the same four stages.

4. People generally find it easier to increase through the stages of contraction than to decrease slowly. So the person can be reassured on this point. The person will probably try to contract too fast initially and not be able to sustain the different levels, but little by little he or she will improve and should be constantly encouraged. The goal of the session is not that the person completes the exercises faultlessly but that the person understands the principle and has seen that progress has been made. The person should also have internalized accompanying sensations identifying different tension levels in order to complete home practice (twice + 2 per day) (as per client manual).

5. The same procedure is followed with the affected muscle. The person tries to increase the tension slowly through the four stages (0, 25%, 50%, 75%, 100%) and decrease it slowly. The person will tend to jump up levels too quickly, but after a practice in both directions of around 15 minutes, progress will normally be made. After 25 minutes, the person will begin to tire. The criteria for success is that the person manages to improve on the exercise by a noticeable degree, and that he or she internalizes and identifies the muscle sensation at 25%, 50%, 75% tied to each stage sufficiently for home practice. During the exercise, the participant can use the non-affected side for guidance in anchoring sensation in the affected muscle, by initially contracting both at the same time. But final practice should be with the tic-affected muscle alone.

6. Another important part of the exercise is to confine as far as possible the use of the muscle to contraction of the surrounding implicated muscles and not to respond with non-relevant muscles or in block. It's not possible to isolate the muscle group completely but distal influences like facial grimaces can certainly be reduced.

7. Five (5) minutes post-discrimination exercises are recorded by again asking the person to sit normally and relax and move as little as possible for five minutes.

Therapist Report

The therapist will give a considered percentage score against the success or otherwise of the following five items:

1. Non-affected side contracted slowly through 0, 25%, 50%, 75%, full 100%
2. (a) Affected side contracted slowly through full 100%, 75%, 50%, 25%, 0
    (b) Affected side contracted slowly through 0, 25%, 50%, 75%, full 100%
3. 20–25 minutes practice with pause if necessary on affected site.
4. Degree of success (in passing through four stages of contraction both decreasing and increasing):

0	10	20	30	40	50	60	70	80	90	100

    0 = no success   100 = complete success
5. Participant identified sensations associated with different levels of tension, and understands rationale for home practice.

The criteria for progressing to the next stage is that the person succeeds in decreasing and increasing muscle tension gradually through the different levels, and practices consistently at home.

▶ Stage 3: Progressive Relaxation Exercises

The aim of the discrimination protocol is to induce flexibility and control over tension in the tic-affected muscle. It may indirectly have the effect of relaxation but it may also increase tension level (see O'Connor et al., 1995). However, the aim of the relaxation exercises is to induce a genuine state of relaxation. The exercises are adopted from the classical progressive relaxation of Jacobson, and address the principal muscles involved in voluntary movement. The person should be in either a comfortable sitting or semireclined position with legs apart and feet in contact with the floor or other surface. The therapist should explain the rationale of the exercises and why there are four stages. Relaxation is a learning process: first we learn to feel relaxed, we then learn to arrive at the state more quickly, and then we learn to apply the learning automatically and in everyday life. Finally, the person can combine the exercises with pleasant or neutral imagery, but the focus is always on muscle relaxation.

The four stages permit acquisition of skill at each stage before progressing to the next stage. A preliminary stage involves mastery of slow respiration. Regulated diaphragmatic breathing accompanies the relaxation exercises. The first stage is to master slow contraction and relaxation in each muscle group, and also to isolate the muscle group in question and combine this with diaphragmatic breathing.

The second stage is only attempted when the person has appreciated the benefits of the first stage. Namely, the ability to distinguish and experience the difference between relaxation and tension, to synchronize breathing with the tense contract cycle, and appreciate whole body relaxation. The second stage achieves this state faster, but without losing any of the relaxation experience, and the criteria for progressing to the third stage is that the person does achieve the same effects from the quicker version.

In the third stage, the person applies the technique in everyday life, and uses it to detect tension and then implement relaxation immediately before tension builds up. The person is still using the tense–release cycle, but can implement it conveniently and without the need for prolonged exercise. Again, it is important that the person experiences the same relaxation effect from this procedure.

In the final stage, complete integration of the exercises is required so that the person can simply say or think "relax" and feel the same experience as in the other stages. The therapist may need to model each stage and, in particular, ensure combination with the respiration.

The four stages are covered over the ensuing four weeks in combination with other steps of the program. However, each week the therapist should check on the relaxation stage to follow up any problems and ensure that the person is achieving effects.

▶ Stage 4: Reducing Sensorimotor Activation

The previous sessions have focused very much on the motor side of activation. We now focus on the sensory side, particularly the sensations experienced with muscle activation in tic-affected sites. The reduction of sensorimotor activation takes two forms. The first form deals with general signs of activation such as tingling or discomfort or ultra-sensitivity to touch or sensation which often leads to motor restlessness or other forms of self-sought stimulation. The second form addresses the premonitory sensation often preceding the tic onset itself.

The person can understand from Figure 7.5 (see p. 170) how his or her reaction to the stimulation or sensation encourages the sensation and leads to a further need for stimulation. The reaction usually takes the same form of motor agitation or restlessness or distraction or avoidance which aims to neutralize the sensation. Tingling, hypersensibility to touch or sensory stimulation and a hypermonitoring of sensation also lead to a focus which attributes meaning and consequence to a normal sensation (see Figure 2.2). The role of this attribution can be illustrated through exercises. For example, the person can be asked to use his or her imagination to create significance. For example: "Focus now on your hand. Do you feel anything there like an ache or a warmth? Now imagine this sensation building and building until it feels real and you need to react to it."

Every time the person feels a tension or urge that might lead to ticcing, he or she should employ the following procedure:

1. Examine immediate reactions. Is the person tensing up in expectation? Does the thought immediately appear that the tic will occur? For example: "Oh no, here it comes again." Has the person started to actively prepare in mind and body for the tic's appearance as though it is inevitable?
2. All the above thoughts should be caught and put on hold and challenged as automated thoughts. The tic is not inevitable. The sensory urge will go away if an urgency is not attributed.
3. The person should ideally immediately initiate a relaxation response with breathing to feel the tension lifting. Any response or posture change, however minor, that may feed the stimulation cycle is avoided.
4. The person should be encouraged to make a decision not to do the tic with the knowledge that the sensation will go if it is not fed by anticipation and focus.
5. Carrying on with everyday goal-directed tasks, paying as little attention to sensation and focusing on external reality will help to speed habituation.

This stage applies particularly to those who have premonitory sensations before the tic, or pronounced sensations during the tic. But the exercise can also help to: (a) explore attributions the person may give to background muscle tension and show how the tension is tolerable or controllable; (b) address any anticipations or vigilance that might lead the person to build up anticipatory tension; and (c) address any safety or protective behaviors that might lead to a build-up of anticipatory tension. The tolerance of the sensation needs to be accompanied by a shift in cognitive focus and in behavioral reactions.

▶ Stage 5: Style of Planning Action

In this stage, the person must first of all understand the link between a tension-producing style of action and specific, experienced muscle tension. It is helpful to locate, using the STOP questionnaire, the actual items pertinent to the person. This item, representing either over-investment or over-activity, can be explored in detail and related to daily examples when the person undertakes a task over-actively. For example, if the person is cramming a lot into his or her agenda, a list of the activities that the person feels he or she must accomplish in a day can be examined and rested for real priority. What would happen if, say, one of the six tasks was put back to tomorrow? Usually, the person will volunteer that it's more efficient and time saving to do them all at once. At this point, a distinction can be made between efficient and over-active, since over-active is the opposite of efficient. These notions can be related to the person's actual experience, whereby the over-activity actually leads to stress and tension. The important point to convey is that doing the activities in a less over-active way is more efficient, not less efficient, since the person is calmer and more able to carry out the tasks in a complete way. The person is likely to be more present in the here and now. Personalized advantages and disadvantages of doing tasks over-actively can be relisted with the person, and, as disadvantages, might include not concentrating properly, too rushed to feel comfortable doing the job, mind always on the next job to be done, feeling worn out at the end of the day. When listed, there are likely to be less advantages, and the advantages are likely to relate to irrational thoughts, which can then, in turn, be addressed later in the cognitive restructuring. For example: "Well when I've got all the jobs done, then I can relax" (in fact, the person is likely to be too stressed out to relax properly, or the person misinterprets fatigue for relaxation, or thinks that he or she can only relax when fatigued), "If I'm rushing, I look efficient and give a good impression" or even, "Well I've always done things that way and it works". There may also be perfectionist beliefs about the need to do more to appear good, and the fear of not doing enough and hence not functioning as well as possible.

These thoughts can be addressed in the next step of cognitive structuring. In the present stage, however, the person is encouraged to try to act in a less over-active way in one or two habitually over-active tasks. The exercise should be treated as an experiment, and the approach to planning and executing mapped out in detail with the person, to make sure that planning, behavior and tension are all controlled in a calm way and that the person leaves no gaps in the time course of the task that can be filled up over-actively. The person practices this new non-over-active routine during the week. The following week, the person reports how he or she felt and how the tasks were accomplished.

Over-active example: I'm going to visit my friend downtown, so I can pick up groceries, return the library book, wash the car and go to the post office before I see him at 2:00. What typically happens? I feel stressed and, inevitably, there is a delay somewhere in the line, so I get held up. Then I get irritated that I'm late and I might not do all I should do and I feel frustrated that I didn't do all I should and I feel tenser.

Calmer planning: I'm going to visit my friend downtown, the grocer's shop is directly on the way and I do need to buy food for this evening, and I should be served relatively quickly. But returning the library book is out of the way and I know there is always a long queue at the post office so I'll leave this to another day. In any case, the return is not urgent.

▶ Stage 6: Cognitive Restructuring

The client will have read the relevant manual section on the importance of beliefs and the realization that certain rigid beliefs can underlie a stressful style of action. The person will also have completed Kelly's grid and have elicited relevant construct evaluations underlying high- and low-risk activities. Further, the person can identify very precisely the link between thought, feeling and action for each high-risk tic activity by completing Appendix 2h. This knowledge should prepare the person for a more general thought restructuring. Following the rationale of the manual, it is always important to tie the change in beliefs with the goal of changing tension and hence tic onset. In this sense, beliefs should always be linked to changes in intentional action in a high-risk situation. This strategy also avoids getting entangled in other beliefs which may address other areas of life not relevant to ticcing.

Cognitive therapy for tic-related beliefs is likely to touch four areas. Firstly, beliefs about the utility of ticcing, or its inevitability. Secondly, beliefs about the way to act in high-risk tic situations. Thirdly, perfectionist beliefs or black and white thinking about the way to organize personal actions. Fourthly, beliefs about self-image and the judgment of others related to appearance, performance or expressing feelings. The beliefs can in part be taken from Kelly's construct grid, which rated opposing evaluations across high- and low-risk situations and so revealed any constructs clearly distinguishing high- and low-risk tic activity. It is worth listing all relevant beliefs and tracing with the person how each belief or evaluation leads to immediate anticipations about high-risk situations, and what alternative behavior could be in place without these beliefs.

The exercise listing the link between immediate and remote beliefs and anticipations should be completed by the client (Figure 7.3, Appendix 2h). The belief cycle can be initially explained with reference to everyday events; for example, how a belief about interviews determines an evaluation of an immediate encounter with a job interview. The link can then be completed more specifically for the tic-related beliefs and anticipation.

The triple-column technique is often the most appropriate for use by the person, since it clearly pits the irrational thought against a more constructive alternative, and then leaves room for clear articulation of evidence for and against the two beliefs. This reality test will, of course, highlight the fact that the belief is usually an untested or half-tested assumption. If the person is able to challenge general beliefs initially, all is well and good. But more usually, specific anticipations about high-risk situations may need to be initially addressed which then, when confronted, lead back to the validity of more general beliefs.

Other cognitive techniques, such as Socratic dialogue, may be useful to tackle other thinking such as dichotomous or black and white thinking, or "either I'm stressed or I'm lazy". These definitions could benefit from becoming more flexible through discussion of their utility. Sometimes cognitive biases such as over-generalization or personalization also reinforce such beliefs: "It happened once so it's going to happen always"; "Yes, but that's OK for others but I can't allow myself to relax, since I'm always blamed." Otherwise, simply arbitrary or acquired inferences may need to be grounded and re-evaluated: "Oh I just always thought that was how to act. Is there another way of acting?" Although most people will view their tic negatively, it is possible, especially with mature clients with TS, that the tic may be perceived as an eccentric part of themselves, and hence may be seen positively in terms of self-image. There is indeed an advocacy group which quite reasonably advises TS and TD to "click with their tic". Such affirmation is excellent to help people to live with their tic and feel proud of themselves despite prejudice. But our aim here is to distinguish the tic from the person who tics. Ideally, this over-identification with the tic would have been addressed at the motivation stage. But if it appears here at this stage, it indicates a conflict over self-image and may require a comprehensive therapy for self-affirmation, which is largely beyond the scope of this manual.

▶ Stage 7: Behavioral Restructuring

The idea of the cognitive restructuring is to facilitate credible motor and behavioral restructuring in high-risk tic situations/activities. Following the model of motor action, if the intention of the action plan changes, so does the planning and both the general and specific preparation for action. In the first instance, a script is devised with the client, describing how the new belief could influence action. The existing link already recognized between the old belief and old tension patterns should provide a guide for the new script. This script should be mapped out in detail from the intention stage right through to the final action stage, covering all the preparatory stages, and behavior and muscle preparation relevant for the task. Integrated into the script should be any motor techniques such as prevention by relaxation, competing response or normalization of the response, which should form part of the restructuring rather than be adopted as isolated techniques. Obviously, the person then needs to put the script into practice. So, at this point the therapist chooses either a low-risk or the easiest of the three high-risk activities (entered in Kelly's grid) and progress hierarchically through the three activities over the next three or four sessions. In children and some special needs population, the restructuring may need to take a very concrete and mainly behavioral form with the cognitive element translated into very specific thinking and feeling events. In children, the restructuring may need to be animated in an appealing form, perhaps using a comparison pet animal as a model for relaxing or behaving differently.

In the script, no parameter of motor coordination should be ignored even if, in fact, it already follows a relaxing pattern, including gait, posture, head, eye position, hand, arm, leg tension. This sounds like a daunting exercise except, as noted earlier, it is essentially a question of aligning stages of preparation and movement with the new beliefs, intention and anticipation springing from a change in attitude towards the high-risk activity. Reference can, of course, be made to behavioral patterns in the low-risk activities to draw inspiration for restructuring, where actions in general take a less tension-producing form already.

▶ Stage 8: Cognitive-behavioral Restructuring

Once the person has mastered and practiced the new behavioral approach, he or she can progress to the next situation in the hierarchy. Often the script for this and the subsequent third activity will be similar to the first activity, particularly if the underlying belief is similar. However, there will be some differences in preparation since it is a different activity. It may be also that other beliefs are in play in different activities, for example, distinct beliefs about being judged, or about competence, or outcome. So these issues may require to be addressed independently for each high-risk activity. The person may find changing behavior all at once more difficult in the higher-risk activities and hence part of the repertoire can be changed gradually. An important point is that the person is consistent in the application and does not let stresses or excuses diminish the application of the new behavioral script in high-risk activities.

The aim is for seemless integration between behavioral and cognitive aspects when restructuring movement. As the person becomes more familiar with the script and is able to apply it, evaluations of the high-risk activities, as revealed by Kelly's construct grid, should change, thus indicating cognitive and behavioral restructuring.

It should be noted that phonic and cognitive tics are addressed in exactly the same way as motor tics. The aim in both cases is to prevent or reduce the state of activation preceding tic onset. Cognitive and phonic tics are often more clearly functionally linked to activity and posture than motor tics, where the tic may be in an irrelevant but nonetheless activated muscle group. In the case of phonic tics, special attention may be focused on tension in the diaphragm and breathing muscles, and the tic-provoking activities, which may seem to focus on these muscles. In the case of cognitive tics, special attention may be directed to thought stimulation and thought activation, using content manipulation of the mental tic to reduce activation (see Appendix 3).

▶ Stage 9: Generalization

The program has deliberately targeted one dominant tic or habit, and usually people with tics, especially with TS, have more than one tic or habit they wish to address in therapy. It is important in treatment that the person stays with the same tic unit throughout therapy, but clearly the therapy can start again for different tics or habits. It is possible that a separate independent tic unit has already shown a decrease in frequency during initial treatment, but most likely, particularly if other tics appear in distinct situations and activities, the awareness, tic activity profile, cognitive and motor restructuring will need to be reworked and reapplied. Since the relaxation exercises involve the whole body, they will not need to be relearned, but they will need to be consistently reapplied in the new high-risk activities. Knowledge of the program and of the success with the previous tic helps technically and psychologically, and the person will feel more confident in applying the program.

Post-treatment Assessment

Assessing final outcome measures is important not just in terms of formal tic measures, but in terms of the responses given in questionnaires and measures directly related to the interventions of the program. For example, if the modification in the style of action has been successful, we would expect a decrease in the STOP score towards less over-activity. If the cognitive and motor restructuring has been successful, then we would expect a change in the evaluations of Kelly's grid towards an equalization of evaluation scores in the direction of the original low-risk situation scores on the original grid (see Figures 7.8 and 7.9).

Likewise, we would expect a significant reduction in ratings of the tic frequency, intensity and increase in degree of control on the daily diary. This reduction can be illustrated in graphic form (see Diary guide, Appendix 4). We would also expect a decrease in the tension questionnaire, and in the negative impact of the tic on life questionnaire. These results can also be presented in graphical or histogram form to convey a permanent and vivid record of achievement to the client. Decrease in such ratings post-therapy has been shown predictive of relapse prevention (see Chapter 4).

▶ Stage 10: Relapse Prevention

In relapse prevention, it is important to:

❏ Recap with the person any achievements and review his or her participation in the program.
❏ Highlight the strategies he or she has found useful and reassure continued use.
❏ Evaluate and rate the person's degree of confidence in maintaining the gains and continuing to implement strategies.
❏ Explore if the person sees an impediment to continued use of the techniques.
❏ Assess how confident the person feels about successful application of techniques in the future?
❏ If there are other tics or habits to change, it will be worth listing them and assuring that the person plans to deal with them realistically one at a time, by going over the relevant parts of the manual.
❏ It is also helpful to make a list of potential new or unforeseen risk situations or activities to prepare the person for future stress. Such risk situations can be extrapolated from Kelly's grid and diary activities.
❏ A plan to modify other stresses or unwanted habits, including lifestyle changes, may be beneficial.

In case of relapse, the person should follow the recommended course of:

• accept relapse as a slip, not catastrophize it as a failure;
• analyze what went wrong, or, more precisely, which strategies were not implemented;

- decide, using the manual, a plan of how best to prepare better in the future and target those sections of the manual that need revising;
- recap past progress to boost confidence in what has been achieved to permit optimism for the future.

▶ SESSION BY SESSION PROTOCOL

This section provides a guide to each session in the fourteen-week, 10-stage program. The sessions and homework run in parallel with relevant sections from the client manual, including exercises. The sessions follow the client manual step by step. The first four sessions deal with awareness training, including diary, video, close other rating and identification of high- and low-risk tic activities. The next four sessions cover the psychophysiological exercises, including discrimination, isolation, relaxation, sensorimotor activation, and the mind–muscle link. The next four deal with cognitive and behavioral restructuring and modifying style of action. The remaining sessions deal with generalization of new behavior to high-risk situations and relapse prevention. Depending on severity and type of tic, and compliance of the person in completing homework, some flexibility may be necessary. It is also possible that someone with a light tic may complete the program sooner than scheduled. However, adequate sessions should be scheduled to ensure covering the complete content of the program. Every step is important.

▶ Assessment Sessions (Pre-treatment)

The aim of the assessment procedures is to complement existing instruments (Table 6.1, p. 104) to arrive at a satisfactory description and history of the TD and its impact on function. A full case formulation may need to await information from self-monitoring and awareness stages.

▶ Treatment Sessions

Session 1

Introduce the client to a plan of awareness training, as follows:

(a) Four weeks baseline evaluation, including diary keeping.
(b) Video monitoring and close other monitoring.
(c) Questionnaires are to be filled in and tic diaries maintained. It is emphasized that this tic monitoring and questionnaire evaluation is also therapeutically important.
(d) The therapy consists of 14 weekly meetings plus 4 weeks of home practice with weekly phone contact.

In the first treatment session, any information required or missing for tic assessment is sought. The overall plan of treatment is discussed, plus the first section of the manual is to be read. The awareness exercises for the first week are explained, using the tic diary manual.

The dominant tic is identified with the person. The person is asked to describe it, and try to reproduce the tic voluntarily. The therapist can imitate the tic with the client's permission to help visual feedback. Feelings associated with the tic and sensations before and after are described as well as a general discussion of the impact of the tic on life. The form of the tic from first urge to final coping strategy is discussed in detail. This may be the first time the person has really described the tic. At this point, any other "coping strategies" or "avoidance" are described. Strategies currently in use to "control" the tic are described. A distinction is made between our use of the word "control" (as given in the diary) and current strategies used to *resist* the tic appearance. These strategies may include containing the tic, suppressing it, camouflaging it, etc. "Control" applies only to strategies other than resisting the tic by tension or suppression (i.e., the type of strategies we will teach to prevent tension build-up in the program).

The client's current model of tics is explored with the help of the tic quiz. The basis of a learning model approach to tics is explained. The learning model implies acquiring new habits and abilities, new ways of controlling movement. Learning to control tics is similar to learning any other skill. Firstly, we must isolate components and then cumulatively learn the components of the skill until it becomes automatic. The course of a learning curve is never straight up but is bumpy and has ups and downs and good and bad days. The key elements of successful learning are: complicity with the guide, compliance with exercises and practice, practice, practice. It is helpful to ask the person to repeat the exercise instructions to ensure understanding, and a realistic expectation. The important point is to attempt the exercises. If there is a problem, it can be discussed at the next session. The exercises will be discussed with the client, and the participant will never be asked to do what is too difficult or what he or she feels unready to do. The aim is to achieve error-less learning. The cumulative effect of errorless learning is improved confidence in learning. A parallel can be drawn with another skill or habit that the person has mastered. Any questions so far are answered. Information on the efficacy of the method can be relayed to the client (see Chapter 4). A general outline of the 10 stages of the treatment is given and how it involves both cognitive emotional and behavioral exercises (see Figure 6.1). The collaborative nature of the program and the person's active participation are emphasized in the first chapter of the book. The feasibility of recruiting a close other is also discussed.

At the end of the first session, the person should understand the aims of the program, the need for compliance, the importance of self-monitoring, the nature of the tic he or she wishes to prioritize. The week's homework is to complete the initial two-day diary as given in the daily diary guide and to read the daily diary monitoring guide; to read the first overview section of the manual and complete the exercises; and to examine the feasibility of recruiting a close other to help to monitor the tics and give positive support and reinforcement throughout the study.

Session 2

Check that the introductory overview exercises have been attempted and the initial two-day tic diary have been completed. Question the participant about keeping the daily diary and cover any problems. Did awareness of the tic increase when keeping the diary? Did the diary keeping affect the tic frequency or intensity? How does the person now feel about keeping a daily diary? The person now progresses to filling out the diary on a daily basis, which should be explained according to the tic diary manual.

The model is discussed in more detail following a review of the person's reading of the introductory overview sections of the manual. How does the learning/habit model fit with the person's prior model of TD? What elements of the model were found to be troublesome? Is the person open-minded about working with the model? The model can be linked to other habits the participant has successfully modified (e.g., smoking). The elements in the model can be enumerated with a résumé of how they will be addressed (see 10-stage schema, Figure 6.1).

The underlying message is that it is by reducing muscle tension and sensorimotor activation that the tic will be prevented from occurring. There are cognitive, emotional and behavioral aspects to reducing the activation that makes the tic likely to occur. The different elements can be named: chronic muscle tension, style of action, over-investing effort, lack of muscle flexibility, all-or-nothing style of thinking – strategies that seem to help but, in fact, maintain the tension. Preventive strategies used currently by the person are discussed and their impact on tension and behavior.

The person will find it difficult at first to accept that there is a problem with his or her thoughts and feelings, believing mostly that the tic is neurological. The triple model triad (Figures 7.2, 7.3, 7.4, on pp. 164, 167, 168) can be illustrated by discussion of normal tension during preparation and how thoughts influence preparation in everyday life. However, a good strategy here is to point to the situational or activity profile of tic occurrence and look at situations or activities where the tic is high and low risk. The person will, in any case, now keep the daily diary, noting high- and low-risk situations and activities. This profile can be discussed with the person. The situational/activity profile is a good demonstration that tics are associated with behavioral functioning. This point can be further emphasized by looking at thoughts and feelings accompanying the high- through low-risk situations, in preparation for completing Kelly's construct grid. The diary tic unit has to be decided and the definition of activity explained.

At the end of the second session, the person should have read and understood information on the tic, including the tic quiz. Doubts about the program and any impediments to participation should have been clarified. The person should be familiar with the stages of the program. For homework, the person continues monitoring the daily diary, staying with the agreed tic unit and noting situational variation in the tic using the forms in Appendices 2d and 2e.

Session 3

Situational/activity profile analysis can now be completed from the diary and high- and low-risk situations chosen. Feelings associated with these situations can also be elicited. The video high-risk situation can be discussed and decided and scripted with the person for the next session. In the unlikely event that a suitable situation cannot be role-played, the person creates the situation in his or her imagination. Taking some examples of high-risk situations from the diary, the problem of teasing out what characterizes a low-risk situation from a high one can be started. What the person feels or does and how he or she evaluates the situation are all relevant discriminations.

At the end of session, three high- and low-risk situations should be identified. The person should understand how to complete Kelly's construct grid and decide which scoring system they wish to use.

Session 4

After reviewing the diary, the completed construct grid and any problems, the entire session is taken up with the video. Firstly, 10 minutes of video is filmed during low-risk activity (e.g. relaxing) either in the presence of the therapist, or the person can be left alone. The video is then filmed under high-risk conditions, for 10 minutes, or until the tic is elicited. The tic is then replayed to the person. If the tic is not elicited, another situation can be scripted or a high-risk scene created and enacted in the imagination. The person may sometimes be distressed by the sight of the tic but it can be explained as over-focus on a small part of the body and not what people see in general. If no video is available, then the person may be encouraged to seek visual feedback from another source, for example, a trusted other person or a mirror.

Session 5

The next four sessions focus on the psychophysiological exercises. The fifth session focuses on discrimination exercises. The person may not feel tense but in the case of chronic tension, the person may not be aware of it. The person will have read the discrimination instructions in the book, but the therapist may need to restate the rationale. If using a biofeedback apparatus, the person will need to understand the principles of operation and that the recording device just touches the skin to detect the underlying muscle activity. The electrodes should be attached in standard fashion to both tic-affected and non-affected muscle groups. The principle of the bar or other graphic display increasing and decreasing with tension accompanies the exercises, and allows the person to see how tensing and relaxing change the muscle state. The first point is to underline the presence of chronic tension and show how the person may not always be aware of it and believe that he or she is relaxed. The tension level can be demonstrated using the biofeedback machine. (The apparatus can usually be obtained commercially.) If a machine is not available, then the hand or a rubber gauge may be placed on the muscle to give equivalent feedback. During the discrimination exercise, movement is limited to the muscles involved and there is no surplus strain or generalization to other parts of the body.

Typically, the person has more trouble reducing the level from high to low than from low to high. The person may experience difficulty in reducing the muscle activity in the tic-affected area completely to zero. The person increases/decreases the contraction slowly, going from 0 to 100 in 25% steps and back again. Exercises are compared between a tic-affected and (if possible symmetrical) non-affected muscle. Practice should not exceed 30 minutes since fatigue may set in. Homework exercises are a minimum of 10 minutes per day of discrimination practice.

If the person has not succeeded in passing through all the contractions, the exercise can be restarted at the next session. The person continues practicing the discrimination exercises throughout the therapy and also while learning relaxation.

Session 6

Relaxation is explained as a learning process but with a very different aim to the discrimination exercises. The aim of the exercise is to achieve a state of relaxation in targeted muscles when tension is detected. Hence, the aim of the exercises is to effect a transition from high to low tension. Respiration is mastered first, and then combined with relaxation. In Stage 1 of the exercises, the person should be able to master the series of exercises on both sides of the body. The therapist can repeat them with the person until the sequence is performed satisfactorily. Relaxation is a course in four stages. Stage 1 is rehearsed with the person in the session. The person practices Stage 1 on both sides of the body separately at least twice per day with at least two repetitions at each practice.

Session 7

In Stage 2, the relaxation exercises are performed quicker but only on the basis of having successfully mastered Stage 1. When the person is able to appreciate the distinction between a relaxed and tense state and is able to effect a transition between the two states in each muscle group individually, he or she can then be encouraged to effect the transition without the counting delay – but including the respiration which takes the form of inspiration cuing tension and expiration cuing relaxation.

Session 8

In Stage 3 of the relaxation exercises, the person progresses to applied relaxation, putting the exercises in practice in everyday life when tensions in the course of a daily stress have been detected. This session might also address relaxation as an alternative to tension in tic-related situations. One can also discuss alternative muscle restructuring during high-risk situations, particularly if the activity requires resting still but with the accent on changing behavioral rather than cognitive features. The person can also be encouraged to pay attention to how tension builds up in the course of everyday planning of activity and how such planning relates to activation. In other words, the alternative strategies of normalization and prevention by relaxation can be applied in each high-risk activity in order to restructure tension.

Session 9

Along with the introduction of Stage 4 of the relaxation exercises – if the person is ready – cognitive restructuring is also blended into the discussion. Stage 4, in any case, is acquiring the ability to think 'relaxation' and bring about a state of relaxation by mental focus. Hence, it provides a good example of how thinking affects tension (in this case for the better). At the same time that positive focus for reducing tension is underlined, the negative vigilance and hyperattention characteristic of premonitory urge can be addressed to help to reduce the impact of sensorimotor activation. The person can also practice exposure to the urges or hypersensitive sensations (where applicable) without performing stimulating or maintaining counterproductive behavior (e.g., moving, scratching, rubbing). A classic habituation graph can be of use here, to demonstrate decline of sensation over time is the absence of maintaining factors.

Session 10

Assuming that the person has successfully accomplished the attribution training and exposure and habituation, the high-risk tic situations can now be addressed with a combination of all the previously acquired skills, through cognitive behavior restructuring.

The cognitive restructuring is implanted seemlessly as the first stage of planning action. The anticipations/evaluations relevant to each tic situation are traced back to more permanent beliefs about judgments and the correct way to act. These beliefs are tested by triple column or other techniques to see if there are alternative formulations, and whether the alternative formulations are more realistic. The implication of the initial chain of thoughts on tension and action are explored in detail. How did a prior belief specifically produce a frustration (e.g. action conflict)? How did conflict produce tension and interfere with smooth execution of action (e.g. advance planning and feedback)? How does the tension provoke frustration, emotion and the urge to tic as a natural development of the foregoing?

It may be that there is a common construct theme running through all three high-risk activities, as revealed by Kelly's grid, but the grid may also give a guide as to which elicited construct among several combined constructs is the most relevant to each high-risk activity. By definition, since the three high-risk activities are noted independently, there will be differences in action structuring in each of the activities. It is important in the restructuring to address all elements of restructuring through cognitive, emotional and psychophysiological changes. There must be no vestiges of the old tension-producing style in any domain.

Mastering restructuring in the first high-risk activities should facilitate application in the other more difficult activities. It is important that the person is persistent in application of the restructuring. If there is an element of the restructuring with which the person feels uncomfortable, this probably means there is still an investment in the old tension-producing habit, and it may be necessary to revisit beliefs and evaluations.

Session 11

Person applies restructuration to second high-risk activity.

Session 12

Person applies restructuration to highest risk activity.

Session 13

After the person has mastered the cognitive-motor restructuring for the three high-risk activities, he or she may need to learn to apply it to some tic-related activities other than the three chosen. This should be relatively easy since the high-risk activities are the more difficult. However, the aim of generalization to leave no trace of the old tension-producing style.

Session 14

This is the last session prior to the four-week home practice. These gains are detailed and the person is encouraged to complete some of the initial ratings and note changes. At this stage, the diary should reflect a significant decrease in tic frequency and intensity. The importance of continuing with practice is emphasized. If there are any problem areas, they need to be addressed. Relapse prevention is covered. Generalization of new habits of thinking and acting is encouraged, not only in tic activities but also in general areas where the style of planning was problematic. The person can be encouraged to confront rigid black and white beliefs in other areas of life using the triple column technique. Also, changing other life habits is recommended, e.g., smoking or leisure activities. If the person has other tics or habits, these can be listed during the four-week home practice. Also, the person should be prepared for unexpected stresses or events that may lead to tension and frustration and tic onset. In effect, the best guarantee of relapse prevention is to keep the knowledge of the manual close to hand.

Sessions 15, 16, 17, 18 by Phone Contact

The goal of the supplementary sessions is to monitor the person during a month of autonomous home practice, in order to see that self-administered control is functioning. If the person has succeeded in eliminating the targeted tic, then the goal is to maintain the new habits and perhaps begin to generalize the program to other tics or habits. If the person has nearly succeeded, the practice period permits the person to arrive at the goal, with reconsideration of what aspects need particular attention. It may be just that more consistent practice is required. If the person has only partially arrived at his or her goal, then the person may need to reapply different aspects of the program more rigorously, or use the period to reconsider the motivation to eliminate the tic. Here, obviously, it will depend on why the person has had only partial success (see trouble shooting). The person may need to recommence the program and return to Session 1.

Telephone interviews for the home practice are given in Appendix 8. In effect, the sessions can also serve as booster sessions addressing blocks and problems and reinforcing the person in his or her practice. The person should continue monitoring the tic and practicing restructuring and tension awareness. The interview also takes account of advances in generalization and other life/habit changes.

At the end of the home practice, follow-up is advised but is optional. Certainly, at the end of the practice, evaluation forms should be recompleted by the person to evaluate changes in style of action, impact of tic, evaluations of risk situations, since these changes have been shown to be predictive of relapse. Recommended intervals for follow-up are six months, one year and two years, during which baseline evaluations or telephone evaluations can be re-administered.

► TROUBLE-SHOOTING GUIDE

► General Problems

Jumping Ahead

The first problem may be compliance with the form filling and awareness stage of the program. The person may wish to rush straightaway into the exercises and feel that evaluation is a waste of time. Equally, the person may wish to skip some steps, believing he or she can pick or choose relevant ones. Clients may consider that they should proceed more quickly. This rush must be discouraged and the person helped to see the importance of a gradual learning process. The therapist can draw the analogy with other learning projects, where time is an important factor in the integration of skills and knowledge. It is essential that the person understands the utility of awareness and detection exercises, and engages in the exercises as a learning experience.

Motivation

Despite the initial assessment of motivation, some people may be more or less inclined to give the program a priority as their interest in other aspects of life waxes and wanes. Tell-tale signs of a drop in motivation are homework partially completed, the diary missed for several days, appointments cancelled at the last minute, and a general complaint about the length or intensity of the program. Motivation in those with HD, especially light HD, often seems to be a greater problem than with TD. Clearly, the answer here is to refer the person back to the introductory chapters of the manual and rediscuss motivation and priorities in a non-judgmental way. The solution may be to defer treatment until another time. It is certainly not recommended to let the person carry out the program if he or she is not motivated since failure will result and the person may be discouraged to pursue future programs.

Abandon Due to Improvement

Another problem is abandoning the program mid-way after a noticeable improvement. In a minority of people, awareness and discrimination exercises can reduce tic frequency significantly. The philosophy here is that since the person has improved, he or she can do the rest without the need to follow the program to the end. The importance of following the entire course of the program needs to be reiterated.

Negative Support

Most partners or spouses offer good support and encouragement. But, occasionally, the home environment may not be therapeutic and conducive to improvement. Either the close other will provide continuously negative feedback, being critical or noticing only when the tic appears and making discouraging remarks about therapy, or the close other (especially a parent) may personally suffer from tics and so set an unhelpful role model in the management of tic behavior. It is also possible that the close other may draw a secondary gain from the client's tic problem and so discourage progress. In all the above cases, if the client is willing, it is important to furnish information to the close other on the program and, where possible, involve the person in the role of co-therapist, giving appropriate encouragement, support and positive reinforcement to the client and also acting as an external rater (see Appendix 2j).

▶ Step 1: Awareness

The person may find the awareness stage and the self-monitoring a challenge. This is why we introduce the person gradually to the full daily diary keeping. When choosing the functional tic unit with the person, it is important to find a monitoring time (not less than two hours per day) which suits the person and doesn't leave him or her feeling over-burdened. Initially, the diary keeping can lead to an increase in tic frequency, but this is just temporary as awareness develops. The effect of awareness becomes beneficial over time as onset is detected earlier.

The tasks of divided attention (see client manual) need to be practiced to help the person to attain optimal awareness capacity. The skill of detecting tic onset needs to be practiced, in particular with the therapist acting as prompt within the session. Accurate description of the tic is important as is choice of the appropriate tic unit, since the person must target this tic throughout therapy. Sometimes as one tic reduces, the person may be tempted to start recording another tic. It may also be tempting for both therapist and client to target a less problematic tic initially, but this strategy risks demotivating the client since he or she will feel that the real problem is not being dealt with. Also, a less problematic tic may occur less frequently and in fewer situations which might derail attempts to assiduously apply functional analysis and restructuring. It is important to target a tic that is significantly distressing to the person. There seems no advantage, as there might be with other problems, to creating a hierarchy and starting with the less distressing problem.

Generally, discovering the situational or activity profile and the emotional and other behavioral associations of the tic is a positive experience, but the focus on the tic can be distressing to the person. This is particularly so when replaying and viewing the video. It is important to explain to the person that in everyday life, people see a person, not a tic, and we are artificially focusing on the tic in therapy.

► Step 2: Discrimination Exercises

The aims of the discrimination exercises are to give some degree of control over an inflexible muscle which generally contracts from all to nearly nothing. The goal is that the person gradually experiences more freedom of contraction of the muscle. The person may have difficulty recognizing and labeling degrees of tension. The reason for starting the discrimination exercises with a non-affected muscle is to anchor the gradation in personal experience of the change in degrees of tension. A major problem is that the person may not practice the exercises long enough or frequently enough or in a slow enough way to receive benefit. Sometimes a client may repeat the exercises in a mechanical fashion, without focusing on the sensation of graded tension through use of the feedback. It has also to be understood that in the exercise the person is isolating the muscle in addition to gradually changing tension levels. Occasionally, people may try to turn the discrimination into a relaxation exercise and contract the muscle more forcefully and more quickly than necessary.

If the feedback is not available from a machine, muscle feedback can be given by a mirror, through lightly placing a hand on the area to tense or from observation by a third person. All these feedback techniques seem equally effective. Some external feedback, however, is essential to accomplish the discrimination. The person should stick to the daily practice protocol, since repeated exercising and contraction may lead to muscle fatigue and a reduction of flexibility. Successfully completing the discrimination exercise can by itself successfully eliminate the tic in rare cases. Certainly, it is one of the most usefully rated components of the program and people should be encouraged to practice it throughout treatment.

► Step 3: Relaxation Exercises

The person may perceive no immediate benefit and so abandon the exercises. If the person does not benefit immediately from relaxation, this is normal since relaxation is a learning process. It may take a week or so of continuous practice to feel an effect. It is important to choose a daily time when the person can successfully and routinely practice. At night and in the morning may be appropriate as the person may then have more time available. Also, relaxation does help sleep. There may be a tendency for the person to short-cut the exercises or to miss out certain muscle groups or to relax both sides at once. It is important that criteria are met before passing to each progressive stage. Combining with the breathing is a good way to ensure that the correct rhythm of the relaxation exercise is maintained.

If the person suffers pains during the exercises, this may be due to over-exertion during the exercise. Similarly, dizziness may be due to over-breathing. The solution in both cases is to stop and recover and then breathe or contract to the correct rhythm. Occasionally, someone may panic at the relaxation response, generally due to a fear of letting go. This may signal the presence of obsessional or anxious traits. The beliefs behind this response need to be examined.

▶ Step 4: Sensorimotor Exposure

A common failure here is inadequate exposure to the premonitory sensation or tension so that the person does not realize that, if tolerated, it will dissipate. The person may also attempt the exposure while focusing on the sensation to see if it disappears – a counterproductive strategy guaranteed to maintain the sensation. Alternatively, the client may tolerate the sensation in some but not other situations, or implement substitute actions or resistances to partially perform the maintaining action or an action that may serve the same purpose. Instead of moving or restlessness, the person may just change position. The person needs to be aware of the contribution of self-fulfilling thoughts about the inevitability of sensation leading to further stimulation, tic onset and the subsequent tendency to focus on the sensations, which highlights and augments the sensation. The vicious circle of how need for stimulation leads to more stimulation and a renewed need for stimulation, means that one has to break the circle at an intellectual as well as behavioral level.

The person can be shown a graphical representation of the exposure and habituation curve and shown visually what to expect if the person tolerates enough and does not feed the sensation. Comparisons can be made with everyday situations where habituation takes place – for example, when habituating to the noise of a fridge in an apartment. The key to success is control over the right exposure and response parameters, and continual practice with no cognitive or behavioral avoidance.

▶ Step 5: Style of Action

A serious difficulty with confronting the style of action is that the person may feel that his or her style of action is efficient, mainly due to beliefs about the correct way of acting. However, without going too deeply into the beliefs at this step, the person can make a list of the conveniences and inconveniences of the person's way of acting to illustrate that it is not so efficient. Pointing out obvious inconveniences, like feeling exhausted and always under pressure, and never really being present in the here and now, can prove effective. Usually, people with tics will score high on at least one major STOP item, loading on over-investment of effort or over-activity. If the person does not score highly, it may be worth exploring how the person interpreted the items since this style of action seems a defining characteristic of TD. If the person has difficulty changing his or her style of action, it probably means that a belief is well entrenched, and hence further modification can be left to the next step of cognitive restructuring. Changing style of action does not mean asking the person to be less efficient or become a jello. It simply means reducing, say, an agenda with six tasks to one of four or five, so taking the strain and conflict out of performance but leaving the healthy motivating stress.

▶ Step 6: Cognitive Restructuring

The approach here is informational and educational, not confrontational. We are replacing automatic thinking with more adaptive thoughts. The person at this stage should understand the model and, with the help of the self-administered triple column technique, the person can replace a habitual thought with a more realistic one and test it out in a spirit of enquiry to see which belief is best supported.

The therapist acts as guide, but it is very important that there is no arguing or disputing with the client. The aim is a non-threatening one of helping to correct maladaptive action plans. We are not seeking to modify deeply held personal beliefs. The model emphasizes the role of thoughts as the first stage in an action plan that eventually leads to tension and tics. The program should logically have led the person to his or her maladaptive beliefs, from the initial awareness of tension through the link of tension to preparation strategy, the vicious circle of attributional style maintaining and style of action, sensorimotor activation, and the association of style of action with beliefs about actions.

Sometimes in restructuring the beliefs about organization, other beliefs about interpersonal relations or other life events arise. If they are not relevant to the tic, they are not addressed in the program. However, asserting oneself more in social situations could be relevant to, say, a facial tic likely to occur socially. So the therapist must use judgment in deciding the relevance of beliefs. As long as a belief can be tied directly to plans about action in high-risk situations, it can be considered relevant to the program.

▶ Steps 7 and 8: Behavioral and Cognitive-Behavioral Restructuring

The behavioral restructuring here follows naturally from the previous challenges and changes in belief. Now it is a question of asking the person what would this belief lead him or her to do in practice. However, the preparation for action has to be broken down stage by stage to make sure the person is aware of a new routine at each stage of the action plan, otherwise he or she might easily step back to an older routine and style of action at certain stages. The person may be tempted to go through the motions while maintaining the same ideas or perform little snippets of the old style of action to help the task to move along more familiarly.

The main benefits of changing the style of action is that the person realizes that he or she has been creating a strain in the approach to action planning and that it is unnecessary and unrealistic. However, although the person feels better, he or she may still be attracted intellectually by the idea of moving fast. Here, also, the stimulation from proprioceptive feedback that follows from swift abrupt action may reinforce the old style. The person's attention may need to be redirected towards the benefits in terms of a calmer, more accomplished result from decreasing over-preparation and over-activity. A lot of back and forth between cognitive and behavioral restructuring, one feeding back to the other, may be necessary.

Successful application of restructuring to one area should encourage subsequent application to other high-risk activities.

► Step 9: Generalization

Although it is essential in the program to deal with one tic at a time, this might be frustrating for the person and his or her entourage, since at the end of therapy, although in one sense the person has mastered the tic, in another sense, the tics are still present. Unfortunately, there is no automatic generalization from the elimination of one tic to the elimination of others. However, if the person has worked to reduce activation by relaxation and restructuring, there may well be some impact on the intensity of other tics, but as the other tics are distinct functional units, they will probably require a distinct functional analysis to discover related activities and emotions and high-risk cues. It is, however, a good idea to encourage the person to apply the method to other tics as soon as possible after therapy in order to profit from the first success, and implement them as new while the strategies are still fresh in the person's mind. Dealing with other tics will also help to strengthen dealing with the first tic, and aid relapse prevention. If the person has multiple tics, the choice of subsequent tics should, however, be one by one, starting with the next most disturbing. Allowances may be required for any special strategies required for phonic tics.

► Step 10: Relapse Prevention

Relapse prevention strategies are standard for all HD. Relapse is possible, and most frequently occurs in the first three months post-treatment. However, it can occur up to two years or longer post-treatment. Relapse is most likely to occur when the tic has not been completely eliminated post-treatment. The home practice and generalization periods are crucial to help the person to arrive at zero frequency. Continued application of changes in style of action seem very predictive of low relapse. Obviously, in the absence of regular therapist meetings, motivation may lag and the person may become sporadic about putting strategies into continued practice after therapy. It may be important to devise and implement with the person's collaboration a positive reinforcement schedule that will encourage him or her to continue practicing; for example, rewards or leisure periods at the end of each day, contingent on practice. Alternatively, a close other can be recruited to provide motivation and support.

Sections of the book particularly relevant to the person's coping can be earmarked for revision. The person should be encouraged to complete the diary and questionnaires at regular intervals as an objective way of motivating continued support and progress. If dealing with the tic has revealed other coping problems, then the person can also at this point be encouraged to seek help for these and other outstanding problems. Positive changes in other unrelated aspects of lifestyle can be beneficial in maintaining gains post-treatment.

▶   CASE ILLUSTRATIONS

▶ Case No. 1171 (Figure 6.2)

Personal History

Julie is a 56-year-old divorced mother of an adult child who is still living with her. Presently unemployed, she is undergoing vocational training and wishes to work in the data-processing field.

Evaluation and Problem Awareness Stages

Dominant tic   Diagnosed with Tourette's syndrome as a child, Julie suffers presently from multiple tics: clearing the throat, sniffing and squinting. She hopes to work on clearing the throat as a priority because it leads to a permanent throat irritation and, according to her, is "bothering other people". For example, her son, with whom she shares a small apartment, often makes offensive remarks when the tic occurs, and particularly at bedtime. Those remarks markedly increase the frequency and the intensity of the tic. Some sensations precede the tic: such as the impression that she has secretions in her throat, "like cement". The client regularly practices relaxation (Schultz method) and tries to relax when her tic occurs, but to no avail. She notes that her throat remains tensed when she does the relaxation exercises. Since she is uncomfortable when her tics appear in front of strangers, Julie hides her problem by blowing her nose to justify the presence of sniffles or takes lozenges to simulate an actual throat ache. She has had tics since she was six years old and blames their origin on her adoption by her stepfather.

We identified together the targeted priority tic unit to be noted in the daily diary. The unit was defined as throat clearing occurring either individually or in series. She agreed to record frequency, intensity and control over the tic for a period of two hours every day.

High-risk and low-risk situations   Julie identified the following situations as potentially increasing the frequency and the intensity of her dominating tic: exams following training sessions, being bored, thinking about her problems, not having slept enough, thinking about unpleasant things she has to do. The low-risk situations are: exercising, going to the movies, and going to a restaurant with friends.

Kelly's construct grid   Kelly's grid, once completed and interpreted, revealed the following underlying attributions and evaluations peculiar to high-risk situations and the occurrence of the tic: being tired, being pensive or preoccupied, lacking self-confidence, being afraid to be judged, failing, feeling helpless and being perfectionist.

Thoughts, emotions and physical activity associated with the high-risk situations   The three high-risk situations chosen by Julie in order to complete Appendix 2h were:

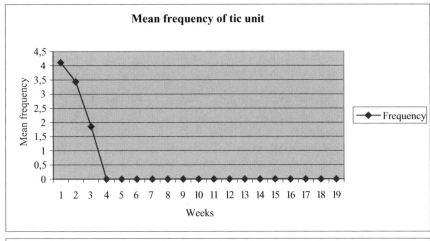

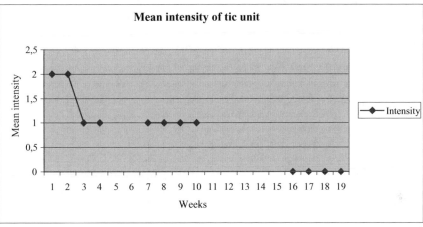

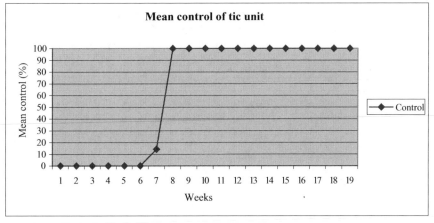

Figure 6.2   Case No. 1171

exams following training sessions, stuck in a problem at home, after having spent an entire sleepless night. The associated cognitions are: "I will fail" (situation 1), "I won't be able to find a job, or better my situation" (situation 2), "I will feel bad for the next few days" (situation 3).

The video recording   We had agreed to film two sequences. The first one, a low-risk situation, had her conversing with the therapist, as usual, at the beginning of the session. The second situation involved a discussion about her financial difficulties and her job search. During the second sequence, the dominant tic was very present and Julie was ill at ease and irritated. When we reviewed the video together, she was not surprised by what she saw, and recognized her numerous tics.

Comments   During the first sessions, Julie seemed sometimes hostile: her gestures were abrupt, her regard was elusive and, as soon as the session was over, she would take her belongings, say her goodbyes, and leave the office rapidly. She often interrupted the session and seemed impatient when addressed by the therapist. Despite her sometimes disconcerting attitude, she seemed very motivated and adhered diligently to the program. By the second session, she seemed to know the manual by heart.

▶ The Therapy

At the first session of therapy, Julie remarked that the tic that we had agreed to work on seemed to have diminished. She explained this by the fact that her son, with whom she fights daily, had left to go to live on his own. In fact, she had noted a link between this tic and her son's remarks about it ("stop coughing"). However, Julie says that other tics were now more frequent (mainly a shoulder movement). Nevertheless, we agreed to start the program with the dominant tic. At the 8th session, we decide to work simultaneously on two tics: throat clearing and a shoulder movement, since the former had almost disappeared and the latter had increased considerably in frequency and did seem functionally related to the throat clearing. (Figure 6.2 shows only the dominant tic.)

Discrimination and relaxation   The biofeedback training (Session 5) involved placing an electrode on the left side of the neck to record the relevant muscle activity. Julie had some difficulty contracting and releasing this area progressively. In the first week of discrimination, training didn't improve and she tried to do the exercises with the muscles implicated in her other tics. She was advised against that and reminded of our main objective. Progressively, even if it remained difficult for her to contract and gradually release the neck tension, she was able to better perceive the tensions in this area. At the eighth session, the client was asked to do the discrimination exercises for the shoulder tic and to try to control the tension through exercise in both tics. The client had an easier time with the muscular contracting–releasing of the discrimination exercises in the shoulder.

Learning the relaxation technique was easy, since Julie was already familiar with this type of approach. After two to three weeks of regular training, she progressed rapidly to Stage 4 and was able to let go of the tension without completing the entire relaxation sessions (contracting–releasing of many muscles groups), what she termed "passive relaxation", i.e., releasing the superfluous muscular tensions in a few minutes while breathing and without contracting the muscles beforehand. With Julie, the use of prevention by relaxation seemed to have been rapidly effective. In fact, by the tenth session, she was able to control her throat clearing through relaxing (it had, in fact, already diminished considerably), and the second tic (shoulder movement) was also decreasing rapidly in frequency. However, even if the client no longer experienced tics, she continued to perceive, for the next few weeks, considerable tension in the neck and shoulder. She continued to successfully release those tensions (and in the rest of the body also) as soon as she detected them, as she had done when the tension led to the tics.

Action styles and underlying beliefs   When we discussed informally ways to be or act that can create tension, Julie said that she had a tendency to keep to herself her anger towards others and, generally, a tendency to repress her feelings. She was also aware that she was doing a lot of things too fast (walking, eating, working, . . .). As a matter of fact, she had to endure many negative remarks from her employers because of the speed with which she would do her work; mistakes were made or some aspects were forgotten. Her vision of the work she was doing and the many training sessions she felt she must attend conveyed a tendency to be a perfectionist ("I am mad at myself if everything is not perfect"). The beliefs that keep her "running" are: "I am doing well when I go fast" and "I am saving some time". We first discussed the utility of doing things rapidly and her belief that by doing so she would objectively save a lot of time. She initially agreed with the "theoretical" idea that the time saved was probably not considerable. She was thus encouraged to test this hypothesis by timing herself on two occasions: when she was shopping for the groceries rapidly and then when she was pacing herself more steadily. She realized that the time saved was very small and she also noticed that by slowing down, she felt more serene, which contradicted her belief that it was essential to do things rapidly in order to feel good. By becoming aware of her problematic action style and of the advantages in changing it, Julie decided to systematically try to do things less rapidly in her everyday life. Progressively, she noticed that she felt better but was no less efficient in her tasks.

In her relationships with others, Julie feared being rejected, which led her to keep her opinions or her negative emotions to herself: "I keep everything to myself". When the inconveniences brought about by this behavior were discussed, Julie realized that they were numerous: interiorized painful emotions and feeling ill at ease; feeling passively subjected to situations and then getting angry with herself; running away from certain situations because she felt she could not assert herself. Nevertheless, Julie mentioned that those inconveniences were less painful than the risk of being rejected or getting into an unbearable argument. She was encouraged to think about the fears and to say that what she feared could realistically happen. Even if her worst fears were to happen, would they be so dramatic? Julie progressively started to lift the cognitive barriers that kept her from expressing her negative affects. She was thus given some assertiveness tools to help her to concretely modify this action style. Two weeks later, Julie mentioned having made a remark to her English course teacher. This contributed to the course being modified and helped Julie to release some anger that had accumulated over time.

Usual ways of thinking   Cognitive restructuring continued and addressed two high-risk situations: her job search and her relationship with her son. Actually, because the first situation considered at risk was no longer present (doing exams), the two situations addressed here were currently those most likely to increase her tic onset. The job search was a constant preoccupation for Julie and she could see a strong correlation between her tics and this worrisome situation. Many automatic thoughts were present: "I will never find work", "all the doors are closing", "making an effort is useless", "life is unfair", etc. The cognitive exercises of finding alternative thoughts were effective and allowed Julie to take some distance from the situation (allow herself to go out and have some leisure activities . . .) and allowed her to see the job search in a more pragmatic way ("Instead of ruminating on the injustice in this world, I have to keep my energy to find a satisfying job", "I will try to better orient my search"). Her son had now returned to Julie's house and she feared that the conflicts would start all over again and would create stress and induce tics. Thus, it was agreed to examine and relativize the associated automatic thoughts. Again, Julie was able to pass from pessimistic and negative thoughts ("he didn't change, I can't talk with him, he doesn't respect me . . . ") to more constructive thoughts ("we have some good moments together but if the situation doesn't get better, maybe we will have to take some distance from each other") and this helped her to face this situation in a more serene manner. Beyond the direct effects observed on those two situations, the fact that Julie implemented this new way of dealing with thoughts to other problematic situations diminished overall the frequency and intensity of the tics. She then used cognitive restructuration in her daily life and was able to notice that her state of mind was better, especially in her relationships with others where it allowed her to express her feelings more easily.

Comments

Julie rapidly gained some control over her muscular tensions inducing the tics, which allowed her to work on her action styles and especially on the automatic thoughts that can, indirectly, increase the amount and intensity of her tics.

Home Treatment

During the four weeks in which we had our telephone follow-ups, progress was maintained and Julie considered that her control over both her tics was around 90%. She continued to "keep an eye" on her muscular tension and was releasing this tension systematically as soon as she could feel it increasing slightly. At the end of the program, she seemed satisfied and confident about her ability to continue her progress and eventually get rid of her tics once and for all. Moreover, she felt less anxious and more able to deal with her daily difficulties.

Her Tourette's Syndrome Global Scale (TSGS) had decreased from 37 pre-treatment to 11 post-treatment.

▶ Case No. 1189 (Figure 6.3)

Personal History

Gerald is a 47-year-old man, married and a father of two adult children. He is an engineer and has been working as a self-employed consultant for some months. He was diagnosed with Gilles de la Tourette's syndrome as a child. He suffered from both motor and vocal tics.

Evaluation Phase and Awareness of the Problem

Dominant tic   At the beginning of the therapy, Gerald suffered from multiple motor tics, centered around the face (eyes, forehead, etc.). When asked to choose the tic to prioritize during the course of the program, he chose, without any hesitation, a tic that appeared recently (about a year ago) and, according to him, has a considerable impact on his life. This tic was to brush the palate with his tongue while moving his lips. The priority tic unit was defined with the client as a movement of the tongue against the palate accompanied by lip movements, whether a brief or long movement and whether in series or alone. The period of observation for the therapy period was four hours per day during which frequency, intensity and degree of control of the tic were recorded in the daily diary. This complex tic was preceded by a "tickling" sensation on the palate ("something that scratches") and Gerald mentioned being more aware of the occurrence of that tic than his other facial tics. This involuntary mouth movement had daily negative repercussions and consequences for his work: it disrupted his pronunciation and affected clients' judgment of him. In fact, when he conducted meetings or when he met a new client informally, Gerald feared that his tics might be interpreted as a sign of nervousness and so reveal a lack of self-confidence, which would be, according to him, a major problem since a consultant should appear self-assured. At the somatic level, the frequent contact of the tongue on the palate provoked its irritation. At this point, Gerald did not have the impression of being able to control his tic. He had tried to disguise and contain the tic by breathing deeply in order to relax (yoga) or by keeping his mouth firmly closed. Recently, he had told people he met that he suffered from Tourette's syndrome and asked their opinion about it ("Did you notice my tics?"). During the first sessions, Gerald seemed very tense and anxious. The contact was not very good. In fact, the client had some difficulty to maintain his attention when spoken to and frequently interrupted.

High-risk and low-risk situations   In the course of the awareness exercises, Gerald identified the following situations as potentially increasing the frequency

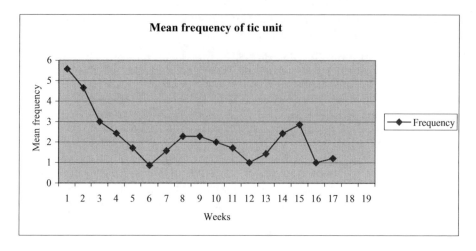

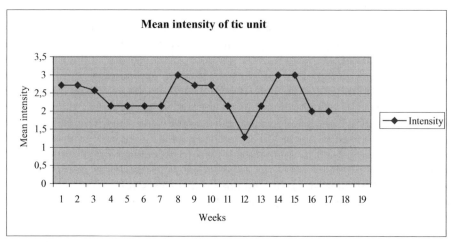

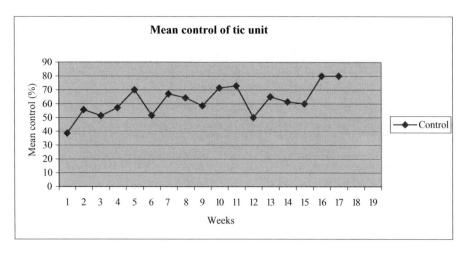

Figure 6.3 Case No. 1189

and intensity of the dominant tic: meetings at work; meetings with new clients; being unoccupied (vacations, etc.); seeing his in-laws; and weekends. The low-risk situations were: doing sports; concentrating on something; practicing yoga; and going to shows.

Kelly's construct grid   The grid, once completed and interpreted, revealed the following attributes or constructs associated with high-risk activities: being tired, staying still, being pensive or preoccupied, lacking self-confidence, being obliged to speak (an aspect elicited from the client himself). Gerald was of the opinion that remaining still, being pensive or being tired are the aspects most correlated to his problem.

The thoughts, emotions and body activity associated with high-risk situations   The three high-risk activities for which Gerald chose to complete Appendix 2h were: conducting a meeting, meeting a new client, doing nothing (i.e., watching TV). He didn't manage to identify the thoughts and emotions for the last situation. The thoughts and anticipations associated with the first two situations were similar and revealed a significant social anxiety. Gerald feared not being able to answer questions and spent many hours preparing each meeting. He also anticipated being perceived by others as incompetent, nervous and lacking self-confidence.

The video recording   During the recording, Gerald was anxious. At the previous session, we had agreed to record two sequences. The first, the low-risk activity, involved the client alone in the room reading a text. The second situation was scripted as a brief interview with the therapist acting as interviewer, where the client had to explain his work and to argue his point of view following remarks and criticism. During the second video sequence, he had great difficulty containing his anxiety and became agitated, interrupting me and trying to control the interview by monopolizing the conversation. The tics were very numerous and intense. The viewing of the filmed sequences made the client ill at ease. He hadn't realized that his tics were so visible. He hence perceived himself as nervous and lacking self-confidence.

Therapy

Discrimination and relaxation   On the fifth session, after some theoretical explanations regarding the discrimination exercises and their purpose, biofeedback training was carried out by placing an electrode on the corner of Gerald's mouth. After a few minutes' practice, he managed to increase progressively and to decrease gradually the tension in the mouth muscle.

During the following five weeks, Gerald practiced the discrimination exercises very regularly (once or twice a day). However, during the first days of training – conceived to help the person better to perceive the muscular tensions and develop the capacity to isolate and grade those tensions – Gerald used discrimination as a strategy to control the tic. In fact, when the tic occurred or when he felt the urge to tic, he contracted his lips and his tongue progressively and repeatedly in order to release the tension gradually. The therapist insisted on the importance of not confusing the discrimination exercises (which allow an increase in flexibility or a prelude to control) with a control strategy that consists of releasing the tension in the tic-affected muscle without first contracting the muscles. With this clarification, Gerald exercised the implicated muscles and felt his control over different tension levels improve little by little. After five weeks of discrimination training, Gerald was more aware of the tensions around his mouth and, even before the tic happened, he often succeeded in reducing the tension level in this area. In doing so, he also prevented or stopped the tic.

Learning the progressive relaxation of Jacobson followed the discrimination exercises (Session 6). Gerald was interested in yoga and on occasion practiced the yoga exercises that he knew. When the relaxation method was proposed and demonstrated, he seemed interested and motivated. Gerald's intellectual curiosity regarding this technique seemed positive and likely to facilitate allocating the required time for learning (two sessions of 20 minutes each day during the course of several weeks). Gerald also understood the importance and rationale of relaxation, namely, that it should help his capacity to perceive excessive muscular tensions in his entire body and to efficiently release those tensions. Nevertheless, over the first weeks, Gerald had some difficulties practicing the training regularly, since the practice periods did not fit with his daily routine: "relaxation takes too much time", "I tell myself that I have something better to do", "I can't concentrate", etc. When the role of those thoughts was confronted (not untypical thoughts for people that suffer from tics), Gerald agreed to "let go" and to invest more time in relaxation. At the end of the therapy, Gerald considered relaxation as a habit and a pleasure. Now at Stage 4, in his everyday life he attempted to function while monitoring and releasing tension in his entire body automatically.

Styles of action and underlying beliefs   Reading the relevant section of the manual and further discussions highlighted a characteristic action style and a way of acting important for Gerald: to do things rapidly. This style could be illustrated by many examples: he talked rapidly because he feared being interrupted; he drove quickly and ate quickly because he anticipated being late for his appointments; and that others had a negative opinion of him. So he didn't want to waste time. Gerald also had some difficulty in concentrating, especially when he had to listen "passively" to someone. He says that he quickly became impatient when the person "didn't get right to the point". In a general sense, he has had trouble concentrating since his childhood.

Even if his schooling was successful and allowed him to pursue his education at university level, he didn't remember being able to listen to his teachers for more than a few minutes since elementary school. He had to work hard on his own, at home. Looking back, he described himself as a "self-made man" and it made him proud.

In his work, Gerald showed some perfectionism related to organization and personal standards and more so when he had to lead a meeting. He would spend many hours preparing himself and felt "competent" only when he felt able to answer all the possible questions that might be asked.

At this stage in the therapy, the belief labeled "I'm wasting my time" was addressed in situations where it occurred frequently: "When I do things less rapidly", "When I listen to someone who doesn't get right to the point", "When I do the relaxation exercises" or "If I don't do many things all at once". The advantages, together with the advantages of alternatively doing things slowly, one at a time, and "taking his time", were considered. This reflection led him to consider the gains expected in terms of the quality of his work, in his relationships with his clients, his well-being (cf. relaxation). The therapist then contrasted the benefits of taking his time to the stress of his perfectionism (for example, when he prepares his meetings "to perfection"), which implied that being calm was a waste of time. He was shown an illustration of an inverted U curve showing how excess preparation can actually impair the quality of his performance by increasing his anxiety. After some work on his beliefs, Gerald modified many behaviors by himself: he tried very hard to do everyday activities more slowly (walk, drive, speak, etc.) and to take some time to relax. In the last three meetings, Gerald's behavior seemed calmer and more poised. He no longer interrupted and spoke more slowly. A little while before the end of our weekly meetings, he told me that he had decided to change the pace of his life and that, from now on, he would work at home as much as he could.

Usual ways of thinking   The three high-risk situations addressed in therapy were: meetings at work; meetings with a new client; and get-togethers with friends or family. Those three situations provoked in Gerald very similar automatic thoughts that can be summarized as follows: "Others can see that I have tics. They then find me nervous or bizarre and deduce that I am incompetent and lack self-confidence. They end up rejecting me either at work or in my personal life." Paradoxically, anticipating ticcing made the tic onset more likely.

Professional situations (meetings, clients) provoked additional cognitions concerning his file management and preparation ("it is important to be able to answer all questions"...). When Gerald was asked, using the triple-column technique, to realistically compare his usual thoughts that generate anxiety and tension, to reality, it seemed that he was objectively perceived by his clients and colleagues as someone who was very competent in his work. In fact, nothing proved that others judged him negatively because of his tics. Rather, his other qualities were judged as important, if not more so, in the evaluation of Gerald as a person and a professional: the ability to interact with others; the quality of his advice; his lively mood; his sense of humor, etc. Presenting a "perfect façade" was not necessary in his relationships with others.

Gradually Gerald, at first a prisoner of his anxiogenous thoughts in his relationships with others, realized the excessive and maladaptive nature of his interpretations in those situations and began to give weight to more constructive hypotheses in order to alleviate the painful emotions he usually felt, and to indirectly diminish the frequency and intensity of the tics.

A little while after having addressed those issues, Gerald led a meeting in front of 25 clients. He felt some anxiety before starting to speak but took a big breath, went calmly towards the microphone and remembered the constructive thoughts that we had identified together. His presentation was very successful.

Other comments   After therapy, Gerald less often displayed the tic we had worked on and considered himself as having it under relatively good control. He also seemed much calmer although his other tics were still present. Gerald, confident because of the progress he had shown, made a list of the "challenges" (i.e., his other tics) that he now wanted to address.

Home Treatment

Telephone interviews were conducted weekly over a month of home practice. During that period, Gerald continued to apply the control strategies taught in the program. He reported maintaining a good control on his dominant targeted tic and was trying to control another tic. However, he had a relapse when he spent many days on vacation at his in-laws. He was both surprised and disappointed because of this. The telephone interview that followed this event allowed us to contextualize this sudden reappearance of the tic and place it in perspective as a slip, not a relapse. Gerald was encouraged to adopt a problem-solving approach and to learn as much as possible from this relapse (i.e., understand what happened, which strategies he could have put into place, etc.). The following week, Gerald said that he had regained control and was still progressing.

His Tourette's Syndrome Global Scale (TSGS) had decreased from 17 pre-treatment to 6 post-treatment.

▶ **Case No. 1142 (Figure 6.4)**

Personal History

Louise is a 36-year-old woman. She lives with her husband and has no children. She works full time as a head of communication. She consulted our clinic in order to diminish the frequency of her tics, especially in the neck, because it was very painful. As far as she remembers, she always had tics. Furthermore, there is a history of tics in her family, her brothers and sisters having suffered from them in their childhood. Thus, Louise became aware of her tics when she entered school. Over the years, the tics evolved and transformed themselves, going from mouth movements to shoulder movements, wrist movements, feet movements and finger movements. She also suffered from simple vocal tics of a coughing type. During the initial evaluation, Louise complained about frowning, eye blinking, nail biting, picking skin around the nails and neck contractions on the right, but without any visible sharp movements. The contractions resembled muscular spasms. They appeared about two years ago and are bilateral. Louise successfully managed to control the left contractions, but the right ones intensified and caused extreme pain. According

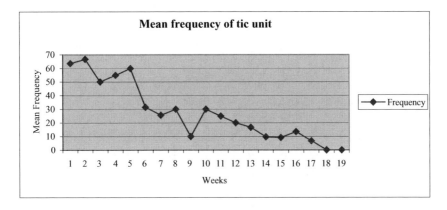

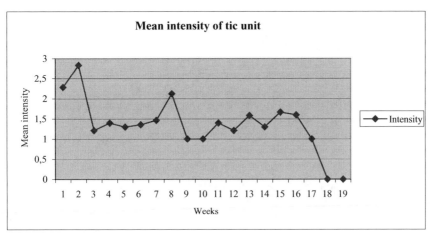

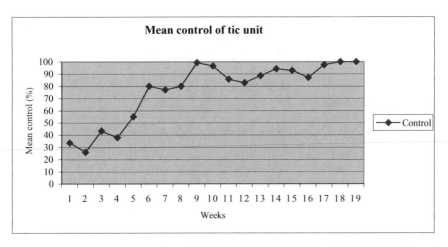

Figure 6.4 Case No. 1142

to Louise, the tics are present at any given time during the day and rarely disappear completely.

In the past, Louise's tics greatly impaired her social and professional functioning. For example, she often refused promotions at work, preferring not to put herself in situations that resulted in more pressure and stress. Moreover, as a child, she isolated herself and for a long time only frequented people that she already knew as she was afraid to be judged. Today, she says that she accepts herself more and manages to do the activities that she likes. She considers she has a lifestyle that suits her. Actually, Louise noticed that her tics diminish when she maintains a healthy lifestyle, i.e., offering herself relaxing moments and taking time to do one thing at a time. She adopted this way of life a few years ago when she was coming out of a difficult time in her personal life and started a supportive therapy. Therefore, she doesn't use techniques to camouflage her tics. She noticed that the more she concentrates on not doing the tics, the more she does them. In order to control them, she only attempts to remain as calm as possible.

Evaluation and Self-observation Stages

Session 1   The first therapy session was entirely dedicated to the evaluation of the problem and explanation of the model. Louise understood the rationale very rapidly and provided many examples to illustrate the extent to which the model applied to her situation. She prioritized the neck tic as the dominant tic. The muscles implicated in the tic were identified and Louise started to reflect upon the situations, thoughts and emotions strongly related to the emergence of the tic. She admitted to not feeling any sign or premonitory sensation when the tic occurs. She undertook the self-observation throughout the day to provide her with more information.

Session 2   Louise's first self-observations permitted her to notice that her tic was less present at the weekend than during the week. She already started noticing that her work brought about an unnecessary muscular tension. The session continued with the enumeration of high-risk situations where the tic usually occurs. She noted the following situations: (1) when she is concentrating on an intellectual task; (2) when she is passionate about something she does; (3) when she has an animated discussion and/or when she has to debate her point of view; (4) when she has emotions that she finds "disturbing" (argument, doubt, panic, insecurity, fear); (5) when she finds herself in a tight deadline and has to reach some specific objectives at work; (6) when she is in the car on the passenger side; (7) when she's reading or watching TV (especially during a film with lots of suspense). She also highlighted some low-risk situations where the tic is less likely to appear: trips, weekends in the country, public transport, restaurant and telephone.

Session 3   At the third session, Louise noticed that the intensity of her tic had diminished slightly. However, another tic that she was no longer doing had reappeared: turning her wrist. But she chose to ignore this tic and to continue to concentrate on the neck tic. By the means of her tic diary, she observed that the muscular movements of her neck now occurred abruptly in series and then subsided progressively. She also observed that her tics occurred mostly at the end of the day. The other goal of this third session was to confirm or discover what was associated with tic occurrence. In the Kelly construct grid, Louise chose three low-risk situations (hiking in the mountains, public transport, and restaurant) and three high-risk situations (being a passenger in a car, television, and at work). In order to better understand how these situations become high risk, she compared high- and low-risk situations and noted how she evaluated both. The grid ratings allowed her to confirm that the presence of the tic was associated with a state of preoccupation, of a lack of confidence and of pressure to perform or finish a project. We returned to the model in order to identify other cognitive, emotional, sensorimotor or behavioral aspects associated to the three high-risk situations. Louise claimed that when she's travelling in a car, she has no tic (or almost none) when she is driving. When she is the passenger, she has a greater tendency to anticipate the gestures of the other drivers. She then has the habit of tensing and looking constantly around her. When watching the television, she has tics when she views subjects that fascinate her or when the intrigue of the scenario is captivating. Once again, she noticed that she adopts a tense position and needs to let go of her attention to her tics to concentrate entirely on the activity. Finally, at work, she realizes that she has more tics when she has to plan or complete a task in a short time. She fears making mistakes or not performing according to her superiors' expectations. Furthermore, she has tics when talking with colleagues whether it is to give instructions, participate in a meeting or have a trivial conversation. In these cases, she fears being judged, not finding the right words, not being able to express herself clearly and wasting her time. In all these situations, Louise realizes that she has a tendency to move for no reasons and to put herself "in a state of tension".

Session 4   Louise continued to self-observe meticulously. This activity motivated her a lot because she realized that her tic was not as continuous as she thought before starting the therapy. The self-observation also provided her with some feedback about the emotions she had during the day. This feedback allowed her to manage the emotions differently when she became aware of them. She also noticed that her wrist tic had almost disappeared, but that the neck tic was still intense and painful. However, she was very proud to have experienced a moment where the control of her tic was about 75%. The remainder of this session was devoted to the video. This video exercise allowed Louise to realize the extent to which the muscular tension is more intense when she is in a high-risk situation (reading), compared to a low-risk situation (discussion with her therapist).

Intervention Stage

Session 5   The intervention stage began with the discrimination exercises. Before getting started, the exercise's rationale was explained to Louise. She already acknowledged that she was unable to recognize the different tension levels in the muscles implicated in the tic. She was under the impression that she had no control over the release of the tension she felt in those muscles. At the beginning of the exercise, Louise had some difficulty in gradually contracting the muscles affected by the tic for two main reasons. Firstly, she had some difficulty in isolating specifically the muscles implicated in her tic. She first had to start by exaggerating the movement in order to identify the specific action of the muscles. She then had the impression that this exercise created an urge to do the tic. We went over the rationale once more before pursuing the exercise. She understood that by releasing the muscles gradually, the tension would have no other choice but to disappear and the tic would no longer serve its purpose. The fact she had previously done the same exercise with non-affected muscle convinced her that it was possible to do this. She understood the importance of taking back control of the tension levels in her muscular activity. After some practice, Louise realized that her muscle can gain flexibility rather rapidly. At the end of the session, she felt her muscle was now quite relaxed.

Session 6   Over the last week, Louise had done the discrimination exercises many times per day and in different contexts (work, home, bus). She had succeeded more easily in detecting the level of tension in her muscles and was finally motivated to have a certain amount of control over the tension level and hence over her tic. The session was then devoted to the first stage of the deep-breathing and muscular relaxation exercises. Louise was very much at ease with those strategies, because she knew them well already. She had learned them while taking some relaxation and yoga classes. However, that was a few years ago and she has not been practicing them, so the exercises were reviewed and practiced in the session.

Session 7   During the previous week, Louise practiced the breathing and relaxation exercises at least once a day. This was mostly before going to bed, but also before going to a meeting. She then realized that, consequently, she didn't experience any tic during that meeting. Her husband also made the remark that she seemed more relaxed and that he was observing less tic. Actually, she made the same observation in her tic diary. She observed that the frequency of the neck tic had decreased considerably. She noticed that it was now more likely to appear when she was in interaction with others (i.e., even during a meaningless conversation) or when she had to make an intellectual effort (i.e., while she was writing a paper, at work or at the movies when she concentrated on the plot). Moreover, she underlined the fact that she had some difficulty detecting her tic when its intensity was weak. Thus, she repeated the discrimination exercises and practiced grading the tension a few times. In addition to moving on to the second stage of the muscular relaxation, the response prevention by relaxation was explained. Because Louise had integrated the model well, she had already started to use this strategy (i.e., before her meeting). Thus she was prompted to use this strategy before entering a situation that was considered at risk, immediately after the occurrence of a tic and when she felt an increase of tension in the muscles implicated in the tic.

Session 8   In order to maintain her motivation, Louise had decided to generalize the prevention by relaxation to all her tics. She then realized how much she has progressed since she now had hardly any tics. Thus, the habit of removing her skin, her nail biting and her blinking completely disappeared even though they had not been targeted by the therapy. All that remained was frowning and the neck movement, where the tension seemed to have accumulated. We decided to gradually increase the efforts in order to eradicate those tics. Firstly, Louise decided to work on all her low-risk situations by: (1) making sure that she was aware of the tic occurrence at all time and (2) applying the strategies systematically without missing one tic. Secondly, the identification of the action styles was addressed. Over the last few years, Louise had already identified and worked on many aspects of her action style. Younger, she had been hyperactive, i.e., she had a tendency of wanting to do too much at a time and felt guilty when she was taking some time to relax. Today, she described herself as very efficient in her time organization. She had a very detailed agenda and did one thing at a time. With years of experience, she learned to do her best and respect her limits. However, she still had a tendency to over-prepare her muscles, especially in situations where she felt pressure to perform or fears to be judged. She was encouraged to continue to do the relaxation exercises at the third stage.

Session 9 Following our discussion of the previous week, Louise noticed that she still had some difficulty sitting still. Thus, she paid more attention to staying still and calm. Daily, Louise observed that she has long periods without tics. Work on the low-risk situations was also fruitful because the tics in her neck and eyebrows became less intense. However, another tic that she had experienced in the past was resurfacing: the movements of the nostrils that open and close. When she detected this tic, she systematically and successfully applied the prevention strategies. In order to maintain her gains and to avoid the recurrence of this tic, she has maintained the work on the low-risk situations. The triple-column technique was illustrated and applied to her fear of conflicts. We chose a situation that arose during the week in which she feared giving her opinion to her superiors because she had thoughts such as: "I could make a mistake", "I could appear tense", "What will they think of me?" She filled in alternative thoughts such as: "Everybody makes mistakes and they are not judged negatively", "I work hard and know enough about the dossier to give my opinion". In fact, having proposed these alternatives, she instantly realized that they were more realistic. Hence, she decided in future to approach the situation more positively and give her opinion more affirmatively.

Session 10 Louise was very proud of her progress, because in addition to observing the decrease of tics in her diary, some family members also made the remark that she had no more tics. Following consistent application of the exercises, the nostrils tic didn't reappear. Her eyebrow frowning also disappeared completely and the neck tension had diminished in intensity. She did, however, feel a "tickling" sensation in her jaw, but she tolerated the sensation in order to avoid the occurrence of another tic. She also monitored peripheral movement such as moving for no reason and Louise noticed that this helped to reduce tension and sensorimotor sensations. After having worked on the lower-risk situations, Louise started to address the high-risk situations. The first one she chose was to control her tics during planning or writing situations at work. She targeted all aspects that increased the risk of the tic occurrence. On the cognitive level, she did the triple-column technique to confront her fear of not having enough time to do everything. At the sensorimotor and behavioral levels, she decided to do the relaxation exercises before doing a task. Moreover, in order to help her to divide her attention and be more aware of her tics during the task, she installed a visual prop (a *Post-it*) on her desk to verify her muscles' tension level every 20 minutes. If she felt a strong tension, she would take a minute to release the tension (relaxation, Stage 4) or take some deep breaths. Finally, to avoid having a tense position during her work (which would increase the muscular tension), she decided to position herself with her shoulders square and her back rested on the back of her seat.

Session 11 Louise maintained her gains from the previous week. Regarding the tension in her jaw, she noticed that tolerating the tension was not enough and began to implement an antagonist response. Thus, if releasing the tension by relaxation was not sufficient, she opened her mouth slightly to relieve the tension. Over the previous week, Louise realized that self-observation had helped her tremendously to apply the strategies. For example, in working on her first high-risk situation, she said that observing herself every 20 minutes was the best technique for diminishing the frequency of the tics. She considered that her tics had diminished by 50% in that situation. She also restarted physical exercise three times a week and has already noticed the benefits because she said she has much less difficulty in releasing her muscular tension. We addressed a second high-risk situation. Because Louise hasn't had tics while watching television for a few weeks now, we decided to work on another high-risk situation. This time Louise chose the situation in which she is in contact with her colleagues (i.e., meetings, courses and discussions). At the cognitive level, she completed the triple-column technique to work on her fear of being judged and of stammering in front of people whom she considers have a better vocabulary. At the sensorimotor and behavioral levels, she decided to do the relaxation exercises before presenting in front of her colleagues. She then had to concentrate on what was happening outside of her as much as possible instead of focusing too much on her physical sensations. Finally, she had to make sure that she did not move or gesticulate needlessly.

Session 12 Louise had a more stressful week because of a family situation. Despite that, she had few tics, but those she had were more intense. The tics were mostly at the neck level, the others having disappeared completely. She noticed that her tics had disappeared in the low-risk situations. However, the high-risk situations that remain difficult were those in which she had to concentrate on a task. We thus talked about the importance of doing the "prevention by relaxation" technique before entering the situation and repeating it regularly during the task. In spite of that, she still considered that her tics had decreased by about 60% at work. We addressed the last high-risk situation: in the car, on the passenger side. Since Louise rapidly generalized the suggested exercises to all her tics and to all high-risk situations, she had, in fact, been working on this situation for some time. Thus, we only covered the strategies briefly. She confronted the belief that she must be vigilant and monitor the driver's driving. She relaxed her muscles when in the car or just before, and remained calm with feedback from the contact of resting her shoulders on the back of the car seat, and placing her hands on her knees. Finally, she decided to concentrate on the road ahead and/or on the conversation she was having with the driver.

Session 13   Louise had experienced no tics in the previous week, but still felt some tension in her jaw. This meeting was centered completely on reviewing the strategies and relapse prevention, especially in high-risk situations.

Session 14   We summarized our weekly meetings during this session. The tension in her jaw was less constant and less intense. She considered that her tics had diminished by 90%. The situations in which she was interacting with her colleagues or in which she had to make an intellectual effort remained at risk. In all the other situations, she only occasionally experienced tics.

Telephone follow-ups   The four weekly telephone follow-ups over the month of home practice showed that the gains were sustained. During the first two weeks, Louise reported her remaining tics had now leveled out, and were not diminishing as quickly as before. On the third week, however, she noticed that she was progressing again. The strategies she used most were: awareness, breathing and prevention by relaxation, and confronting stressful thinking. Despite a stressful situation in her family, Louise's progress was sustained. She noticed that if she did not put herself in a "tension mode" when she had a problem, her tics were almost non-existent, but she was also aware that she had to continue her work.

Session 19 (post-treatment)   Louise reported that she had tics, only rarely, in stressful moments when she was very tired. She felt that the efforts she had to make were not as great as when she started the program, although they were still quite demanding. She rated her global improvement at about 90%.

Comments

Louise showed exemplary motivation during the whole program. It was clear that she had already started some work on her style of action before coming to the Center. The program implementation has thus been greatly facilitated. For example, she already knew the progressive muscular relaxation technique. Moreover, she had already identified and worked on her action style for many years now. One of her main difficulties was to deal with the fact that her tics kept moving from one place to another over the weeks. However, because of her motivation, she managed to maintain a sustained effort and to address one obstacle at a time.

Her score at the Tourette's Syndrome Global Scale (TSGS) went from 15 (at pre-treatment) to 3 (at post-treatment).

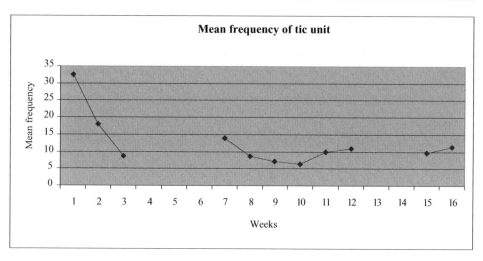

Figure 6.5   Case No. 1118

► Case No. 1118 (Figure 6.5)

Personal History

André is a 20-year-old man. He lives with a room-mate and studies full time. He has been diagnosed with Tourette's syndrome since he was nine. Since then, he has been taking medication to control his symptoms. His tics consist of abrupt and rapid back and forth head movements. He touches objects, hits the table or the walls and stretches his right arm to touch, with his little finger, the walls or people. He also presents some nail biting and some skin scratching. Finally, he suffers from vocal tics: throat clearing, echolalia, coprolalia and screams. André says that rarely can he spend a day without any tic and that his room-mate mentions that he can do many tics in a single minute. André realizes that his tics tend to increase when he is tired and to diminish when he is very focused on a task.

André's tics interfere greatly with all aspects of his family, social and school life. He says that he is bothered by his tics because he fears being unable to meet a girlfriend and to make new friends. Thus, he has a tendency to isolate himself and only to frequent people that he knows well. He uses techniques to camouflage his tics. For example, he puts his hand in his pocket, he clenches his fist or he crosses his arms to avoid touching others or hitting the walls. He bites his lips or tries to think about something else to avoid blurting out a word or repeating what just been said. It is important to note the fact that André also suffers from obsessive-compulsive disorder (OCD) and hyperactivity. However, these symptoms seem well controlled by medication.

Evaluation and Self-observation Stages

Session 1   The first therapy session is entirely devoted to the evaluation of the presenting problem and to establish a first contact. During that meeting, André has many tics (head jerks and echolalia). He identifies them one by one and ranks them going from the least disturbing to the most disturbing. He chooses to give priority to his tic of touching objects and people, even although his head tic is the most disturbing (because it leads to significant pain in his neck). Actually, he knows that this tic can bother people around him and it makes him uncomfortable and shy. He says that he doesn't feel any premonitory sign or sensation before the tic occurs. André seems very motivated to start the program and agrees to monitor the tic unit throughout the day.

Session 2   André says that he had great difficulty with the initial self-observation exercise because he is rarely aware of his tics. Thus, we establish that he will start his self-observation only when he is at home. It will then be easier for him to divide his attention. Moreover, he identifies the muscles implicated in his tic: the tension goes through his neck, towards his arms, his forearms, his hand and his fingers. The cognitive-behavioral model is explained. André is surprised to know that tension is provoking the occurrence of a tic. He feels that the model applies to him, especially in regards to the increasing muscular tension prior to onset. As he pays more attention to the tic, he notices that his tics are provoked when he is under a lot of tension. André lists the situations in which the probability of the tic occurrence is high: when his room-mate seems annoyed, when he moves a lot or when he asks him a lot of questions at the same time, in the metro, in the classroom or when he studies. André also notices that that the tics mostly occur when he is angry, nervous or tired. Finally, he mentions situations in which the probability of the tic occurrence is low: when he sleeps, when he takes a walk, when he is doing sports, when he is talking to a pleasant person and when talking to a person one on one.

Session 3   André found it easier to observe his tic over the previous week using the daily diary. Actually, he noticed that he only touches people with whom he feels at ease. While going over the model, he understands well that he has to learn to release tension in another way, but remains skeptical as to the efficacy of tolerating the sensorimotor urge to do the tic. He fears that the urge will increase to the point where he will burst out in a fit of anger. The Kelly construct grid allowed us to confirm that the following aspects were associated with the tic occurrence: tiredness, preoccupations, lack of self-confidence, fear of being judged, anger and nervousness. The constructs were elicited on the basis of three low-risk situations (talking to a nice friend, doing some sports and taking a walk) and three high-risk situations (studying, being in a course and being with his room-mate).

Session 4   André continued his self-observation and even took down some notes while he was in class. He says that he is becoming more aware of the occurrence of his tic and, since then, notices that he does it a bit less. The rest of the meeting was then devoted to the video. André chose to read a schoolbook as his high-risk situation. He performed one tic repeatedly: the head movement.

Intervention Stage

Session 5   The goal of this session was to introduce the discrimination exercises. The rationale behind the exercise is explained to André. He was motivated to see if he will be able to recognize the different levels of tension in the muscles implicated in the tic. However, he has doubts because he says that the tic can occur without warning. The biofeedback machine allows André to acknowledge that even when he tries to stay as calm and still as possible, the tension level is still very high in his tic-affected muscle. After establishing the baseline, André starts to contract and release the muscle. He has some difficulty to avoid doing abrupt movements. He gets discouraged easily and gets upset for not being able to get it right at the first attempt. He then does some exercises with another muscle that is not implicated in the tic to establish that he is capable of using the machine. We also address the fact that the muscles implicated in the tic have lost a lot of their flexibility and he will have to do the discrimination exercises many times before seeing any changes. He thus restarts the exercises with the muscles implicated in the tic. After a few attempts, he already notices that it is easier to contract the muscle gradually. Even though releasing the muscle remains difficult, he will continue to do the exercises over the next week.

Session 6   André has practiced the discrimination exercises every day. He says that he now detects more easily the different levels of tension. In order to encourage him, the exercises are repeated using the biofeedback machine. He is very proud to see that the tension is not as high compared to the baseline and that contractions–relaxations are done more gradually. The remainder of the session was devoted to the deep breathing and muscular relaxation exercises. André performed the exercises seriously and diligently. Once again, slowly releasing the tension of each muscle is what he found to be the most difficult. At the end of the session, he felt very relaxed and noticed that he had not experienced many tics during our meeting.

Session 7   André did the breathing and relaxation exercises every night before going to bed. He says that this helped him to fall asleep. In addition to moving on to the second stage of the muscular relation exercises, the response prevention by relaxation is explained. We establish that he has to keep his arm as relaxed as possible. He has to release the tension before entering a situation that he considers at risk. He will do the same immediately after the occurrence of the tic and when he feels an increase of tension in the muscles implicated in the tic. Because André still had difficulty in becoming aware of his tics, he had decided to use a visual prop to help him. Thus, he decided to stick some stars at certain places (in his agenda, on his fridge, on the table and on his desk) in order to remind him to check his level of tension. Finally, we discussed certain action styles associated with tic occurrence. In his case, André pointed out that he found it difficult to stay calm, to organize himself and to concentrate. He also said that he is disorganized, impulsive and quick-tempered. He noticed that when he had many repetitive and intense tics, he was usually in one of those states.

Session 8   André had some difficulty using the prevention by relaxation technique, because he had the impression that his muscles were never completely relaxed. Hence, the discrimination exercises were repeated to enable him to gauge again the different levels of tension. He decided to practice discrimination twice each day over the next week in addition to moving to Stage 3 of the relaxation exercises. To help him, it was decided that, initially, he would apply prevention by relaxation only in the low-risk situations. On the other hand, André noticed that it was sometimes his thoughts that were inducing the tics. For example, when somebody irritated him, he had thoughts of insulting this person and of blurting out some vulgar words. He then got so angry that he became very tense. The increase in tension in his whole body resulted in motor and vocal tics. In such cases, it was only after performing a series of tics that he felt he could calm down. Thus, these beliefs were addressed using the triple-column technique. We went over some examples with some thoughts that he had during a conflict with his room-mate. In reviewing the conflict, André had many thoughts about the injustice of his room-mate's remarks which led him to aggressive thoughts. But in looking at the situation objectively, he saw that the room-mate's reaction might have been reasonable and could have been resolved by compromise. He realized that if he had calmed down by taking some deep breaths and by applying the triple-column technique, not only would he have avoided doing that many tics, but might also have found a solution to the conflict.

Session 9   André felt more in control of his tics over the previous week. He carried out all of the recommended exercises. He was better able to discriminate between the different levels of tension and he continued to do the exercises. However, he noticed that although he sometimes was able to identify the increasing tension in his muscles, the urge to do the tic in order to feel "relieved" was still intense. We discuss the importance of tolerating this sensorimotor urge in addition to releasing the superfluous tension by other means (e.g., relaxation). The more he succeeded in tolerating this urge, the less intense it became. He also used the triple-column technique during two conflictual situations and felt more competent to deal with conflict by confronting his thoughts about the situation.

Other cognitive, emotional, sensorimotor or behavioral aspects associated with the three high-risk situations were identified. André said that when he studies, he anticipates the amount of time it will take and fears being unable to understand or will make mistakes. During those study periods at home, he often becomes frustrated and stressed. He then has the habit of tensing his body and hitting the table. When his room-mate asks him many questions at the same time or is agitated, André also has motor tics and swears. Once again, the emotions that surface are anger and stress. He also feels guilty because of his thoughts. He then moves around with no purpose, gets up and gets worked up. In his courses, he anticipates not knowing the answers, being slower than other students or not having good marks. He then becomes frustrated and stressed. He remains seated, but tics or fidgets on his seat.

Session 10   André's motivation was really greatly affected this week by the remarks of another mental health practitioner. He told André that it was impossible to diminish tics with an approach like the one used in the program. André feels discouraged, having invested so much effort into it. In order to put the comment made by the practitioner into perspective, André lists the pros and cons of pursuing the program. He comes to the conclusion that the cons are null, except for the effort to invest, and the benefits can be considerable if he commits himself. He decides to pursue the program because he feels that his tics have diminished about 60% in the low-risk situations and those in which he doesn't feel intense emotions.

Before pursuing the session's main objective, we do a cognitive restructuration exercise of a conflict with his room-mate. André is happy with the result and is even eager to solve this situation. Afterwards, we start working on the high-risk situations. The first one that André chooses is when he is in the classroom. He then targets all the aspects that can increase the probability of the tic occurrence. On the cognitive level, he does a cognitive restructuration exercise to confront his fear of being slower than others. He decides to use the triple-column technique as often as he might need it, especially if he is experiencing strong emotions. On the sensorimotor and behavioral levels, he decides to make sure he relaxes his muscles before entering the classroom. Moreover, he will try to verify his general tension level as often as possible during the course. In order to help himself, he will use visual props. Thus, if he feels some tension, he will try to relax his muscles as much as possible. In terms of his posture, he will also have to make sure that he doesn't move without a reason.

Session 11   André integrates the model into his behavior, he adopts a posture more in line with his thinking, plus he tolerates the urge to do the tic more and more. André estimates that his tics diminish by 25% when he is in class. We address a second high-risk situation. This time, André chooses his study sessions. On the cognitive level, he applies the triple-column technique to work on his fear of running out of time and of not being able to succeed at the first attempt. When he has moments where he feels discouraged, he realizes that he will have to take some time to calm himself and to use the cognitive restructuration remedy instead of becoming upset. On the sensorimotor and behavioral levels, André decides to do the relaxation exercises before studying. He then has to regularly monitor the state of tension in his muscles. Finally, he has to make sure that he monitors himself to prevent automatic movement or restlessness for no reason.

Session 12   André is aware that he is progressing, but still finds it hard to control his tics when he feels strong emotions. In spite of that, he considers that his tics have diminished by about 25% when he studies. We address the last high-risk situation: during conflicts or possibility of conflicts with his room-mate. André anticipates that this situation will be very difficult to work on because the conflicts have increased recently. We start by doing some problem solving to see if it is possible to decrease the stress in the environment. André comes up with many solutions. He also knows that he has to remain as calm as possible, to work on his thoughts with the triple-column technique and to say what he thinks without aggressiveness.

Session 13   André considers that his tics have diminished by 30% during the conflictual situations and is very proud of this result. His own efforts to decrease conflicts with his room-mate have contributed. He notices, however, that although his vocal tics and his tic of touching others have diminished, his head tics are still present. Thus, we try to do some generalization by going over all the techniques, and how they might apply to the remaining tics.

Session 14   An overview of the progress is made in this last session. André is very happy with the progress he made even if there is still some work that remains to be done. In order to help him to integrate the model and all the techniques, we make an *aide-mémoire* of the techniques and he will keep that with him wherever he goes.

Telephone follow-ups   During the four weekly telephone follow-ups, André said that his tics were still diminishing. He was continually using the "breathing and relaxation", the "prevention by relaxation" and the "triple-column" techniques. During the last follow-up, André said that his head tic had also started to diminish.

Session 19 (post-treatment)   André is very satisfied with the therapy, because he feels that he has improved by about 60%. He knows that he will have to pursue his efforts and to continue to monitor his emotions (anger, irritation and stress).

Comments

The main difficulty for André lay in the frequency, intensity and presence of many different tics. He could have become discouraged because we had decided to only work on one of his tics, but his motivation helped him to complete the therapy. Actually, he even managed to generalize his gains to his other tics at the end of the therapy. In addition to diminishing the frequency of his tics, the program also had an effect on his self-esteem. Despite the many pitfalls he had to face in life, he felt optimistic at succeeding, and this sentiment was encouraged by the fact that he felt he was now able to control his tics.

His score on the Tourette's Syndrome Global Scale (TSGS) reduced from 69 (pretreatment) to 22.5 (post-treatment).

Chapter 7

CLIENT MANUAL

▶ INTRODUCTION: WHO IS THE MANUAL FOR?

The manual covers the complete range of tics: motor, vocal and mental tics. It also applies to other complex repetitive movements termed "habit disorders", the most common of which are hair pulling, nail biting, scratching, teeth grinding, skin picking and neck or knuckle cracking. These are repetitive movements that are often associated with a stimulus, situation, activity or mood which can be very distressing and self-mutilating and may result in serious destruction to tissues.

A distinction has to be made between manual play (or twiddles) and tic habits. A manual twiddle or twirl could be any repetitive movement to idle away time, such as twirling a paper clip or twiddling fingers on the table. A vocal twirl could include whistling or smacking the lips. These may or may not serve the same function as tics but they are easily controlled by noticing and stopping them. Tic and habit disorders cannot be controlled so easily and can cause severe distress and impairment in function.

▶ ABOUT TICS

▶ Definition of Tics

Tics are defined as repetitive non-voluntary contractions of functionally related groups of skeletal muscles in one or more parts of the body. Tics occur over all cultures, and have been reported anecdotally since classical times. Currently, the fourth (revised) edition of the *Diagnostic Statistical Manual of Mental Disorders* (DSM-IV; American Psychiatric Association, 1994) distinguishes transitory tics from chronic tic disorders (TD) and Gilles de la Tourette's syndrome (TS). In TD, one or several motor or phonic tics occur daily or intermittently for at least one year and appear before age 18. TS is recognized in the DSM-IV as a separate diagnostic category with multiple tics including vocal (phonic) tics occurring several times per day, appearing before age 18, and causing marked distress.

Cognitive-Behavioral Management of Tic Disorders by K. O'Connor.
Copyright © 2005 John Wiley & Sons, Ltd.

► Simple Tics

Tics may be simple or complex. Simple tics include blinking, cheek twitches, head or knee jerks and shoulder shrugs. Tics are mainly confined to the upper body and the most common occur in the eye, head, shoulders and face. Tics can also be vocal and include coughs, tongue clacking, sniffing, throat clearing, hiccing, barking and growling. Some recurrent involuntary somatic sensations are classified as sensory tics. These are identified as heavy, light, warm or tingling premonitory sensations, often muscle focused, leading to muscle tension.

There are also mental tics which take the form of playful or stimulating thoughts or scenes turned over in the mind. A premonitory urge frequently precedes a motor tic. The premonitory urge can be identified with one or several cognitive and physiological states and may take the form of an anticipation, a tension or other feeling. Motor, mental and phonic tics can also occur in the absence of a discrete premonitory urge.

► Complex Tics

Tics are classified as complex if there is a contraction in more than one group of muscles. Complex tics may involve sequences of movements, and may take the form of bizarre mannerisms involving limbs, head or extremities. Some complex tics can look like maladaptive normal responses. They may exaggerate a normal action, or include a redundant aspect in a normal action, for example, by involving an irrelevant body part (e.g., turning the head whilst extending the arm). Complex tics may take the form of self-inflicted repetitive injurious mannerisms such as head slapping, face scratching, tense–release hand gripping cycles, or dystonic postures. Complex vocal or, more precisely, phonic tics take the form of repeated sounds, words or phrases or swear words and, in rare cases, swearing (coprolalia). Normal actions and words of the person may also be repeated, and copying others can itself evolve into a complex repetitive movement either by motor mimicry (echopraxia) or by repeating others' words, phrases or sounds (echolalia). Complex tics can resemble habit disorders (HD) such as hair pulling (trichotillomania), teeth grinding (bruxism), skin scratching or picking (scabiomania), and nail biting (onychophagia), which are, however, classified among the impulse control disorders. Sometimes people with tics also suffer from different types of HD. Examples of tics in different parts of the body are given in Table 1.1 p. 3.

► Habit Disorder

HD is a term covering a variety of destructive impulsive habits including: trichotillomania (hair pulling), bruxism (teeth grinding), onychophagia (nail biting) and scabiomania (skin scratching or picking). Both TD and HD can be preceded by premonitory sensory urges rather than obsessional thoughts, and respond to distinct pharmacological and behavioral interventions. There are similarities between

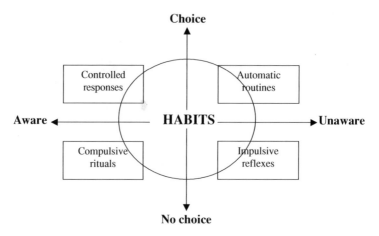

Figure 7.1   Reflexes, routines, rituals and responses

the two disorders in the tension–release cycle of motor action, and in a similar beneficial response to behavioral treatments. Tics and habits have, together, been classified as nervous habits, and although, in both cases, emotions associated with the onset of the habits seem more related to frustration, dissatisfaction and tension, they may sometimes be associated with more complex mood, such as depression.

Technically speaking, complex TD and HD are distinguishable from stereotypies and compulsive rituals, routines and habits, since tics are neither completely conscious purposeful rituals nor totally nonsensical repetitions. In fact, the term "behavioral stereotypy" is usually applied to abnormal rhythmic actions associated with organic loss and mental deficiency. In practice, however, it is sometimes difficult to distinguish tics, rituals and repetitive movements. The diagram in Figure 7.1 illustrates the distinction between habits, tics and routines, in terms of two crucial dimensions of *awareness* and volitional *control*. In normal automated routines, there may be little awareness but there is overall volitional control. In rituals, there may be awareness but no control. In reflexes and tics, there may be neither awareness nor control (see Figure 7.1).

▶ Secondary Distress

Tics are seldom life-threatening except in rare cases where they may provoke automutilation. Psychosocial distress, however, in this group can be considerable and can involve secondary phobias, depressions and social anxieties and worries over self-image, very low self-esteem and relationship problems. In our estimation of the interference of TD and HD in daily activities, we found problems ranging from unemployment, marital conflict, interpersonal difficulties, employer relations, travel restrictions, problems attending social or public functions, performance worries (e.g., about driving, speaking, teaching, dancing, sport), all of which were perceived (by the affected person) to be a result of the tic habit. Such problems multiply for those with multiple tics, as has been documented by the Tourette association (in literature available from Tourette's Association). People with tics often experience low self-esteem and are (or become) hyperattentive to the judgment of others, with consequent low self-satisfaction. Ironically, the very anticipation of experiencing a negative self-evaluation can provoke the tic.

You might now like to fill in the questionnaires given in Appendix 1b to see how your tic impacts on different aspects of your daily life.

► How Many People Have Tics?

The incidence of TS in adults is about 0.1–1%. The lifetime prevalence of TD is not known but estimates vary between 5 and 10% of the population. Other recent estimates have placed the prevalence of TS at 1% and TD at 10% of the population.

► Are Tics Associated with Other Disorders?

Tics occur together with attention deficit hyperactivity disorder (ADHD) in about 20% of children. Adults with tics frequently have another type of HD. About 25–63% of people with tics also suffer from obsessive-compulsive disorder (OCD), and about 17% of adults with OCD also experience tics. There is no evidence that people with tics are more likely than others to suffer severe mental disorder.

► Rationale for Tic Treatment Program

The program has been developed and tested over a number of years at the Fernand-Seguin Research Centre in Montreal, Quebec. It is a behavioral program, which means that we aim to regulate your tic by asking you to complete behavioral exercises. The reason we consider this useful is because we see tics as behavioral habits.

As you will discover over the course of the program, although tics seem like reflexes, they can be viewed as over-learned responses, sometimes developing from normal responses learned a long time ago or tied by association to what you do at present. The aim is for you to unlearn these behaviors step by step and discover how your habitual way of thinking and acting influence your tension level and maintain the tic habit.

The program is organized into 10 separate stages and takes 14 weeks to complete, together with a month's further home practice. Although the program can be self-administered, better results are obtained when used in conjunction with a professional trained in cognitive-behavioral therapy (CBT) who should be available through local professional organizations. The program is planned and streamlined for maximum effect, and as each step is very important, you must not skip any stages or sessions. You may feel at the beginning that a lot of time is invested in evaluating your tic. For example, we ask you to fill in forms and to monitor your tic by observation – if possible by video and by a daily diary. These exercises, also called "awareness training", are an *essential* first step to controlling your tic. Do not feel you are wasting your time doing these exercises or that they are just a chore and are not the real therapy. In fact, establishing the patterns of behavior against which your tic takes place is crucial to develop an idiosyncratic profile of your behavior, your tic, your emotions, and all aspects of your activities that can create tension. As we point out in a later exercise, thoughts, especially anticipations, can have a considerable impact on behavior, tension level and emotions, and therefore on the tic habit.

Another important reason for awareness training is that, in our model, we place a lot of emphasis on preventing the tic occurrence. In effect, this means becoming aware of several processes preceding tic onset, processes even as distant as lifestyle and ways of planning and preparing actions. These are processes that you can only identify through monitoring them yourself since they are peculiar to you. In many ways, through the course of the therapy, you will become your own expert on your own tic problem and your own behavior. Unlike other types of therapy, behavioral approaches encourage autonomy of the client, not dependency. We want you to feel empowered enough at the end of therapy to control the tic by yourself. This is also your greatest insurance about relapse prevention. If you think of other skills you have mastered in life, such as cooking or swimming, you will note that these skills very seldom leave you since they have become automatic. Our research shows that once people have mastered the strategies in the program and achieved the crucial goal of reducing all sources of unnecessary nervous tension, relapse is very unlikely, and actually improvement can continue after therapy in other related behavioral areas.

▶ What Is a Habit?

A habit is defined for our purposes as an automatic action or sequence of actions that cannot be consciously controlled but involve muscles that are otherwise under voluntary control. Facial muscles are usually under our control but, in the case of an involuntary tic, the cheek and corner of the mouth may twitch uncontrollably. Shoulder muscles are usually at our command to contract or relax as we wish, but when tension develops, muscles may react despite our wishes. Fingers are usually under our finely controlled command, but where we find them playing with our hair or rubbing together involuntarily, they seem to have a will of their own. In this way, habits lie somewhere in the middle of response preferences, reflexes and compulsions, but are not identifiable as any one category, as is illustrated in Figure 7.1. A compulsive ritual is a sequence of actions that are performed consciously by the person, purposefully to achieve a goal or to gratify a need, even though the person may not like what he or she is doing but has no control over the action. A reflex generally occurs in muscles termed "smooth muscles" which are never under conscious control. A preference is clearly where there is a choice of action, and is a voluntary action directed towards gratifying a need. Actually there is a relationship between the four types of movement listed in Figure 7.1, and habits are often a mix of these four types. Habits can be preferences or routines and may include both rituals and reflexes, but in this manual, we are excluding rituals which are termed obsessive-compulsive behaviors and problems resulting from abnormal biological drives.

▶ Who Develops Habits?

Everybody, including psychologists, which is just as well since habits are essential to our lives. Unless we had the capacity to develop some automatic strategies, we would not be able to perform any of the complicated skills necessary to life. Every action has an automated component. Imagine trying to drive a car while paying attention to every individual movement of gear stick, wheel or brake. Automated subroutines that allow your hands, eyes or legs to get on with complex actions by themselves are very useful. The ensemble of habitual ways we do things make up our style of life, and are part and parcel of our personality. We all have our own ways of eating, talking, laughing - it's part of being human. The problems arise when an automated action outstays its welcome, or gets into the wrong sequence, or is unhelpful, or conflicts with another subroutine, or was never properly mastered in the first place.

Frequently, habits get left over from some past reaction, or develop peripheral to the main action we wish to perform. They are superfluous and unhelpful, but we are not always conscious of it.

▶ What about Nervous Habits?

As we said, everybody has habits and they help us to function but it is obvious that some habits are not serving any purpose and seem out of place with the rest of us. People term these their "nervous habits", but this is really not a correct description. It is probably correct to say that the habit is more likely to appear when the person is stressed or nervous, but it may also appear when the person is tired or fatigued because at times of stress or fatigue we tend to fall back on automatic (unthinking) patterns of responding. In fact, many habits disappear when people are aroused and occupied, but reappear when they are relaxing or not doing anything in particular. However, it is possible that the nervous habit once served a function. Frequently, habits get left over from past reactions or become superfluous to the main action we are performing. We may not even be conscious of doing them. Sometimes these "nervous habits" are normal reactions that were never learned properly. But often the habits have developed independently of their original usage and have now taken on a life of their own, perhaps becoming more of a nuisance in the process. Some tics do have a neurological origin and are not related to behavior, but unless you have a diagnosable neurological disease, it is more than likely that your habit forms part of a learned skillful response, perhaps a part that persisted or developed while the rest of the habit ceased to be useful.

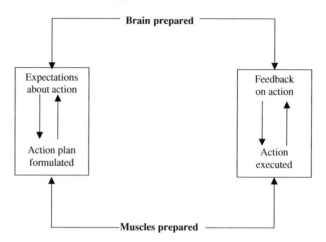

Figure 7.2   Flow of movement organization. The elements in boxes determine how the brain and muscles respond

► When Do Habits Develop?

As soon as we are born, and maybe even before that, we start to develop complex movement patterns. Some basic building blocks are pre-programmed in the infant, in particular, reflexes like blinking and some basic movements like reaching, grabbing and staring. But all the actions we recognize as a repertoire develop gradually through interaction with the environment. Through various feedback operations between muscle and brain, action plans are installed and, when initiated, activate certain muscles to perform the job. When the job is completed, the message gets back to the brain and the action plan is cancelled or develops into another program (see Figure 7.2). The first few years of life are a fruitful period for development, since the muscles are plastic and much tuned to developing new connections into maturity. Unfortunately, the other side of the coin is that many of our habits develop during childhood when we lack sophisticated coordination. As a consequence, the child's response to, say, traumatic events often engages much more of the body than would an adult's more mature response. A young child, for example, pays attention with the whole of the body, not just the eyes. In other words, the child's system over-responds. There is also a tendency for the child to generalize actions to situations that are emotionally similar but substantively different. For example, a child told to sit still in a certain way for a certain occasion may generalize this over all occasions where sitting is involved. Many of our redundant habits develop from childhood even though they go through changes in the meantime. We should also emphasize that habits are not only about moving, but also about inhibiting movement. Doing one thing, of course, always means not doing something else. Habits develop as ways of stopping, as well as ways of executing, movements. For example, some people have developed the habit of holding their breath when under stress.

▶ You Are Not Alone

Make a list of your unwanted habits. About 1% of the population have unwanted tics. If we include repetitive movements, it's about 20%, and if we expand unwanted habits to include awkward posture and unwanted tension, this figure rises. So an unwanted movement habit, in one sense, is not unusual. One of the most distressing aspects of any problem is feeling that you're the only one who suffers from it and that everyone else is different from you. This is particularly so if you have a severe tic and you think that everyone looks at you. You might find you avoid certain situations where you feel vulnerable. However, in a way all movement habits, including tics, are related to tension. So, whatever your problem, you're in good company – and similar approaches can help all tics and movement habits.

In fact, studies and clinical work suggest that people with tics in general are no more likely than anyone else to have severe psychiatric problems. However, they do have certain habitual styles of action. Of course, having a tic may itself cause psychological distress.

▶ A COGNITIVE-BEHAVIORAL MANAGEMENT APPROACH TO CHANGING HABITS

The phrase cognitive-behavioral management of tics may be the most appropriate to apply to our approach to the control of tics and movements, since it is by managing aspects of our behavior, including thoughts and actions, that we can facilitate or impede the movement we wish to change. We control much of our involuntary physiology in this indirect way. We adopt a certain posture or have a certain expectation and this makes it more likely that a involuntary reflex can occur. When the reflex occurs, it seems to us as though we had little control over it, but in some way we ourselves managed the set-up. Next time you're waiting for your kettle to boil, try to intently anticipate the whistle or click-off. Focus on the muscles that are tense. How do you react to the boil? Now contrast this reaction with your reaction when you are not anticipating the boil. The way we habitually approach a situation in body and mind can often determine our later "involuntary" responses to it. So, in this manual we include exercises aimed at directly changing muscle activity but we also pay a great deal of attention to managing the background behavior, against which tension, movement and tics occur.

▶ Avoiding Coping Strategies that Maintain Old Habits (False Friends)

People with tics and tensions often develop strategies to suppress or disguise their problem. These seem to help for the moment but do not help in the long run.

Example, a patient with a chronic neck tension, leading to a slight tremor of the head, adopted the strategy of moving his arms and shoulders when speaking to hide the tremor. In fact, when he stopped doing this during conversation, the tremor was worse. When he just kept still, the tremor was better, all the moving about produced tension.

Other people react to tics and movements by tensing up everywhere to resist and block the movement – so creating more tension, or they try to hold their movements in, even more. Other more general strategies are to avoid certain situations, so creating even more anticipatory anxiety when the situation occurs. Sometimes, there is the problem of substitution. As a result of tensing, some people find that the "urge" to do the habit remains even if this does not result in an overt tic, and if they do not tic, that it is replaced by another tic. The "urge" in this case is preparatory tension, which has not been relaxed enough. One client who had control over a nose tic found she would close her eyes forcefully if she didn't do the nose tic, since the tension still needed to be relieved. Here the problem for her was a raised level of preparatory tension that still required a tic response. Appendix 1h lists some of these coping strategies. **Perhaps you can add some more of your own**.

▶ Habits Are Active

People tend to view tic habits as annoying baggage that comes along independently and interferes with their flow of action. In fact, as we have pointed out, several habits have their origins in an active movement initiated in the past but which has outstayed its welcome or lost its purpose. Any movement, even an involuntary tic, requires active preparation on your behalf before it can occur. *In fact, muscle tension is active preparation to do something, and that's all it is.* It may be a surprise for you to realize, but you are always actively involved in your tensions and movement and actively maintaining, or at least nurturing, your tic habit. Of course, this nurturing is indirect and you are not aware of it, and even if you were aware, you couldn't just control it by saying "stop". Your problem is the result of a whole series of embedded interlocking maneuvers involving your style of planning and anticipating action, and also your emotional responses. Another aspect about the "alive-ness" of tics and movements and tensions is that they are always developing in new ways, and changing in variations of themselves over time and according to the activity you are performing. You will notice this more when we come to the section on self-observation.

An exercise that will help you to imagine your problem in a more active light is to try to think of a situation in which your problem *would be* an appropriate and relevant response. Imagine that the mime artist Marcel Marceau is doing your tic action and you have to fit a relevant physical context around it. Supposing you have a blink tic, in what context would it be appropriate to blink strongly and repetitively – perhaps if you had something in your eye – or were trying to protect yourself from intrusion? Or if you have a tension in your shoulders, when would it be appropriate to tense your shoulders in that manner? Perhaps it would be appropriate if you expected a heavy weight to be put on you.

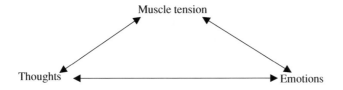

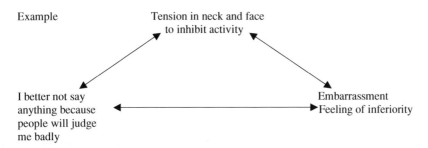

Figure 7.3   Triple link between thoughts, emotions and actions
Note: The triple link is reciprocal in all directions since tension can also produce thoughts and emotions.

The client we mentioned earlier, who had a small head tremor that was produced by a chronic contraction of the back, neck and jaw muscles, recalled that he had adopted a similar posture in school when in the class of a master who was in the habit of slapping boys unexpectedly about the face. His head was held ready to resist a slap coming from any direction.

However, the aim of the exercises is *not* to discover or link a past context to your action. By using your imagination, you will view your problem in terms of an active preparation and this will give you a more active perspective. This will help us when we plan "active" management of the problem. You may gain other insights into your movement from the exercise that help your understanding, for example, you may realize that it is an exaggeration of a normal response or that it is an old response that has persisted. Perhaps your tension has no meaning at all, but nevertheless, by doing this exercise, you can see how muscles can be used to prepare for some expected reaction (Figure 7.3).

► The Tic as a Habit

Tics are muscle or vocal or mental habits which temporarily reduce tension (see Figures 1.1 and 7.5). They are over-learned so they have become automated and reflex-like, and occur involuntarily. Tics, of course, don't feel like habits, they feel more like involuntary reflexes, and, indeed, they are like uncontrollable reflexes when they occur. But tics occur as a result of tension, and tension can develop as a habit. What is the evidence that tics are acquired habits? (1) They occur only in certain parts of the body, not everywhere. (2) They are worse in some situations

(a) A high level of tension makes the tic more likely to appear
at a low level; the muscle is below the tic threshold because it is more relaxed

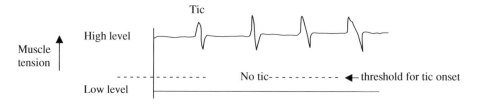

(b) Treatment program addresses processes preceding the apparently isolated tic onset

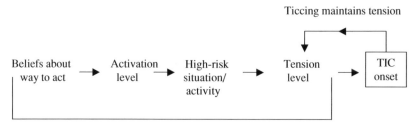

Figure 7.4   Model of processes preceding tic onset

than in others. (3) They form part of a tension–release cycle and so serve a function like all habits, and you feel better temporarily if you tic. (4) Tics are linked to background muscle tension and activity which, in turn, is linked to the habitual way you behave. Typically, after you have ticced or performed your habit, you feel temporarily relieved; but not for long, because unfortunately in ticcing you have maintained your already high tension level. You are caught in a perpetual tension–release cycle whereby high tension produces the urge to tic and the tic itself maintains the tension (see Figure 7.4[a]). Other strategies you use to keep in or hide the tic or habit (see Appendix 1h) also produce tension, and so maintain the vicious cycle. Obviously, we need to break the tension–release habit cycle by learning a less tension-producing way of acting.

► OVERVIEW OF TIC MANAGEMENT MODEL

► Learning a New Habit

The model we adopt on this program is a learning model. Essentially, this means that you can learn to control your tic by learning strategies to control your behavior. A learning method is different from taking a pill or having a surgical intervention. Learning is a process you are actively involved in and, of course, learning takes time, step by step practice, and you can have good days and bad days. Each step is important and, as you go along the steps, your learning will accumulate until you feel more confident and in control. In order for learning to take place, you must be an active collaborator. In effect, you are the most important element in the process. If you are not motivated, not practicing or otherwise impeded from following the program, it will not succeed. This doesn't mean that you need to bring anything extraordinary to your participation. All that is necessary at the beginning is that you have an open and willing attitude and that you follow the exercises. The exercises will always be fitted to your ability and we progress at your rhythm, so you will always be able to follow the exercises.

► Our Treatment Approach

You will notice that our model puts a lot of emphasis on controlling the tic by preventing its occurrence. We see the tic as an end result of a series of behaviors that have become habitual ways of acting, and our studies suggest that it is by changing these ways of acting that we can best control the tic onset. This is different to the strategies you currently employ to control your tic. The strategies you use currently consist of trying to resist or hide the appearance of the tic once it has recurred and lead to more stress and tension. Such tension-producing strategies are listed in Appendix 1h. On the contrary, in our program, controlling the tic means staying calm and preventing its occurrence. It does not mean resisting or fighting the tic.

As you can see in Figure 7.4(b), although tics appear to come out of nowhere, the real control of the tic starts way before its onset. It starts with the style of acting you adopt when planning activities. It progresses through the way muscle tension mounts, and the specific way in which you anticipate and prepare for certain reactions and situations. When we are talking about controlling behavior, we include all aspects of behavior. This means thoughts, emotions, as well as actions. These are all important components of behavior.

There are several elements of the program that you may find difficult at first to accept. The most difficult to accept may be the psychological element of the program. However, from a habit point of view, this is the most important part of understanding tic behavior. You will discover that your tics are worse in some situations and activities than in others, and this situational profile tells us a lot about the way you prepare for tic-related versus tic-unrelated situations. Part of how you respond in a situation depends on how you evaluate the situation. Do you see it as boring, fulfilling, anxiogenic? Some of these evaluations do consistently relate to tic onset. For example, tics are often more likely when people are bored or dissatisfied. Often, the evaluations of a situation build on each other and together cumulatively produce tension. For example, seeing a situation at the same time as demanding, unpleasant and unfulfilling will produce more tension than just a demanding task. Another important psychological aspect is anticipation. Anticipating tic onset can produce it, like a self-fulfilling prophecy. This is often because when we anticipate something, we tend to actively prepare for it "as if" it has arrived. Some people with tics have a tendency to invest more than necessary in both their emotional and physical preparation. This excess preparation itself produces tension. Another tension-producing aspect is the tendency to try to attempt to do too much at once. People with tics can also be perfectionist, particularly when it comes to their own personal organization, standards and appearance. They tend to feel that they should be doing more than they are, and often more than is necessary or realistic. Sometimes, they feel they are lazy if they're not occupied. This over-active style of action, together with the tendency to invest too much, is important to address to help to reduce an accumulation of tension. Do you recognize yourself? **Please complete the questionnaire in Appendix 1c on tension level and Appendix 1e on style of planning action**.

► Our Model

Our essential model is given in Figures 7.4 and 7.5. Basically, your tic arrives because your level of muscle tension in your tic-affected muscle is at a higher than normal level of activation. Think of a guitar string that is stretched so tightly that it easily vibrates. Your level of muscle tension is such that it facilitates the tic. But if your level was lower, you wouldn't be emitting the same tic, just as the guitar string would not emit the same note if it was less taut. In other words, your tension sets you up to tic. A good comparison is to think of the knee jerk reflex evoked when you place one leg over the other and so create enough tension and freedom of movement that when you hit your knee muscle your leg swings up. But if your leg is placed on the ground or if you stretch it in front of you, there is no reflex action because the tendon muscle is not properly positioned. Various researches, including our own, have shown that tic-affected muscles are tenser and less flexible than other muscles. You may not be aware of the tension because it is so habitual. If you have a vocal tic, the tense muscle involved is the diaphragm and throat area. If

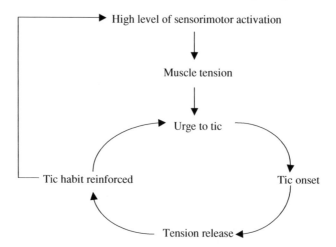

Figure 7.5 Tic tense–release cycle
Note: High background level of activation including chronic muscle tension level leads to the urge to tic which afterwards gives momentary release but reinforces the tic habit as means to regulate tension. The more frequent the tic, the higher the tension level, which in turn maintains the background high central and peripheral sensorimotor activation level.

you have a habit, such as hair pulling, nail biting, scratching or teeth grinding, the tense muscle may be the hand or arm or in the mouth, but the above principle and Figure 7.4 still apply. It may sound strange but, in fact, the way to control your tic is to put *less* effort into your behavior. Throughout the program we will be asking you to lift off or abandon old tension-producing thoughts and habits. The goal of the program is for you to learn a series of behavioral, thinking and physical exercises to reduce the tension and better control the tic. This does not mean you become a jello! It means we take the edge off your tension and activation levels enough for you to control the tic, and because you are less tense and more flexible in thought and action, you will, in fact, be more, not less, productive in your life.

The tension level in your tic-affected muscle is brought about by the way you behave and plan actions as well as the way you think and relate to events. In the program, we will be addressing all these elements to help you to control your activation and control your tics. The programme is divided into 10 stages over 14 weeks and covers three main training areas:

1. *Awareness training*, where you learn to be aware of and detect your tic. You may be surprised to know that your tic is worse in some situations than in others. Awareness is a key step in learning conscious control and making the tic less automatic, and this stage takes about four weeks to learn.
2. *Psychophysiological training*, which is the physical side of the program and involves training your tic-affected muscles to be more flexible. As you can see from Figure 7.4, the typical tension level of people with tics is artificially high, and there is not much flexibility in the tic-affected muscle. It is difficult to reduce this tension without special training. This training, with the help of special feedback equipment, helps you to control contraction in the muscle. You also learn how to reduce your overall tension level by relaxation exercises, which also take four weeks to learn.
3. Finally, in *behavioral training*, we look at how you approach and plan activities in high-risk tic situations and the strategies and beliefs that guide you to plan action in a tension-producing way.

We try to modify your approach in one activity at a time, until you adopt a less activating and more adaptive approach. We then give you advice on how to achieve or maintain your gains over your home practice period of four weeks. The therapist and the accompanying manual will describe each of these stages in more detail. Although the package is standard, it is also personally tailored to your individual problem. **We ask you to evaluate the progress of your treatment in the course of the program by completing forms and evaluations** (see Appendices 1a–1h). This continuous monitoring is also to your advantage since it guarantees quality control and fine adjustment of the program to your needs.

▶ Common Questions

What specific strategies do I use in the program?   You use different types of strategies, including: awareness, physiological exercises, learning to detect tension, planning action more flexibility. Other exercises involve thinking of the way you react and plan actions, and challenging some beliefs about how activities should be done. We also include behavioral strategies which involve doing things the opposite way to your normal habitual way, and letting go of some unhelpful behaviors.

But I already have some control of my tic.   Most of the exercises people use to *control* their tics are rather ways of *resisting*, containing or disguising the tic and lead generally to more tension (e.g., holding in tics, disguising them, delaying them) (see Appendix 1h). Genuine control means preventing tic onset by reducing tension, not creating more tension.

How do I learn to control my tics when I'm not even aware of their occurrence?   The first stage in the program is to make you more aware of your tics by monitoring them each day for a period of time. You may also record a video or use a mirror or close other to model your tic to enable you to observe your tic and become familiar with its form. Sometimes, just being aware of a problem behavior gives you more control.

So, if I become aware of my tic/habit, what next?   Part of being aware of your tic is to identify emotions and thoughts associated with tic onset. For example, tics are often associated with frustration and boredom. By knowing the behavior or feeling or thoughts associated with tics, we are able to address the background behavior-producing muscle tension.

I understand that muscle tension might provoke tics, but what on earth have my thoughts to do with tension or tics?   Thoughts affect tics in different ways. Firstly, our anticipations link up with our muscle preparation. Typically, we intend to do an action and our muscles tense up to prepare us physically for the action we thought up. But thinking can also affect the activities we undertake. For example, some people don't believe they have the right to relax, others believe they must always be on the move. Finally, the way we evaluate our tic, its appearance, its impact on others and the way we anticipate its arrival can also affect our tension level and so make the tic more likely to appear.

What is meant by "higher than normal activation"?   Tics respond to the motor activation system of the brain and body. When activation is high, there is more tension and tics. There is evidence from several studies that people with tics have higher activation levels than normal and this affects their reactivity. But this activation can reduce after behavior therapy, and changing behavior can itself change not only tics but also associated brain activity.

I don't feel I'm particularly tense or over-active   Tics require muscle tension to occur. As we noted earlier, the tense–release tic cycle produces and maintains tension although it may seem subjectively to reduce tension (see Figure 7.5). People with chronic muscle tension may not be aware of their tension since it is so habitual, but one of the key awareness exercises you will learn is to detect the level of your muscle tension and recognize when it is really high or low.

Can the high activation level be changed?   The overall aim of treatment is to reduce the many ways by which your motor system is kept in a state of over-activity.

When this activation is reduced by behavioral, psychological or other means, tics are much less likely. In our model, we see tics as embedded in everyday behavior. It is an ecological approach which means that we take a larger window on tics, seeing them not as isolated jerks but as part of the behavioral repertoire of the person. In some sense, ticcing serves a tension-reducing function in everyday life. The function is generally tension–release although tic habits may also impact on other emotions. However, in all cases the tension is better reduced by addressing the whole behavior, not just the tic.

But isn't this saying my tics are just psychological?   Many older people with tics will have an aversion to the idea that psychology could be involved in tics. During the 1950s and earlier, many children were told authoritatively by medical experts that tics meant repressed hostility to their parents. This opinion followed the psychoanalytic view that tics represent intrapsychic conflict. We are saying that tics are behavioral habits and you need to learn behavioral techniques to control them. Thoughts are also part of behavior and link up with our behavioral repertoire, so it's normal in order to change behavior that we change thought.

What's the difference between behavioral psychology and psychoanalysis?   Behavioral psychology is distinct from psychoanalysis and based on completely different premises and modes of intervention. It is very down to earth, grounded in the present and deals with everyday reality. It deals directly with the tic problem. It is considered to be the treatment of choice in dealing with anxiety and related disorders and changes thinking and behavior patterns in the here and now.

What are the principles of behaviorism?   The behavioral model sees all habits as actively maintained by behavior and sometimes by the very strategies which the person supposes are controlling the habit (e.g., tensing up to keep the tic on hold – see Appendix 1h). Behavior can be self-reinforcing so that the more often you do a behavior, the more you must do it. It's a bit like eating one peanut and then wanting to continue eating the whole bowl. Also, bad habits can be self-reinforcing since they produce a short-term relief which is either stimulating or tension releasing, so this encourages the continuation of the habit even if it produces long-term tension problems.

I don't understand how I maintain my tic   All behavior is dynamic and is maintained by what we do. If we wish to saw wood, we must maintain tension in our hand and arms to do this action, otherwise the wood will not be sawed. Here, our active role in creating tension is obvious, but we often get into an automatic habit of doing things a certain way and it becomes so automatic that we don't realize we are putting effort into maintaining the habit. It seems easier to keep automatically reinforcing your habit than stopping it, because stopping feels strange. Sometimes, we set ourselves up to experience what initially seems like an involuntary act. Remember the earlier example about crossing our legs, so that our leg will react reflex-like to a tendon hammer. The tic seems involuntary but our background behavior sets it up and creates the right tension and opportunity for the reflex, just like us crossing our legs to permit the knee reflex. Learning about background behavior and how this perpetuates tension is crucial to the program and forms part of the awareness training.

What if I have more than one tic?   We advise dealing with one tic at a time, since each tic identified by our evaluations is a separate tic unit, so it will be responsive to at least the slightly different processes that maintain it. Therefore, if you focus on one tic, you're less likely to be confused. In any case, once you have mastered one tic, other tics or habits will be easier to control.

Are tics and habits like hair pulling or nail biting similar?   Both are learned or acquired motor habits and are treatable by the same methods. However, there are differences in both the thinking behind the habits and the type of situations and feelings that trigger the habits. Habits are more complex and more conscious than tics, and may reflect other emotions and not just release tension. They may be triggered by more diverse emotions like depression. However, our program accommodates both tics and habits and has proven equally successful with both disorders.

But I thought tics were all neurological   For many of you it may seem strange that we are proposing a method of controlling your tics by controlling your thoughts, emotions and behavior. You may have heard many times from many experts that tics are a neurological problem. The fact that ticcing involves neurological and neurochemical mechanisms is undeniable. But we should be clear exactly what this means. In one sense, any behavior can be considered neurological since you cannot act or even think without producing changes in brain chemistry or nerve function. Your central nervous system acts very differently when you are out jogging than if you are reading; but it is you who decides to jog or read, not your nervous system. When neurologists talk of neurological problems, they are generally referring to disorders such as Parkinson's disease or Huntington's chorea where we can detect structural abnormalities either in the central nervous system or the brain. In both tics and Tourette's syndrome, there is no *consistent* evidence of any structural abnormalities of the brain. The word consistent is important here since often isolated studies may show peculiar results, but if they are not consistently replicated, then the chances are that the results were serendipitous. If there were consistent characteristic, neurological or neurochemical abnormalities, then these would form the pillars of diagnosis as they do in cases of brain damage. But as you will know from your experience, TD are diagnosed on the basis of clinical interview and observation about your history and behavior. There are, indeed, some physiological reactions of people with TD which are reliably different from normals. We have already noted that people with tics show higher sensorimotor activation levels. But these are reactions that can be modified. They are functional not structural differences. Often these differences may result from the fact that the person has tics, so modifying the tic will naturally change the reaction. Tics are a functional problem, in that they vary during everyday functioning and are often better or worse depending on what you are doing. In everyday functioning, the traffic between brain and muscles is two way with each modifying the other through interaction.

Please now complete the tic quiz given in Appendix 7 (but do not look at the answers) and discuss your answers with your therapist.

► MOTIVATION

The first important question to ask concerns your motivation for completing the program. As we noted in the program overview, the program does require your active collaboration. This means regular practice and persistence and self-discipline, which is particularly hard if you are working on your own. The stages of exercises are designed to follow each other. Any one exercise or stage is not sufficient in itself to control the tic but cumulatively they are effective since they address distinct components. They require continued practice, however, and since they are cumulative, you need to follow all steps of the program until the end.

It is not a good idea to pick and choose the stages that you find more convenient, or to begin the program but then abandon it after a couple of weeks because dealing with your tic is currently not a priority. So, in order to prepare yourself for the program and ensure that dealing with your tic is a priority, we have prepared a motivational interview in Appendix 1f, and a "beliefs about tics" questionnaire in Appendix 1d listing questions to ask yourself which we consider important in the decision to take the program and follow it as **a priority**.

As we said earlier, from our experience, unless eliminating the tic is a priority in your life and you are willing to accord the program priority, then you should reconsider motivation. Generally speaking, people who seek help to please others or because others wish it are less motivated since they may resent seeking treatment. Other major stresses, positive or negative, new job, new family, new home, can interfere with collaboration in the program. If you are dead set against the idea that you can benefit from therapy, this belief might interfere with active collaboration since you will see no point in it. Obviously, the proof is in the pudding and we don't expect you to accept the model before you've tried it, but equally if you are closed off due to a belief in a magic pill solution or just against behavior therapy, this will be demotivating. Very occasionally, people also get positive benefits from ticcing, and they may feel it's a part of their personality and makes them into a character. One young man reported that girls seemed more sympathetic to his advances when they saw he ticced. Usually, such benefits are illusory in that tics usually prevent people from fully realizing their personal potential, but if you strongly believe tics are part of your identity, you may wish to question your motivation and commitment to decrease their presence.

If you feel that you are not motivated to try the program, PLEASE DO NOT START IT. There are no half-hearted successes and if you abandon the program without benefit, you may be even more discouraged about controlling your tic. If the motivation problem is one of priority, leave the program to a later time when it can be a priority. If the low motivation is due to perceived benefits of ticcing, **complete the inconvenience review sheet in Appendix 1g**. Tics always impede functioning and increase stress and it helps to become aware of their true impact on life. The young man who thought tics helped him find girls also discovered that the tics became annoying later in the relationship. **Please consult your therapist about how to deal with other motivational issues.**

▶ MIND OVER MUSCLE

Since movement is active, then we need to attend to the components that engineer activity in the brain and beyond, including anticipation, planning, emotion, feeling the movement and evaluating its consequences – all are important in modifying the movement.

There is a three-way link up between mind, emotion and muscles tension (see Figure 7.3). In a certain posture, you are more likely to think and feel in a certain way; conversely, anticipating an action in a certain way will lead to certain types of movements, and the kind of emotion you are experiencing can determine both thoughts and movements.

You can demonstrate this link up for yourself by thinking of something, then changing your posture or even just raising your little finger and seeing if it changes the quality of your thoughts. In certain postures and positions, it's easier to think of pleasant scenes than in others. Try lying on your back relaxing and thinking of a pleasant scene – now try thinking of the same scene standing on one leg. Now stand in front of a closed door and imagine that the door you are about to open is very heavy. Your brain will prepare your muscles for this and when you open it, it will seem lighter than usual and your emotion may be one of pleasant surprise rather than tedious effort.

People who are depressed find it difficult to smile or to walk quickly. Adopt now the muscular appearance of someone who is happy. Smile, let your chest open and maintain this posture for about 10 minutes. After a while you will feel a little happier.

These exercises show you that there is a three-way interaction between muscle, mind and emotion. This three-way intersection is relevant to movement problems. Awareness of this connection of muscles and brain in behavior is essential, and is a part of gaining more intimate awareness of your habit. We spend the first section discussing how to develop *awareness* of your habit. There are three stages to developing awareness: *information*, *observation* and *feedback*.

▶ General Information on the Nervous System

All operations of the body are controlled by the nervous system. This system is divided into four principal parts: the brain, the spinal cord, the roots of the nerves and the nerves that transmit the messages coming from the brain to the muscles and the internal organs like the heart and the stomach. These messages indicate to the muscles and the various organs when and how to react.

The nervous system includes two branches: the voluntary nervous system and the involuntary or autonomic nervous system. Whereas we can exert much control on our muscles, our various internal organs function rather in an autonomous way. The voluntary nervous system is responsible for the contraction of the muscles. We describe it as voluntary because it's possible for us to voluntarily decide to contract or relax a muscle. The autonomic nervous system is responsible for the operations of the internal organs. This system is not under voluntary control, it rather functions automatically. This is very useful for us because, for example, if we had to think of making our heart beat, we would have no more time to do other things. However, these automatic operations, which escape our voluntary control, can also cause problems because our system can start to react in a way that is contrary to how we would wish.

The autonomic nervous system is divided into a sympathetic and parasympathetic nervous system. The sympathetic system is responsible for the production and use of energy while the function of the parasympathetic system is to save our energy. The sympathetic system is in charge of providing us with the necessary energy to achieve our various activities. According to the quantity of energy we need, it signals our body to work more or less. In the case of a runner, blood circulates more quickly, blood pressure increases, and breathing accelerates to enable the body to receive more oxygen. There is, moreover, an increase in perspiration to eliminate the excess heat created. The sympathetic system is thus responsible for providing to the muscles the necessary energy for their activities.

The sympathetic system has also a role to play in anxiety problems. Our system assumes that all that irritates us or makes us feel afraid represents a potential danger and thus we will need a greater amount of energy to face it. If we are in front of a dangerous animal, for example, our body quickly produces energy that we will use to fight or escape. There are, however, everyday situations that can be perceived to be stressful, such as an interview for employment where to fight or escape do not represent suitable reactions. But our system, nevertheless, will start to produce energy and we will then be able to witness the appearance of various physiological symptoms, such as: palpitations due to the increase in the rate of heartbeat; puffs of heat or dizzy spells caused by an increase in blood pressure; respiratory problems (short breath, irregular breathing, feeling of suffocation) produced by the acceleration of breathing; and a feeling of hot, moist hands, because of the increase in perspiration. These various manifestations of the sympathetic autonomous system are also accompanied by an increase in muscular tension, which can cause tremors, repetitive movements, voice tremors, or butterflies in the stomach. In addition, noting these various physiological symptoms of anxiety and interpreting them as the sign of an imminent danger can cause an increase in the level of anxiety. These kinds of thought can involve the person in a vicious circle which can result in anxiety attacks or even lead the person to flee to avoid the stressing situation.

Perceiving a situation as being stressful or dangerous can thus have the effect of activating the sympathetic system, even if we do not need more energy, and can produce various physiological symptoms, indicating high anxiety or stress. If it is true that our thoughts have an effect on the physiological system, it is the same for our behavior. A person who always runs, and so tightens the muscles unnecessarily, forces the body to produce a surplus of energy constantly. Anxiety and tension burn a lot of energy and, in the more or less long term, it can lead to physical or psychological exhaustion (especially if sleep is disturbed). Anxious people often have the feeling that something terrible will happen, and imagine the worst. This feeling can vary from one day to the next, often without apparent reason. Moreover, the capacities of concentration and memory can be affected. Tasks normally found easy become major problems. In this case, the person may excessively activate the system. Conflict, confusion and the feeling that things are out of control can also result. The appearance of these various problems in a person indicates the need to lower the level of stress and anxiety. Stress is also cumulative, and can build up unawares over time. If a person has stress after stress, sooner or later he or she is no longer able to face the problems that arise. The last problem to have occurred may have been unimportant, but with the addition even of a small stress, it could be sufficient to bring the level of stress higher and above the highest tolerable limit. In order to avoid this point, it is important that the person learns to monitor the stress regularly and to correctly guage the necessary energy to face the next stress situation.

Nobody can completely avoid stress in life; however, it is possible to learn how to exert a control over stress. As we saw earlier, muscular tension accompanies the various physiological demonstrations (palpitations, hot flushes, etc.) and is dependent on stress and on anxiety caused by the activation of our sympathetic system. Although it is not possible for us to exert a direct control on the autonomic system, it is possible to do it via the voluntary nervous system. By slackening tension in muscles, we tell our body we do not need a surplus of energy and we thus allow the parasympathetic autonomic system to enter the action. We should remember that the function of this system is to save energy. By activating the parasympathetic system, we replace symptoms of anxiety and tension by calm and relief and we thus preserve our energy. When we have more energy, we are less tired, more calm and it is easier to face various problems of life.

To exert more control, it is necessary to learn how to relax the tension of the muscles. But it is firstly necessary to learn how to recognize the presence of tension in the muscles. With practice, we become able to detect tension as soon as it builds up. Once we are able to identify where the tension exists, we can learn how to slacken the tension through muscular relaxation. As with acquiring any skills, we will need practice to learn the skills of relaxation. However, it is a good investment of time because we will have a tool that will be useful to us for our entire life.

▶ How You Use Your Muscles

Muscles, of course, do the work of the body, but they also in turn work the body. In Figures 7.2 and 7.3, we present schematic diagrams of the reciprocal relationship between muscle, output and feedback to the brain.

An important task of the muscles is their feedback function which gives the brain not only information on location and orientation of the body but also influences expression of emotion; this is particularly so for facial muscles. Moving a muscle requires an action plan in the brain which initiates the movement of preparing the muscle. This preparation turns into enactment of what is planned. Control of the action is maintained through feedback from the muscles which signals the brain during movement, giving information on location and also on tension levels. The flow of movement depends equally on the state and flexibility of the muscle as on the coherence of the action plan. In other words, the way we plan action, the way the muscles prepare for the action and how we interpret feedback on your action are all *equally* important in any movement.

▶ Principal Muscles Involved in Tics and Movements

Following the diagram, you might like to test out and experiment with recognizing your own muscle use. Muscles can be in a variety of states: they can be relaxed or tense, and they can also be in a state between tension and relaxation. They can be flexible or inflexible, ready or unready, efficient or inefficient. Muscles are not just levers or marionettes operated by nerve strings, they are sensitive instruments, responsive to even a slight change in intention on your part. In addition, they are always part of a pattern or profile of action. This is why it is difficult to give the function of any one muscle in isolation since, in performing any task, a series of muscles will inevitably be involved, even if they don't move. In Appendix 2g, we list a number of muscles involved in everyday functional actions. When you move around, try to focus on the muscles you use and your tension levels.

▶ Are You Using Your Muscles Efficiently?

Practice some of the exercises in Appendix 2g and examine what you do, when sitting or rising. If you do not know whether a limb is moving or not, place your hand on it to identify its state. The first point to notice is that it is impossible to move one part of the body without other parts being involved. Even a small movement involves a larger background of support tension to carry it through.

In Appendix 2g, we identify muscles that are habitually involved in common actions. Ask yourself if your distribution of energy is appropriate. Are there parts of the tension that do not contribute to the action? For example, do you over-tense your biceps when you throw a switch? Does your face tense up when you lift up a suit-case? Do you write tensing your tongue as well as your hand?

Some of this superfluous action may relate to the degree of anticipation or preparation that you are investing in the action – a point that goes back to what we said earlier about brain and body being related. Because the body must prepare for the future and the future is unknown, the preparation may not always be appropriate. You might be using the same arm action to throw a switch as to open a door, or putting on a summer jacket the same way you'd put on a winter anorak, or preparing to address a crowd when you are talking to a single person. Compare your responses in similar tasks which require more or less energy and see if you are adequately discriminating between them in your muscle use.

▶ Check Your Breathing

Now examine your breathing. People often stop breathing when they move, or start breathing in an irregular fashion. We deal with this later under relaxation. But list here situations where you notice you change your breathing. Do you breathe during your problem?

▶   AWARENESS TRAINING

Now that you have read basic information on how your muscles work, and explored a little your own experience, we can begin to increase your awareness of your specific movement problem, and study it in more detail. But first we must deal with the habit of awareness itself.

▶ Assessment Instruments

Your therapist with your collaboration will have already noted frequency, intensity, complexity and anatomical site of motor, sensory, phonic tics, and also interference in other areas of life. In Appendices 1d and 1e, we give other questionnaires which assess impact on your life and your style of activity. We now come to directly monitoring the type and form of your tic.

▶ Measuring Tic Behavior

There seem to be three preferred types of observing and assessing the tic itself: video rating, self-monitoring and external rater assessment and feedback.

▶ Awareness as a Habit

There is more to awareness than we are aware of. Awareness is a kind of pilot of the mind's eye. When we pay attention to something, our awareness extends beyond the object itself. Awareness places our attention within a whole series of events going on around us. At any moment, I might be concentrating on a particular arm movement but my awareness of this movement includes the social, geographical, physical and emotional context in which I am performing, as well as many other finer and more personal points of information.

Now some aspects of this awareness are themselves automatic so that I may be habituated to seeing and describing my habit in a certain way, say, as a nuisance, or of simply ignoring it or accepting it. In other words, in some way or other, I have got used to living with the problem. A first important step involves changing this habitual awareness. Luckily, awareness by its nature is tuned to changes in the here and now and is adaptable. It is really only necessary to focus on some new information about your habit and, providing you are persistent, the background awareness and appreciation of your habit will change – by knowing more about it, you will see it in a different light.

▶ Awareness and Attention

When your awareness of something changes, then your feeling about it also changes and your thoughts change as well. We can demonstrate this through an exercise. Take a room you know well. Suppose you are about to leave it for a long holiday. Your awareness of it now will differ compared to when you are coming in to clean it. You notice different points about the room, depending on your awareness. Now take the same room and find something in the room you hadn't noticed before. Noticing a new fragment in detail can change your overall awareness of the room as well, so while awareness affects current attention, current attention can also affect awareness.

▶ Dividing Attention

In fact, the way to change awareness is by first and foremost changing the details you habitually attend to in your action, and this is what we work on in the first part of the program. But it requires effort in developing the ability to concentrate on your tic or tension while doing other activities – in other words, dividing attention.

When you perform an action habitually, you pay attention to some but not other parts. We want to change that by observing other new points about the action in detail. Put your hand out to reach for something; now repeat the action focusing attention on your foot. Difficult! Especially if the action you are following through is complex. It is difficult because it is difficult to divide attention in a new way. Yet we divide our attention all the time. It's just a question of habit. Attention capacity is adaptable. When driving, you are able to pay attention to different information – for example, road, dials, conversation. Dividing your attention in new ways is a question of practice, not capacity. In order to complete the next step of self-observation, we ask you to divide your attention between two activities: the tic and whatever else you are doing.

▶ Observing Your Tic Habit

Please refer to Appendix 4 for the daily tic monitoring guide which, together with the daily tic monitoring forms in Appendix 6, explain in detail how to record your chosen tic unit. In the program, we address one tic at a time and the tic chosen must be an important one that occurs frequently and can be described in detail. Once you have chosen the tic, you may like to artificially produce the tic yourself to form a clearer idea of its appearance. Equally, the therapist could imitate it while you watch. The first diary exercise is to keep count for two days of the number of times the movement occurs. If the tic occurs only on certain days, then extend your observation to include these days. If you have trouble noting down or remembering, then it is best to make a mark and tick off the response when it occurs as a line on a piece of paper or a hand counter. You can carry the paper or counter around with you. We will eventually require you to monitor your tic, its frequency, intensity, and your degree of control daily throughout the program.

You may have difficulty at first in recognizing when your problem movement begins and the tension starts. This will become easier after you have done the discrimination exercises but for the moment the best strategy is to focus on the muscles most involved in your problem. Direct your attention onto the large area of the muscle. As your concentration on the muscle persists you will discover that your focus becomes more and more sensitive and narrow and your feeling for the movement also sharpens. You will not succeed in concentrating all the time, but after a while, dividing attention between the movement will become well installed and you won't have to exert so much effort.

After you have successfully completed the diary for two days, we ask you, with your therapist, to decide on a regular time period each day when you can monitor the tic. This monitoring must be consistent throughout the program and can be completed by photocopying or downloading as often as necessary, the diary forms in Appendix 6. Now having developed some awareness of your habit, we can begin to explore its variations. What we are looking for are situations or activities in which the tic occurs more or less frequently, where it varies in degree of intensity and your degree of control. Identifying all of these is essential to our management program. Also, sometimes the movement comes in a series and sometimes it comes individually. Note down all variations of your problem. Mark all this down on the diary cards you have copied from Appendix 6. Keep these cards for a week to allow you to cover a wide variety of situations and activities.

Try to identify activities in which there is a high and low risk of the problem happening. Try to be specific about this. You may think that it is due to stress but be specific about the type of activity that produces the stress or the type of relaxing situations, and try to note down exactly what *you* are doing, what activity you are engaged in when the problem arrives. Please be specific in describing tic-associated activities.

▶ Involving Another Person as Collaborator

Your therapist will ask your opinion on involving a third person who you know and trust to help you with the program. If you are in agreement, the person can help to provide feedback on the nature of the tic and on your progress. The collaborator can, for example, observe your tic to help you to describe it, and can provide support and encouragement throughout the program by complimenting you on progress and providing rewards for your efforts. The person may be able to help when you feel discouraged by boosting morale and helping you to overcome a difficult exercise through discussion of the rationale. It is important that this person meets the therapist and understands the program to avoid adopting any critical or negative attitudes. The collaborator will also provide outside objective feedback on the tic and other changes at the end of the program.

> ▶ **IDENTIFYING HIGH- AND LOW-RISK ACTIVITIES,**
> **AND ASSOCIATED THOUGHTS AND FEELINGS**

In this part of your self-evaluation, we ask you to identify concrete situations or activities that are high or low risk for your tic appearance. You will have already noticed how the strength of your tic or even its occurrence varies over the day and with performing some, but not all, activities. We now need to know what these situations are and what thoughts, emotions or behavior characterize them.

Tics vary with activity. People are used to thinking of their tic or movement as a nervous problem, but for some the problem occurs when they are doing nothing and for others when they are occupied. It is extremely important to be precise and choose three of the worst situations or activities where the tic occurs in terms of frequency, intensity and control, and the three best situations or activities where the tic does not occur (Figures 7.6 and 7.7). Obviously, these must be waking activities.

How to Choose High-risk Activities?

You have now completed the daily diary and Appendices 2a, 2b and 2c, listing situations likely to provoke the tic. You have also kept the daily diary continuously over a period of one week. Look carefully at these records and choose a situation/activity where the tic is most likely to occur. This should also be an activity that repeats itself daily and is unlikely to change. If you are in the habit of avoiding your high-risk situations, you might choose this situation but obviously you must now no longer avoid it. When you describe the activity associated with the tic onset, try as far as possible to be precise and accurate and don't worry if it takes a complex description – for example, putting "morning" is less helpful than "making breakfast with the family".

Next, we ask you to choose an activity where the tic is less intense, less frequent, and you have most control. We ask you here to exclude situations where you are obviously prevented from doing your tic by other factors, for example, when you are sleeping, when the tic-affected muscle is otherwise occupied, when you are deliberately holding in the tic to disguise it. We want, rather, situations where you genuinely feel less likely to do the tic.

Now just to complete the range of variation, we would like you to fill in four other activities which are in-between the two extremes. Two may be classified as high risk, that is, the tic is likely to be present but not as frequently or as intensely or as out of control as the most high-risk activity. Similarly, insert another two low-risk situations, which should be activities that are less likely to provoke the tic but are not as low risk as the most low-risk activity. Again, please be as precise as possible in describing these activities (see example in Appendices 2d and 2e).

	Activities						
	Low risk			High risk			
	A	B	C	D	E	F	
	Cooking for self	Knitting at home in the evening	Reading by myself in bed	Waiting for an appointment	Driving in a traffic jam	Socializing with a group of friends	
Likelihood of tic absent (1–3)	2	2	3	6	7	7	Likelihood of tic present (5–7)
Stimulated	2	3	2	6	7	5	Bored
Active	2	2	5	7	6	4	Still
Concentrating	1	2	2	5	5	3	Unfocused
Socially at ease	3	1	1	5	4	7	Being judged
Confident	3	2	4	6	5	6	Unsure of myself
Alert	5	4	5	4	7	4	Tired
On my own	3	2	1	4	2	7	With other people

Figure 7.6   Example of half-completed Kelly's grid for classifying low- and high-risk activities with illustrations of evaluative dimensions elicited from a participant as appraisals of low- and high-risk activities
Notes:

- Identify three activities at low risk and three activities at high risk of producing the tic or habit. Rank these activities 1–7 according to their degree of low (1–3) or high (5–7) risk.
- If the activity is no more or no less likely to be associated with tic onset, it will score 4, in the middle of 1–7.
- Rank each activity (1–7) according to whether it represents one of the poles of the evaluation dimensions given in the left- and right-hand columns. You may add your own descriptive dimensions relevant to distinguish low- and high-risk activities until you have exhausted all possible evaluations that might be relevant to low- versus high-risk activities (see text).
- If you find rating 1–7 too laborious, you can rate each activity 0 or 1 depending on whether the tic is likely to be absent (0) or present (1) or $\frac{1}{2}$ if the tic is equally likely to be present or absent.

▶ Evaluations Associated with High-risk Activities

In order to identify evaluations associated with tic onset, we use an instrument called a "grid" developed by a psychologist, George Kelly, in the 1950s (Blowers & O'Connor, 1996). The idea of the grid is that there are elements in the world (real people, events, activities) matched with feelings, thoughts, evaluations which are peculiar to them. The grid is so constituted that we can also see the degree to which the personal way you construe events or activities relates to the likelihood of the tic onset. Obviously, all this serves later on to help us to modify and restructure your approach to these activities.

Photocopy or download Appendix 2f and fill in the six activities in the columns representing the three high- and the three low-risk situations/activities. An example of a half-completed grid is given in Figure 7.6. You will see that in the

	Activities						
	Low risk			High risk			
	A	B	C	D	E	F	
	Cooking for self	Knitting at home in the evening	Reading by myself in bed	Waiting for an appointment	Driving in a traffic jam	Socializing with a group of friends	
Likelihood of tic absent (1–3)	2	2	3	6	7	7	Likelihood of tic present (5–7)
Stimulated	2	3	2	4	5	4	Bored
Calculation:	2 −2	2 −3	4 −3	6 −4	7 −5	7 −4	
Difference scores for each activity:	0	+1	+1	+2	+2	+3 = 9	Total difference score summed over all activities

Figure 7.7   Example of calculating difference in rating between an evaluation dimension and likelihood of tic onset

grid, there are rows and columns. In the first row, we have written likelihood that the tic is present or absent. The high- and low-risk tic activities are listed in the columns and, in the first row, we ask you to mark each activity according to whether the tic is likely to be present or absent. There are two ways to do this, either you can rate the situations 1–7 according to their likelihood, or you can simply mark 0 or 1 denoting whether the tic is likely to be present or absent for each of the six activities. Rating 1–7 is preferable since it confirms the degree to which the tic is present during each activity. Now, in the spaces below each of the six activities, between tic absent and tic present, we want you to fill in your evaluations of each of the high- and low-risk activities. The most "high risk" scores 7, and the most "low risk" at 1. The other four are graded at 2, 3 for the low risk, and 5, 6 for the high risk according to which activities you judge to be more or less high risk and which of the two low-risk situations you judge as more or less low risk. The more the tic is present in the activity, the nearer your score is to 7; the more absent, the nearer to 0 by degree. If the tic could be equally present or absent, the score is in the middle, 4. Or if you are using the 0–1 scoring scheme, then 1/2 indicates equally present or absent.

Now we progress to your evaluation of the six high- or low-risk activities. When you come to evaluating the six activities, we are interested in how you see each activity and how you feel about it. Obviously, you are familiar with doing the activity so you don't usually think about it, or you take it for granted. But with reflection, you can ask yourself: "How do I feel about this activity?" "How do I feel in the activity?" "What's typical of this activity?" "What's my opinion of it?" For example, you may find the activity disagreeable and useless, or frustrating and boring, or pleasant and rewarding. Now look at the low-risk activities. How do you feel about these activities as a group? What's your opinion of them? Do you feel the same as when in the high-risk activities or different? Maybe you feel differently in different degrees between high- and low-risk activities or maybe completely different. A helpful method is to ask yourself: "What is different about the way I evaluate the three high-risk activities as opposed to the three low-risk activities?"

In contrast to the detailed description of each of the activities, it is best if the evaluation of the activities progresses one idea at a time. If two evaluations seem relevant to the same activity, then place them separately in the rows and rank them separately. Probably, in the first instance, you will think of one term, e.g., tiring or boring. Place this term in the space in the column at the right-hand end of the second row in the grid. Let's say you decide that the high-risk activities are more boring than the low-risk ones. Now ask yourself: "What is the opposite of this (boring) evaluation (e.g., interesting or alerting)?" When you have found the opposite evaluation (in your own terms) to the first evaluation, place it in the column at the left hand of the second row. These two terms form a dimension along which you can now rate each of the three high-risk and low-risk activities.

Now rank each of the six high- or low-risk activities according to how close it is to being boring, or the opposite. If the activity is closer to boring (the high-risk evaluation), then it will score 5, 6 or 7. If it is closer to the opposite (the low-risk evaluation), then it will score 1, 2 or 3. If there is no difference, it will score 4, or $\frac{1}{2}$ if you are using just 0 or 1 (presence or absence).

You can now find other evaluation dimensions by looking at just two high-risk activities and asking yourself what they have in common, then asking: "What is the difference with a low-risk activity?" For example, you may see that in the high-risk activities you are always occupied while in the low-risk activities you have nothing to do. These evaluations then could form another dimension to rank activities. Not all the evaluative dimensions you think of will be equally related to high- and low-tic onset. In fact, you may find that a combination of dimensions relates better than just one dimension. It should be said that, in our research, we have found wide variations in the activities in which people tic, so if your activities don't match the idiosyncratic example in Figure 7.6, this is not a problem.

In the example in Figure 7.6, we have provided three low-risk activities (cooking for self, knitting at home in the evening, reading by myself in bed), and compared them with three high-risk activities (waiting for an appointment, driving in a traffic jam, socializing with a group of friends). In the example, the person considers being bored the opposite pole to being stimulated, and she is more stimulated than bored when cooking and knitting. However, when we look at how she feels in the high-risk activities, she is more bored than stimulated, since she has ranked the activities in the 5–7 range of the scale, indicating they are more associated with this end of the pole. This first dimension of evaluation came from reflecting on what each of the three high- and low-risk activities had in common, and then rating all activities on this evaluation – boredom and its opposite, stimulation. In looking at what else the high-risk activities have in common, she realized that in all the high-risk activities, she was moving very little or sitting still, as one does when caught in a traffic jam or waiting for an appointment. The opposite of not moving for this person was to be active and so "active" was placed in the left-hand column because it best represented the low-risk activities. When the client ranked each of the activities according to whether she was more immobile or more active in these situations, we can see that the high-risk activity grouped around inactive and the low-risk activities grouped around active.

She now looked to see if there were any further evaluations, reactions or opinions about the activities that might distinguish the high- and low-risk activities by comparing any two high-risk with a low-risk to tease out differences, a method called "triadic sorting". She realized that, generally, in the low-risk task she was more focused intellectually than when in the two high-risk activities. The opposite of being concentrated for this person was being unfocused, so at one end of the row she placed "concentrating" and at the other end "unfocused", and ranked the high- and low-risk activities as to whether they were more likely to be concentrated or unfocused. Another evaluation the client elicited by means of comparing one high-risk activity, "being in a group", with two low-risk activities, "cooking" or "reading". She felt she was more likely to be judged when in a group than when knitting or reading alone. The opposite pole to being judged, for this woman, was to be socially at ease, and she was more at ease when in the low-risk activities. A related dimension was elicited by comparing "waiting for an appointment" with "cooking" or "reading". She felt she lacked assurance when waiting. The opposite to lack of assurance was having a lot of self-confidence, so this formed the opposite end of the evaluation pole, and the high- and low-risk activities were ranked accordingly. A further way of eliciting evaluations is to simply ask yourself: "What is the difference in how I perceived activity A compared to activity D, or between activities A and B compared to E?" and so on until you have compared all activities.

Of course, not all evaluations, reactions, attitudes to the activities elicited in this way will necessarily be relevant to tic onset. For example, in comparing "driving" with "reading", the person realized she was usually more tired when driving, so she constructed a dimension from "alert" to "tired", but when rating each activity on this scale, she noted that for most activities she could be either alert or tired and this dimension scored 4, so did not really discriminate between high- and low-risk activities.

Try to extract as many different evaluative dimensions as possible and score the extent to which each evaluation pole is present for each activity either from 1 to 7 or between 0 and 1. Often, an activity will be complex and relate to more than one relevant dimension. In the grid given in Appendix 2h, we have given as a guide sample constructs which we have found commonly associated with tic onset and which may or may not link up to your tic. But underneath we have left space for your own personally elicited evaluation dimensions. Please add as many as you can elicit.

The next step is to see which of the dimensions relates to the presence of tic activity. One obvious way is simply to compare the scores in each evaluation row to those in the first row (likelihood of tic present or absent) which then reflects the likelihood of an association of this evaluative dimension with tic onset. A more systematic way is to look at the difference between the scores in the first dimension (tic present – tic absent), and each subsequent evaluation dimension separately, and add up the

	Activities							Total differences score
	Low risk			High risk				
	A	B	C	D	E	F		
	Playing sport	Leisure activity	Talking with a group	Watching television	Cleaning the bedroom	Driving in the car		
Likelihood of tic absent (1–3)	1	2	1	5	5	7	Likelihood of tic present (5–7)	
In shape	1	1	4	4	6	4	Not feeling active enough	9
Doing	2	2	4	7	5	7	Watching	6
Relaxing	4	5	2	4	4	5	Attending	11
Calm	1	2	2	4	4	7	Preoccupied	3
Confidence in performance	1	1	2	2	2	1	Insecure	14

Figure 7.8   Evaluation grid for low- and high-risk activities (pre-treatment)

difference in each case. In the example, the first low activity received a score of 2 to indicate that the likelihood of a tic was low in this activity, and it also received a 2 to indicate how unlikely it was to be evaluated as boring. So, the difference between these scores is 0. On the other hand, the next activity is rated 2 in terms of tic present–absent but 3 along the stimulated–bored dimension. So, there is a difference of 1. If one continues along the row of activities for this one dimension, one ends

	Activities							Total differences score
	Low risk			High risk				
	A	B	C	D	E	F		
	Playing sport	Leisure activity	Talking with a group	Watching television	Cleaning the bedroom	Driving in the car		
Likelihood of tic absent (1–3)	1	1	1	1	1	4	Likelihood of tic present (5–7)	
In shape	1	1	1	3	5	2	Not feeling active enough	8
Doing	2	2	4	7	3	2	Watching	15
Relaxing	5	5	2	7	4	7	Attending	21
Calm	1	1	1	1	1	6	Preoccupied	2
Confidence in performance	1	1	1	1	1	1	Insecure	3

Figure 7.9   Evaluation grid for low- and high-risk activities (post-treatment)

up with six difference scores, as given in Figure 7.7. The total of these difference scores is 9.

Calculating total difference scores between the first tic onset dimension and all the six evaluation dimensions gives us six different total scores. The less the difference score, the more likely the evaluation dimension is to be associated with the tic. Conversely, the greater the difference score, the less the two are associated. From our experience, as a rule of thumb, total differences under 10 usually signal some connection, but obviously the lower the score, the more important the dimension. If two or more dimensions score equally, then, as mentioned previously, they may be equally associated with the tic. Obviously, the test of validity for this calculation is for you to ask yourself if the connection between the tic and the evaluation makes sense to you. Figures 7.8 and 7.9 give completed grids for another client pre- and post-treatment showing how evaluations can change.

▶ Connecting Evaluations to Specific Thoughts and Feelings Associated with Each Tic

The connections, perhaps, also help to convince you that you have some indirect role in tic onset. Obtaining these connections is very important since it allows us to see how you view and evaluate high-risk compared to low-risk activities in practice. It also allows us now to go further and specify exactly what emotions, tensions, attitudes and behaviors are identified with the different dimensions of evaluation. This exercise will require a little bit of thought but it gives us insight into specific and subtle differences between each high-risk situation in terms of the way you think, act and feel.

Take all the evaluation dimensions that are relevant to tic onset, put them together and ask yourself what insight they give you about the way you think, feel or behave during your movement problem. For example, if the dimensions "with other people" and "unsure of myself" are important, try to think of the thoughts that would come before you entered these situations, how these anticipations would translate into feelings about yourself, and how this might lead to certain muscle tensions and postures. If you photocopy or download Appendix 2h, we have provided space for you to note specifically the emotions, thoughts and tensions (as far as you are aware) that are associated with each of the three high-risk and low-risk situations.

1. For example, when I am waiting for an appointment, what exactly are my thoughts, anticipations, expectations? Perhaps I'm worried about results, or I'm wanting to get it over as quickly as possible.
2. What are the emotions experienced in the same situation: apprehension, nervousness, impatience?
3. How is my evaluation reflected in my physical attitude? Am I agitated? Do I sit hunched up? Is there tension in my legs and shoulders? How am I breathing?

For a cooking activity, my thoughts may concern accurately following the recipe, focusing on the cooking time, thinking of guests arriving. The emotions may be pride in my work, excitement, perhaps unease in case the recipe doesn't work. The tension may be mainly in the forearm if I'm doing things with my hand, or in my eyes if I'm paying attention. Complete this section in as much detail as possible because it will feature prominently when we come to devise new strategies to restructure your actions. You now have a general idea of how frequently your tic habit arises, the situations/activities likely to provoke it, and the associated thoughts and feelings. Now we continue the exercises by increasing your awareness of your muscles' action.

▶ MUSCLE DISCRIMINATION EXERCISES

Here, we begin the exercises to directly influence muscle activity and we start with the principal muscle or group of muscles involved in your problem. By now you should have identified the muscle principally implicated in your problem and any other muscles you consider involved.

The aim of the discrimination exercise is, as the name implies, to better discriminate distinct states of tension in the tic-affected muscle. But doing the exercises also inevitably changes the nature of the muscle's movement and produces several other benefits.

In order to *discriminate* different states of muscle contraction, you must learn to *isolate* the muscle, and then flex and relax it *slowly*, moving from a state of tension to one of relaxation, passing gradually through the different stages of tension. In doing this slowly, you will gain more flexibility in your control of the muscle since you will be able to identify its different states. The muscle itself will also become more flexible. We have found that muscles implicated in tics and habits tend to be less flexible, show less control over contraction than other muscles, and their owners have, therefore, more problems moving them slowly and regularly.

In most people with tics, the tic-affected sites are usually located more on one side of the body than on the other. We suggest that you practice the discrimination exercises on both sides. You will find the less-affected side easier to control. If both sides are equally affected, choose a non-affected muscle and practice the exercises on this site – as a reference guide to compare with your affected muscle.

▶ Identifying Action of Muscle or Muscle Group

The procedure to follow in discrimination is, firstly, to contract and relax the muscle as slowly as possible. If you have an eye twitch, try to open and close the eye as gently and as slowly as possible. If you have a shoulder twitch, raise and lower the shoulder slowly. If you have a fidgety habit, relax and slowly contract the hand involved. To begin with, you may exaggerate the movement. After you have mastered this, try to isolate the contraction as much as possible so that only the muscle directly relevant is being moved. Also check that no other muscles near or far are involved, other than those that are necessary.

Try to identify when the muscle is completely tense, half-tense and then fully tense (roughly). When you have mastered this, try to find the mid-point between relaxed and half-relaxed and between half-relaxed and fully tense.

▶ Rationale and Procedure of Discrimination Exercises

Remember that our muscles are within our voluntary control and we can thus decide to voluntarily contract or relax them. Thus, by releasing tension in the muscles, we give the signal to our whole body to relax, and we can then replace the symptoms of tension by subjective calm and relief.

However, before learning how to relax muscular tension, it is initially necessary to learn how to recognize it. The exercises of discrimination hence represent a significant element in your relaxation training. It is by practicing these exercises that you will be able to detect the difference not only between the presence and absence of tension, but also between the various levels of tension.

Each day, for the three next weeks, you will have to practice the exercises of discrimination. You will concentrate on two groups of muscles, those involved in your problem and a group that is not involved.

In order to do your exercises, you should install yourself comfortably in an armchair and follow the instructions. Each exercise will be repeated twice. The muscle contraction should be maintained for 5 seconds, $1-2-3-4-5$, and the relaxation gradually carried over a 10-second period, $1-2-3-4-5-6-7-8-9-10$. Remember that you must, as much as possible, associate breath expiration with the muscular relaxation. Moreover, as you relax, try to be aware of the various feelings connected to the various levels of tension, and, in particular, notice the difference between tensing and relaxing.

During the exercises, you must respect the 10-second period to ensure that you do not relax too quickly. In order to help you, we will practice twice for the correct time, before passing to the exercises themselves.

In a moment, you will be asked to contract the muscles of the right forearm by tightening the fist. We encourage you to record the following instructions yourself on a cassette. You will contract these muscles by supporting your elbow against the arm of the armchair.

Now, concentrate on the muscles and contract in the following manner:

Contract	$1-2-3-4-5$
Relax	$1-2-3-4-5-6-7-8-9-10$

Now repeat this same exercise. Concentrate on the muscle and try to identify when it is: (1) relaxed; (2) $^1/_4$ contracted; (3) $^1/_2$ contracted; (4) $^3/_4$ contracted; (5) fully contracted. Then slowly relax the muscle passing slowly through $^3/_4$, $^1/_2$, $^1/_4$ contraction to full relaxation.

Contract	$1-2-3-4-5$
Relax	$1-2-3-4-5-6-7-8-9-10$

We are now ready to begin the exercises for the first week.

Let us start with the non-tic-affected muscles. These will be muscles opposite to your tic-affected site (e.g., if your right cheek is affected, then your left cheek should be chosen) or a muscle or muscle group near to the affected muscle.

Concentrate on the muscle and identify 0, $^1/_4$, $^1/_2$, $^3/_4$ and full contraction then decontract slowly to 0.

> Contract (5 seconds)
> Relax (10 seconds)

Once again. Concentrate . . .

> Contract (5 seconds)
> Relax (10 seconds)

Let us pass now to the tic-affected muscles. Concentrate on the muscle and identify 0, $^1/_4$, $^1/_2$, $^3/_4$ and full contraction, then decontract slowly to 0.

> Contract (5 seconds)
> Relax (10 seconds)

Once again. Concentrate . . .

> Contract (5 seconds)
> Relax (10 seconds)

▶ Practice Criteria

The discrimination exercise should be repeated until:

(a)   you can accurately detect level tension in the muscle;
(b)   you can contract and relax the muscle slowly, smoothly, and only that muscle;
(c)   you are more conscious of the muscle tensing before the tic or movement arises.

We have now finished the discrimination exercises. Do not forget to practice them twice a day. Repeat the exercises with all the relevant muscles related to tics or repetitive movements. We will then be ready to begin the relaxation training.

▶   RELAXING IN THREE DIMENSIONS

Now that you have become more aware of different states of tension and relaxation in your affected muscle, we will cover general relaxation exercises for dealing with overall levels of tension. As we mentioned earlier, although the problem occurs in one muscle, in fact the whole of your body is involved in the problem, at least in a supporting role. Often, a general feeling of tension precedes the onset of the tic in a specific muscle.

▶ What Is Muscle Relaxation?

Most of you will have heard of muscle relaxation of some kind. The traditional Jacobson form is based on the idea that by contracting and relaxing the muscles individually in different parts of the body, the person experiences calm. Actually, the body can never be in an absolute state of relaxation, and furthermore, many other states of the muscle beside relaxation such as stretching or warming can seem equally relaxing. Relaxation is also about feeling comfortable with your posture and with the way different muscles are coordinating with each other, and how the action is flowing. It is not always necessary to work at relaxing each muscle absolutely, so we recommend an applied relaxation training which involves using muscles in a relaxed but active way in a variety of everyday postures and situations – while nonetheless following principles of slow, graded contraction and relaxation muscle action.

The method involves:

1. Learning to breathe better and mastering breath control.
2. Learning to isolate tension and relaxation in different muscles.
3. Learning to detect tension as soon as possible to prevent its build-up.
4. Applying the relaxation even when you are active and in motion.

We begin the relaxation exercises with attention to breathing.

▶ Breathe Better

When they get tense, many people find that they also stop breathing or breathe in an irregular fashion. Have you noticed how you breathe when your tic occurs? An essential part of relaxation is breathing fully and freely. There are two elements to consider: (1) the ratio of breathing in to breathing out; (2) the muscles you use when breathing.

The aim of breathing, as you know, is to take in oxygen which is converted into energy. A functioning system takes in what it needs and expels what it does not need. Optimally, the lungs should be full after inspiration to allow efficient absorption. When we are stressed, we often breathe shallowly because everything around the throat, neck and shoulders is constricted. Just by filling your lungs you can ease some of this tension, and, in any case, establishing a normal flow of air relaxes you. When you breathe in, notice that your ribcage expands; particularly notice that your upper back expands since this is where the lungs are located. Then

> Breathe in to the count of 1 – 2 – 3 and pause
> Breathe out to the count of 1 – 2 – 3 – 4 and pause

You can make a noise on the out breath to give yourself feedback on the slow count. Repeat this deep, slow breathing six times and do this exercise twice a day before we begin the full relaxation exercises.

You might feel dizzy at first, so stop if you do. With gradual practice of the exercises, the dizziness should clear, but if it continues, this may mean that you are breathing too quickly or inhaling more than you are exhaling. If you have a vertigo problem, you may wish to seek medical advice on the exercises. Whenever you find yourself breathing irregularly, repeat the exercise to improve the breathing and calm yourself.

▶ Relaxation Exercises

The aim of the relaxation exercises is for you to become more and more conscious of when the tension begins to build up so that you can prevent it before it starts. The key point here is: *the tension starts before the point you first detect it*. After following the exercises, you will begin to detect the tension coming earlier and earlier and realize that what you thought was the onset of the tension was, in fact, the mid-point in the build-up of the tension.

The relaxation exercises progress in four stages. Firstly, they are practiced as slow, gradual contractions and relaxations. Secondly, the passing from contraction to relaxation is made faster; the person need only check whether he or she is relaxed or not to achieve the desired state. Finally . . . when practicing the exercises, it is important to be attentive to the following points:

1. Make sure you are tensing the muscle in the correct way and do not *over*-tense it or you may get aches or cramps.
2. Ensure that you are in a comfortable position free from distraction and that you are able to direct your thoughts entirely to the exercises.
3. Check that you are breathing correctly during the exercises.
4. Practice the exercises for the times given, do not over-practice, particularly when you are just beginning.

In the following pages, we list the principal muscles and how to tense and relax them. The initial tension–relaxation exercises in all muscles involve two cycles.

Cycle 1

1. Breathe in.
2. Tense muscle, slowly counting to five.
3. Keep tense for a further 5 seconds.
4. Relax muscle slowly over 5 seconds, and breathe out at the same time.

The exercise in this cycle is similar to the discrimination exercise and it is important for you to recognize the difference between tension and relaxation.

Repeat this cycle six times; you will soon become familiar with it and will feel more relaxed.

Cycle 2

1. Tense the muscle again but now check how many other muscles are also tense, either near or far to the muscle you are tensing.
2. Repeat the tense–relax exercise as in cycle 1 but isolate the activity as far as possible to the one muscle involved.

Repeat these two cycles for each muscle listed below in upper and lower body, twice per day.

Forearm (right and left individually)

> Cycle 1 – Tense: Clench fists with thumb outside.
> > Relax: Unfold fists till fingers are loose.

> Cycle 2 – Other tensions: check biceps, shoulders, jaw and legs.

Upper arm (right and left individually)

> Cycle 1 – Tense: Bring forearm up to shoulder and press upper arm close to your body.
> > Relax: Let arm hand down loose.

> Cycle 2 – Other tensions: cheek, mouth, chin, neck, shoulders.

Shoulders I

> Cycle 1 – Tense: Raise both shoulders towards the ears, trying to get them as high as possible.
> > Relax: Let them drop again and hang a little forward.

> Cycle 2 – Other tensions: jaw, mouth, abdomen.

Shoulders II

> Cycle 1 – Tense: As in Shoulders I, but as you lift, rotate the shoulders a little to the back.
> > Relax: As you relax, rotate them to the front.

Neck I

> Cycle 1 – Tense: Press chin down until back of neck is stretched, push chin back so that head moves backwards.
> > Relax: Lift chin up so that head goes back and down and head is hanging back on the shoulders.

> Cycle 2 – Other tensions: face.

Neck II

Repeat Neck I, but lean head left to one side at an angle, and then repeat with head leaning right at an angle.

Jaw

> Cycle 1 – Tense: Push jaw up to mouth, creating tension in muscles next to the ears.
> > Relax: Open mouth, let jaw drop and waggle it about left–right, back and forth.

> Cycle 2 – Other tensions: rest of the face and neck.

Mouth

> Cycle 1 – Tense: Purse lips together and force tongue against the roof of the mouth.
> > Relax: Smile and let tongue drop to floor of mouth.

> Cycle 2 – Other tensions: jaw and eyes.

Cheeks (right and left)

> Cycle 1 – Tense: Raise cheek and corner of the mouth towards the eye.
> Relax: Bring cheek back to mouth.
> Cycle 2 – Other tensions: forehead, eyes.

Eyes

> Cycle 1 – Tense: Close eyes, bring cheek towards eyebrows.
> Relax: Open eyes wide.
> Cycle 2 – Other tensions: cheek, forehead.

Forehead

> Cycle 1 – Tense: Frown and wrinkle forehead, bringing eyebrows together.
> Relax: Show an expression of surprise and raise eyebrows.
> Cycle 2 – Other tensions: cheek, mouth.

Lower leg (right and left)

> Cycle 1 – Tense: Place feet on the floor and try to push feet together (but without moving feet).
> Relax: Feel feet resting on the floor with no effort.
> Cycle 2 – Other tensions: feet, upper leg.

Upper leg (right and left)

> Cycle 1 – Tense: Keep feet on the floor and try to lift knees up (but without moving them).
> Relax: Keep legs still and planted on the floor, making no conscious effort.
> Cycle 2 – Other tensions: buttocks, lower legs.

Buttocks

> Cycle 1 – Tense: Try to press the two buttocks together.
> Relax: Lean back in the armchair so there is no weight on your buttocks and they are loose.
> Cycle 2 – Other tensions: upper legs.

Abdomen

> Cycle 1 – Tense: Pull abdomen in and up until you feel a "knot" there.
> Relax: Let the abdomen expand out as though it has a balloon in it.
> Cycle 2 – Other tensions: buttocks.

Posture

> Tense: Stand up feet apart, tense all limb muscles at the same time.
> Relax: Then untense the limbs, and imagine a string through your centre pulling you up. You should ideally be balanced about your center of gravity and not tilting forwards or backwards.

Cycle 3

Practice all these relaxation exercises in total twice a day (at end and start) for one week until they have become familiar. Then speed up the tense–relax cycle to just one or two seconds in total for each muscle for the next week. Finally, at the end of the week, instead of doing the exercises, just check that each muscle is relaxed and just repeat a word like "relax" to yourself to ensure that each muscle is in its proper relaxed state.

If there is a particular scene or image that you associate with relaxation, you may use that to help to relax you instead of a word.

Cycle 4

The final stage is to move from identification when the muscles are static to when they are dynamic and the body is in everyday motion. Practice the ability you have developed to detect tension and relax, while performing the actions given in Table 1.2. It's more difficult when you are moving about or doing a task to focus on the state of your body, but it's just a case of dividing attention as we discussed earlier. Eventually, checking that you are relaxed will become automatic.

▶ REFOCUSING SENSATIONS

In this exercise, we combine the skills you have acquired in relaxation and awareness to address other aspects of unnecessary activation and stimulation. Although our feelings and movements are separate events, they are often tied together so that when we feel bad or irritated, this affects the way we move around.

In the case of sensations, the same connection applies. Many people with Tourette's syndrome describe a hypersensibility to sensation or touch or experience uncomfortable tinglings or warm rushes in their limbs and elsewhere. For example, Jane would frequently experience tickling feelings up and down her legs which made it difficult for her to sit still. Other clients report suddenly being aware of focus spots or tensions which appear prior to or at the same time as tics. Some clients also experience what are termed "premonitory urges", which are like rising tensions that either predict or lead on to the tic. These can occur some time before tic onset or they can occur immediately preceding tic onset. Many interpret this as an urge to tic. In either case, after experiencing the urge, the person is likely to feel that the tic is inevitable and react accordingly. But if we look at the reaction, we see that in many ways the reaction to the urge makes it a self-fulfilling prophecy. People tense up, or try to suppress the sensation, or act and prepare as though the tic onset is inevitable.

Similarly, when experiencing a tingling sensation, there is a tendency to move around, fidget or change position to try to contain the movement. Recall what we said earlier about viewing as false friends any behaviors that maintain the tension level. These reactions to sensations fit into this category and maintain higher chronic levels of activation, so you are likely to experience a vicious circle. The more you feel obliged to act, react, tense and move to these sensations, the more you will feel the need to move, since movement actually reinforces the need for stimulation. However, if you just stay calm and relaxed when the sensations arise, the sensation is more likely to decrease and you will feel less need for further movement and stimulation.

This section covers exercises known as "exposure" to help you to tolerate better these sensations or premonitory urges. The first rule of exposure is the law of habituation. This law states that the longer you are exposed to a stimulus or sensation, the more you will get used to it, providing, of course, it is not a dangerous stimulus or that you are not investing effort in maintaining its importance. For example, if you go on holiday, you often hear strange noises on the first night like the apartment fridge clicking on and off, but at the end of the two-week holiday, you have got used to or "habituated" to the noise. Knowing that you will habituate is very useful since it allows you to tolerate the noise better. If you didn't know that eventually you might habituate to the fridge noise, you might pay attention to it all night, cursing and getting irritated. If you did this, apart from being tired, you would impede your habituation.

If you do not react aversely to the sensations, they will go away of their own accord. If you feel it is useful to pay attention to the sensations, remain vigilant and try to put effort into reacting to them in order to diminish their impact. This will make the sensations more significant and more annoying and you become more tense. So, the way to diminish the irritation and importance of the sensations is to ignore them. You can accomplish this result by exposing yourself to the sensation and by (1) not reacting behaviorally to it, (2) not tensing physically, (3) not dwelling on it mentally and, in particular, (4) not saying to yourself: "Oh no, here it comes again, I wish it would go away, I'm never going to feel better, this is a terrible feeling, I'm not normal, etc." Such thinking will also exacerbate the problem since you are giving the sensation a great menacing power which it doesn't really possess unless you provide it.

It is also important to realize that the power you attribute to the sensation has become a thinking habit, so the thought is likely to pop up automatically even before you are aware of it. For example, you may find yourself consciously monitoring your sensation by being vigilant to it long before it appears. In effect, the best way to ignore the sensation is to do absolutely nothing special when it arises. Just carry on with your routine and do not react even a little to the onset of the sensation. You must be careful not to let slip any little old habits, such as making even a small change in limb position to accommodate the sensation. In particular, distracting your attention from the sensation with your routine will ensure that you are not inadvertently feeding it with thoughts like "Has it gone away yet?", "Is it still here?", which mean you are still giving it special attention.

▶ Description of Sensation/Urge

For your own benefit, make a note, in the following style, of your attempts to modify the intensity of your sensation or premonitory urge by changing reactions, thoughts and behavior.

> Old reactions: When my sensation arises, I have the habit of:
> Behavior: . . .
> Emotional reaction: . . .
> Attentional reaction: . . .
> Thinking about it: . . .

You can then make an agreement such as: "Today I will systematically tolerate the sensation until it decreases and go about my daily routine and eliminate my usual reactions to the sensation." Afterwards, estimate your degree of success in eliminating your reactions (0, not successful; 100, very successful); record the length of time the sensation was tolerated; then add your comments.

▶ Preventing the Problem

You will now have enough strategies to prevent the build-up of chronic tension and associated sensations at source. Prevention is the best cure. You must:

(a) remain aware of your state;
(b) practice both the mental and physical exercises to relax your state of activation;
(c) persist in regular practice for the next few weeks.

Once you have practiced sufficiently, preventing tension build-up will become automatic and you won't have to exert conscious effort.

▶   THINKING IN ACTION

▶ Relaxation and Planning Action

You will be aware now of how tension builds up, and how it can develop in everyday life. Although tension is most evident while you are executing movements, the initiation or planning stage is just as important to relaxation. The way in which you plan action can determine whether and where tension builds. An extremely important element to planning is what you anticipate will happen when you act. In the same way that you became aware of the tension that relates to your problem and how to prevent its build-up, so it is essential to become aware of anticipations that precede your problem.

Earlier we identified, along with the high-risk activities for your problem, evaluations of your thoughts and feelings about the activities. Go back to Kelly's grid and Appendix 2h and identify these again. It is these thoughts that lead your muscles to prepare in the way they do for the high-risk situation and we must change your thought habits in the same way that we changed your muscle habits.

▶ Changing Expectations about Actions

Anticipations and expectations are always in the future. So, we use our imagination to predict what we believe is most likely to occur. The problem is that our expectations may be strongly biased by some irrational element or by some episode in the distant past that has no connection with current reality. But this expectation will cloud our judgment and make us prepare for the action inefficiently. In Appendix 2h, you identified the thoughts that precede your problem. Suppose the main worry before you enter a high-risk situation is about being judged by others. Firstly, be specific. Ask yourself exactly what you believe you are being judged on. Why do you think you are being judged like this? Does this relate to some feeling of inadequacy you have had in the past, perhaps as a child? What evidence do you have for thinking others are judging you? Have you had concrete feedback? What are the alternative reactions that others may make besides judging you? Which of the alternatives is more likely than your anticipation of being judged?

▶ The Triple Link between Mind, Body and Emotion

Before we address change in style of action, we need to return to the link between mind and muscle. We noted previously the important role that thinking plays in the management of your problem, and we are now in a position to illustrate this role more precisely. It is not easy to make a clear distinction between mind and body since both are affected by our actions. For example, when we pay attention, it is not just with our mind, but with our eyes and our whole body. If we exercise, our physiology changes and so often does our mood and thinking. In fact, type of thoughts can specifically influence brain activation. Doing a mental calculation will affect a different part of the brain than playing a computer game. Athletes and top performers often practice their performances by visualizing in the mind and this mental practice affects the same physiology as physical activity and can improve performance. However, this triple link between mind, body and emotion (see Figure 7.3) is most evident in the process of preparation for an activity. Such motor preparation is important in our approach to tic management.

Unless you suffer from a neuromuscular disease or have muscular atrophy, all regular tension in your muscles is likely to reflect preparation for action. Now, in the case of, say, opening a door, the preparation is obvious and conscious, but due to a habitual attitude, we can also be unconsciously or habitually preparing for a vague reaction. Such attitudes can also be chronic and some people walk around convinced they need to perpetually prepare themselves for all sorts of eventualities and with muscles tensed like armour. Chronic tension problems will develop in those parts of the body that are most affected by this attitude.

Preparation for action goes through several stages. Firstly, there must be a goal in view; secondly, the person must intentionally plan action; thirdly, the planning must take the form of active preparation to complete the action. Finally, the action is executed, and its outcome determines future action. During all these stages, the relation between brain and muscles is two-way, and the muscles through various sensors give the brain feedback on the status of the action.

Muscles are not just marionettes of the brain, their degree of tension is crucial to effecting and executing a good response, and the tension is partly determined by central impulses and also by external demands and forces. Without a muscle's ability to regulate its tension, effective action can be compromised. Feedback from muscles then helps the brain to regulate its goals.

There are various systems that give feedback on our movement position. Our visual system is, perhaps, the most obvious. We see where we are going and visual cues allow us to adjust movement where necessary. As we've already said, muscle tension can also give feedback on the appropriate force to use in a task. Another system feeds back our feeling and sensation about action. Most of the time, these systems all work in harmony but they can conflict. Indeed, there have been a number of experiments showing, for example, that visual information can trick us into believing we have moved. A good example here is feeling yourself move when you see a train alongside moving away. This conflict is resolved when you ground yourself in your actual feelings of being still. Alternatively, the force with which you throw an object can lead you to believe you have thrown it further than is the case until you look. Strong habitual associations between visual and motor phenomena can also create illusions that if one system is stimulated, so is the other. If an image is paired with a thumb twitch over hundreds of times, eliciting the thumb twitch can elicit an illusion of the image. An action carried out quickly and abruptly is a distinct experience from one more slower and nuanced, and gives a different feel to its action. We've all had the experience of judging by feel that an action was on target, but then finding that it was not so accurate.

However, to complicate the feedback picture, there is another type of control over movement termed "feedforward". In feedforward, we control the future of the movement by planning ahead for what we might encounter later. Our planning carries us forward to action, and a change of plan leads to a change in the preparation for action. The type of movement planned has a great impact on how we guide it and the feedback methods that control it. Movements can vary depending on how automated or controlled the action. We spoke earlier in the book about the important function that habits play in allowing some of our actions to run on automatic pilot. However, even within an action, some aspects are automatic and some more controlled, which means we need to balance these two modes of action in the preparation and execution of action. For example, if I decide I need to pick up a mug of coffee and drink it, the action of picking up the mug might be more controlled than the subsequent sipping which may be more automatic and permit my mind to be occupied with other tasks.

There are various reasons why a task may be done in a more controlled than automated fashion. One reason may be its novelty, another may be the complexity of the task demand itself, a third may be the importance of the task, or the importance of the consequences if it is not done properly. The advantage of automated mode is that since it is automated, it can be carried out quickly, without much attentional effort, or feedforward adjustment, and pass through all feedback stages to feedback on execution. The disadvantage is that automatic actions reach a point of no return much earlier than controlled tasks and are much more difficult to inhibit.

However, although some subcomponents, even the majority, in an action may be automatic, all automatic actions form part of a larger intentional action or movement. I may, for example, drive to work each day on automatic pilot, but this action is part of a larger intentional action decision to go to work. In a similar way, muscles never operate in complete isolation of one another, and the activity in one muscle often depends on the activity in other muscles remote from the site of action. The principle applies particularly to reflexes which require a certain planned level of activity in surrounding muscle groups in order to occur.

Heart rate and respiration are automatic reflexes generally beyond my control, yet the way I approach a situation can determine their rate. Similarly, my posture can affect the intensity of knee or spinal reflexes. On the other hand, even the most controlled action must arrive eventually a split second before its execution at an automated point of no return. So, in one sense we could say that every apparent involuntary action is set up by a preceding or surrounding voluntary behavior, or, conversely, that even the most controlled action must, in order to function, contain reflex-like subcomponents. In normal action, we try to keep a balance between all these aspects of action, automated, controlled, feedforward–feedback, planning and executing, visual versus feeling feedback. However, several aspects of use can cause conflicts in the normal flow of action.

At the planning level, we can be preparing action for two distinct and often conflicting goals. For example, to perform a task both as quickly and as accurately as possible, or to be as automated and controlled as possible. I could be preparing to do a correct action in the wrong way since what to do and how to do it are separate stages of motor operation. I could prepare the wrong muscles, or prepare more muscles than necessary, or put too much effort into preparation. There could then be problems with feedback guiding actions in the course of movement. The wrong modality of feedback could be used as information, or modalities of feedback could give conflicting information. The movement system could inform the brain that body position is fine, but the visual system could signal that the position needs correction, while the feeling system could be saying that the feel of the whole task is not correct.

There could be conflict between feedforward and feedback systems, the feedforward preparing for a stage of action not yet reached, while the feedback system feeds back information from a previous stage. Then there is conflict between an automated action wishing to advance quickly to the point of no return, the controlled system holding back saying "not yet". For example, if I carry out a complex action too quickly and forcibly, I may not have the chance to correct the subtle eye–hand coordination, and I will experience more a "feeling" type of feedback. A small amount of these conflicts is not a big deal since, in any case, it is impossible to just activate one muscle or one mode of action in complete isolation, and there is likely to be some redundancy of movement and interplay of conflicting sources in all our actions.

But excessive conflict in muscle use and preparation can lead to suboptimal performance. In the worse case, it can paralyze movement or lead to chronic sustained tension. Subjectively speaking, when we do not perform as we intend, we often experience impatience, frustration or even rage. This emotion, of course, then further compounds the blocked action since we are likely to try to force our action and hence make the system more unstable and out of control. In some circumstances, particularly where too much effort is applied or there is a conflict of goals and planning does not lead naturally to execution, the muscle system needs to try to correct itself. This correction most effectively takes the form of tense–release cycles and these, when over-learned and habitual, can become tics (Table 7.1). There is evidence that people with tics tend to over-invest in their movement, often they exert too much effort in a task, or they use irrelevant muscle groups to complete the task or they try to do too much, or try to carry out two tasks at the same time. Such conflict produces chronic tension which, in turn, leads to tense–release tic cycles to release the tension.

For example, Frank, who suffers a mouth tic, is determined not to be late for an appointment, but, on the other hand, he hates to waste time, so he wants to do as much as possible before leaving for the appointment and does not want to arrive too early. So, he uses his time until the last possible minute before leaving for the appointment. He ends up rushing to the appointment in automated fashion, but in this automated mode, he is not well equipped to deal with unforeseen events

Table 7.1   Example of negative belief leading to frustration–action tic cycle

Tic	Head and neck tic
↑	
Frustrated action	I'm not sure exactly where to turn and what movement to make next
↑	
Specific preparation	I'll also get ready to leave in case the going gets tough
↑	
General preparation	I'll keep myself generally tensed, ready for any unforeseen response
↑	
Forward plan	I'm going to keep to myself and monitor all my actions
↑	
Anticipation	I feel very uncomfortable going to parties
↑	
Belief	People are always judging others

on the way. He finds it difficult to negotiate a correction in his action plan due to a road closure or an accident. He cannot easily implement a change in attitude, since he has the idea that he must arrive on time and must reach his appointment as quickly as possible. His feedback mode is relying on feel rather than visual environmental cues, so he gets into a frustrated action cycle rather than reorient and revise his action. The frustration makes him try harder to adapt his circumstances to his plans of rushing to the appointment, and he becomes even more tense. As a consequence, his mouth muscles tighten, perhaps because he feels like cursing or complaining. But these muscles are not useful in his rushing mode, so they just stay tense and prepare for action. The tension leaves the face muscles in a stage of constant preparation which eventually leads the muscle into a tense–release cycle to maintain the preparation. This quick tense–release cycle becomes the tic and its role is to recalibrate the muscle tension to permit it to remain tense and prepared. The frustration–action conflict then can be set up by an initial attitude, "I must do things this way", "The time cannot be changed", "It's impossible that I am late", which subsequently confounds the feedforward intentional stage of planning action.

▶ Exercises

Monitor yourself when you perform actions during the day to see if any of the motor strategies given in Appendix 2g apply. When you are performing everyday actions, are you investing too much effort? Are parts of your body doing jobs they need not do? Is your face or tongue helping you to lift up a suitcase? Are your legs helping your hand to write a letter? Are your shoulders helping your eyes to read a book?

The following are more active exercises to test your economy of movement.

1. Stop an action, such as getting out of a chair, or writing, and freeze in a time frame. Then monitor all the tensions present in your body. Are they all relevant to the task?
2. Imagine yourself about to perform an action and see which muscles spontaneously tense up.

3. Perform an action under time pressure, then without time pressure, to see the difference in tension level.
4. Deliberately tense non-relevant muscles in an action to see the difference in performance compared to a time when these non-relevant muscles are relaxed.
5. Perform an action that is usually automated such as knitting, playing the piano, tying up your shoe lace, and then stop mid-way and focus on each element of the task to make it a more controlled action. How does this affect the performance and the feeling?
6. Try to prepare to do two different tasks where normally you would only plan for one, for example, writing with a pen, but also holding it as firmly as possible. What effect is there on performance?

► RETHINKING YOUR THINKING

As you will know from our model, the most important aspect of the program is to prevent the appearance of the tic by restructuring the background behavior associated with tic onset. In this sense, our program differs from other programs such as HR in that we try to avoid implementing more strategies to resist, contain or impede the tic once it has occurred. In order to change your style of action, we need, in accordance with the motor model of action discussed earlier, to consider all preceding stages of movement prior to the tic onset, including planning and intention, in order to modify the movement and tension. Movement involves several stages: contemplating, planning general preparation, specific preparation and execution at the point of no return.

So, let us start with the thinking stage. Thoughts are also habits; they can become automatic and rigid and we can enter into a pattern of thinking, without really consciously thinking about our thinking. For example, we may go to see a colleague or friend and immediately thoughts about him or her will come into our head (e.g., a negative memory from the last visit) and may determine our attitude to the visit. So, our first task is to look at any automatic thoughts associated with performing high-risk activities.

In the previous exercises, we identified and linked thinking, emotion and tension associated with each high-risk activity. Now we need to capture the thinking more finely. As noted earlier, automatic thoughts come into our head naturally and we assume that they are the only way of thinking and are essentially correct. Obviously, the thoughts encourage us to plan and act and so experience in a set way, to which we also habituate. The problem sometimes is that one thought chains onto another thought and before long, if we accept the validity of the first thought, we become further and further embedded in the credibility of subsequent thoughts which may be far from valid.

Imagine you are with a group of strangers and the thought comes into your head automatically that they could judge you badly. Perhaps this is a fear you've had since childhood. Anyway, as a consequence of accepting this thought as valid, you begin to be vigilant to see if others are watching you. You see a group talking and looking in your direction. You interpret this to mean they are talking about you. This thought makes you even more nervous and uneasy. You try to compose yourself and act normally, but this only encourages the feeling that you are being watched and you begin to feel tense and worked up. Subsequently, you may develop an anticipation for all similar situations, and this will make you tense and nervous even before you enter the situation.

Your anticipations about an action, then, are a crucial guiding factor for all actions. They decide the intention of your activity and affect its outcome. We already noted earlier that an action depends on feedforward, that is, purpose and intent to achieve its goal. This is largely influenced by psychological factors, reflecting, for example, degree of confidence in outcome, but also anticipation of the consequences of action at different stages.

Frequently, if we anticipate too much, we can almost live and repeat the action to its conclusion in our mind, before we have even started. This can have good or bad effects. Frequently, in sport, it is helpful for sports people to anticipate and visualize their action to perfect their real performance. But, of course, this could work negatively; if you are always anticipating negative outcomes, this may discourage your planning and preparation since you think it can only lead to negative outcomes.

Anticipations are essential to guide actions, so we need to use them in the correct way. However, anticipations, although they guide the outcome of our actions and lead the body to prepare in a certain way, are themselves linked to wider beliefs we hold about actions. Whereas the anticipations are automatic, the wider beliefs may be consciously held but are nonetheless habitual. They may also be irrational and based on selective subjective impressions we have built up over the years which do not really reflect present reality.

Table 7.2 shows the link between irrational beliefs and negative anticipations. You can see how a general belief determines an activity-specific anticipation which leads to a negative behavior: inability to relax; feeling ill at ease; difficulty communicating. You can probably add in your own chain of thoughts relevant to your tic behavior. Begin with the way you experience the tic activity, and trace this back to the anticipation. Now ask what wider belief the anticipation fits into?

Table 7.2 Example of how irrational beliefs affect anticipations of action through generating negative consequences

Irrational belief	Negative anticipation	Negative consequences
People who take the time to relax are lazy	Even if I try to relax, I won't be able	I am never able to relax
One must always appear perfect to be respected	Others will judge me stupid if I make the slightest error	I feel ill at ease in the company of others
Pleasing other people is more important than being yourself	If I say what I really think, I'll lose all my friends	I watch what I say and never express my opinions

▶ How Can I Change My Thoughts?

In Appendix 2i, you will find a form with three columns. This technique, an adaptation of the triple-column technique from cognitive therapy, allows us to highlight the irrationality of our thoughts and modify them. Let's say you believe that relaxing is a waste of time. Photocopy or download the appendix and write your habitual belief in the first column. In the second column, you confront your belief by testing out its validity. "Is the belief true in all situations?" "Is what I believe supported by others?" "What led me to believe this?" Finally, the big question, "Is there another way of viewing events in a less negative way? For example, couldn't I say that people who take the time to relax are more efficient?"

Now, the new belief that you place in the third column is new to you and you probably don't really believe it. However, now you must seek evidence to support each belief. For example, can you find people who relax who are efficient? What evidence is there that relaxing is lazy? What do others believe? Often, just articulating a less negative alternative will help to highlight the inadaptive nature of the first belief. Try to do this exercise for each belief derived from the evaluations identified with each high-risk activity. Then, in your copy of Appendix 2i, fill in appropriate anticipations and consequences following on from the *new* alternative belief, and compare these with the original anticipations. Which set is the more desirable?

▶ Example of Catherine

Catherine, who has a face tic, plans has to attend a reception. She gets tense just thinking about the strangers she will meet and who she must talk to. She is convinced that she won't feel well and that she won't feel well for the whole evening and she'll have difficulty concentrating. She won't be able to say or respond as she wishes and her tic will appear often. She is convinced that she looks odd and that people judge her badly and talk about her. She has, behind this anticipation, a strong belief that people always judge others critically, that they always notice defaults, and that the least error causes people to think others are stupid. Consequently, since she's not perfect, they will find her stupid.

She realizes that this is a belief she has had since childhood, without really challenging it. When she was young, her parents were very critical of her, often highlighting her negative points at the expense of her positive points. However, recently with her current friends and social circle, she couldn't recall one instance where she had been openly criticized. However, she was still continually anticipating this reaction. So, she felt it was time to replace this belief with an alternative that "people do not constantly look for errors in others to judge them badly". She tested out both beliefs by getting feedback from friends, going over her experience to see which belief fitted best, and she came down in favour of the new belief. The new belief led to a new set of anticipations and expected outcome. She anticipated people to be less focused on her and more respectful of her comments, and this led her to expect herself to feel more open and comfortable. When she adopted this new belief, she found immediately that she was more relaxed in anticipating social events, since her tic was abating and she wasn't jumping to negative conclusions. She also found that she was more able to focus on what others were saying, so profiting more from the encounters and reinforcing her new view that people were friendly and non-judgmental.

▶ BELIEFS RELEVANT TO PLANNING ACTION

We now cover in detail some typical beliefs that we have found particularly relevant to tic experiences, and how to cognitively challenge them. Most of these beliefs have a particular relevance to the way people with tics organize actions, as identified from the STOP questionnaire. Let's take some typical items you may have identified as relevant to your style of action. For example, the tendency to try to do too much at once. Do you have a tendency to try to fill up your agenda as much as possible? Or if you are going out to visit a friend, do you try to fit in as many other jobs on the way? Maybe you tell yourself it is more efficient like that. We live in a high-stress world and we have to get as much done as quickly as possible. For sure, some tasks need to be done quickly, but is it necessary to try to do many tasks at the same time? Some beliefs underlying this style might be: To be efficient, I have to be always on the go. It's important I appear to be efficient by doing a lot. If I don't do a lot and keep busy, I won't be able to function.

Again, it is easy to see how each of these beliefs could lead to an anticipation of how to act in a daily situation where there are several jobs to do, and consequently induce high tension levels associated with activity. Frequently, people who are always on the go are too stressed to appreciate the acts they are completing. Often, they are not centered completely in the present but more focused on the future task ahead. So, in everyday functioning terms, being always on the go is not necessarily efficient.

Each of the three sample beliefs above can be challenged by a more appropriate belief about prioritizing actions, completing them properly and not being rushed. A related organization problem is always feeling the need to move, whether in an activity or not. The person may feel incapable of paying attention, performing or concentrating on activities properly unless he or she is moving legs, body, or otherwise being stimulated by loud music or distractions. In terms of our model, the person is feeding the stimulation level by offering more stimulation rather than reducing the degree of activation, and so reducing the need to be aroused. Accompanying beliefs are often: I will fall asleep if I'm not stimulated. I won't be able to concentrate properly unless I'm active. The job is too boring and I need to be fully occupied to be attentive.

However, these are also usually beliefs that have not been put to the test and, of course, are self-perpetuating because the person never acts otherwise. But if you believe that calming yourself will help get rid of the need for stimulation, you can attend in the following fashion.

Focus on relaxing your muscles and breathing properly. Direct your eyes, head and body towards the aim of your attention. Immerse your attention visually in the task. If thoughts come in to distract you, do not yield to them but keep your attention fixed, keeping a distance from the distractions. Another problem linked with continuous movement and activation is the inability to relax, or, more correctly, we should term this the lack of permission to relax. In such cases, even when people try to relax, their mind won't permit it and it often feels as though their head is racing with ideas. People sometimes have a black and white notion of relaxing, saying either, "I am active, busy and productive" or "I am a 'jello'". In such a case, it may be that relaxing is considered a waste of time, almost sinful.

Some people also have difficulty staying still. They feel the need to be constantly in movement. They often say that they feel tingling or a sensory discomfort if they do not move all the time, without realizing that the movement may well produce this sensation. One client had what appeared to be involuntary vocal sounds coming out of her throat every minute or so. This turned out to be an exaggerated burp, brought about by her constant fidgeting and gulping during meals, and an inability to keep still. The belief here was, "I must keep moving, otherwise I will feel uncomfortable, ill at ease, irritable", but such constant agitation only raised her muscle tension. Unfortunately, usually when such people try to keep still, they do so by tensing and resisting muscle movements. But, actually, it is better to practice resting calmly without moving, to pay attention and monitor the parts of your body that move, to focus on relaxing them or putting them into contact with a surface that gives you sensory feedback on movement and allows you to appreciate the stillness (see Table 4.4).

Are you always trying to do tasks too quickly? Are you always anxious to be finished before you have begun? Perhaps you begin several tasks at once because you become impatient with the speed at which tasks are done. Do you talk or walk too quickly, or try to grab things too tightly and quickly and knock them over? People who rush tasks generally do them less well, and make themselves stressed at the same time. You also have less control but, more importantly, you lose out on the process of accomplishing and experiencing the moment of performing the task. People often believe they have to get over such jobs as soon as possible and then they will feel all right. But slowing down the rhythm of performing relieves the tension and also leaves you feeling more relaxed with a feeling of accomplishment and well-being.

▶ Perfectionism

People with tics often have very strict expectations about themselves and sometimes others, mainly about their personal standards, organization and self-image. They are not so perfectionist about performance or making mistakes. Perfectionists are generally not satisfied with the way things are organized, and are always pushing themselves to be more punctual, more tidy, more organized, and to do more during the day. They are very severe with themselves and feel they must take responsibility for unforeseen events that are outside their control. They are often very intolerant of any change in plan or the unexpected. Perfectionism can lead to a fear of doing the job and the person may avoid it, or deliberately rush it, in order to be able to say they weren't themselves when they did it, and so disclaim responsibility for not being perfect. They also set the bar at too high a level and have a tendency to magnify any defects.

The triple-column technique can be useful to change beliefs about "perfect" performance by replacing "perfect" with "human" and accepting a functional definition

Table 7.3 Perfectionist beliefs relevant to tic disorders

- People who look relaxed appear lazy
- If you are not on the go all the time, you are not performing well
- Wasting time is terrible
- Cramming as much as possible into a day means looking efficient
- If you are not quick, you appear stupid
- Doing several things at the same time is being productive
- Either I'm active all the time or I'm a jello
- People are judging your performance all the time, you can't let up for a moment
- I feel under pressure to make a good impression and can never be myself
- It's important to always look ahead to the next job to be well prepared
- I need to invest more effort than others to be good
- I feel under pressure to please people or they will get annoyed and irritated
- You need to take into account as much as possible every aspect in your planning

of perfection as a task done as it needs to be done. Do you like your affairs to be just so? Do you get irritable if objects or people are not completely in your expected order? People who are perfectionist sometimes feel they must control everything. In practice, we cannot control other people or events; we can only make sure that we are prepared to adapt optimally to what occurs.

People with perfectionist tendencies often think they will be held responsible for all sorts of events that are really out of their control. They invest enormous effort to ensure that the future is 100% under control. Ironically, this perfectionist attitude leaves such people less and less in control of their lives, since they invest a lot of time and concern with ordering events and feelings and less on what really matters. They may also live in chaos since they will not attempt to finish a job unless they feel it will be 100% perfect (see Table 7.3).

Try to challenge your perfectionist thoughts by asking yourself: "Am I taking on too much responsibility?" "Are the consequences of my actions really as I imagine?" "Why is it important for me to always organize myself just so?"

▶ Inhibition

People with tics often have problems with inhibition. This may take the form of over-preoccupation with inhibition at one time when they are unsure of responding, and not being able to inhibit at another time, when jumping into tasks too quickly with fast automatic styles of action. Sometimes, people with tics also inhibit emotions and expressions, and this can lead to tensions (Table 7.3). Certain tense–release tic movements can be provoked by chronic inhibition. This was the case with Paul, who moved his mouth and contracted his lips rather than say what he felt. Other people may just hold themselves rigid, afraid that they will perform inappropriate acts or gestures. There is a belief often in people with tics that they do not have permission to be themselves, and not just because they have tics. It's a more general belief that they may be judged or criticized or be considered odd and stupid, or will deeply hurt others, as they are often sensitive to others' feelings. But this inhibition only leads to frustration and, frequently, the person with the tic will become super-frustrated with his or her own inhibition and feel the need to let

Table 7.4   Examples of everyday styles of action

- Attempting to complete six appointments in the same day, resulting in late appointments, rushing around and frustration
- Wanting to give the impression of efficiency by never taking a break, and taking on several jobs at once
- Tensing all muscles when paying attention on driving, so causing muscle ache
- Speaking too quickly for fear of appearing unintelligent if speaking slowly
- Moving around and changing posture when working for fear of falling asleep
- Keeping mind always busy with thoughts due to feeling, otherwise will be bored or not on the ball
- Feeling need to maintain high activation level through stimulation
- Unable to be present in the here and now due to daydreaming of other or next situation
- Experiencing conflict over which job to start first and feeling all should be done immediately
- Trying to watch oneself do a task at the same time as doing it, trying to see oneself as others see you
- Feeling you want to leave the present task or situation but being unable to do so
- Feeling all the time under pressure to not do or say all you want because you can't be yourself

it out. Rather than keep emotions pent up, it's better to communicate and express them, since what you fear will seldom happen in any case. If you express yourself correctly, you will be better received and real feedback is always better than what your imagination conjures up if you keep it suppressed.

Do you have difficulty expressing yourself? Some movement problems, as we discussed earlier, result from over-inhibiting yourself. We gave the example of Paul who moved his mouth a lot, instead of speaking his mind. Are your actions a result of keeping emotions in? Is this your style of interaction? Do you let things simmer inside rather than express yourself? Again, start off by going back to the thinking exercises in Appendices 2h and 2i. What do you believe will be the consequences of expressing yourself? What feedback have you had on these consequences? Try expressing yourself in a reasonable and appropriate tone and see what happens.

Communication is always better than building up a spiral of frustration on the basis of what you think might happen. The frustration gets bigger and more imaginative and the reality gets further away.

► MOTOR AND BEHAVIORAL RESTRUCTURING

Now that we have challenged the beliefs associated with the high-risk situations, and replaced them with more realistic beliefs, it becomes easier to construct an alternative way of behaving, which is in accord with the new belief. If you now think people are friendly, you can enter a situation calmly, be yourself and look a person in the eyes. So, every aspect of the planning and preparation can be revised.

We return to the behavioral elements of action to see how they can be revised in accordance with the different goals of movements. When you decide to approach the high-risk activity, you will be changing your behavior globally. This begins with your belief about the situation, your anticipation and your intentional movements. An important point is that your movements should be in accord with your intentions, there should be no conflict, no hesitancy. The larger movements like posture control the smaller movements because they permit the movements to take place.

Basically, your best bet is to prevent the tic arriving by avoiding the tension and, hence, the behavior producing the tension. In other words, you act in a manner antagonist to your old tension-producing habit. The aim, of course, is that you have more flexibility, options and control in cognitive, muscle and behavioral systems, which leads you unnecessarily into a tension mode. At each stage of your action, you have the degree of freedom to rethink and reorient your action plan. We now list some techniques that can help you to see how you can change your habitual responses.

► Prevention by Relaxation

The first technique is prevention by relaxation. Before you enter the situation, focus on relaxing the muscle that would normally be involved in your tic. Make sure you keep it at a relaxed level (remember the discrimination exercise). Focus on keeping as wide an area of the muscle relaxed as possible. If you feel it becoming tense, immediately relax it, and don't forget to breathe normally. If the tic seems to be on the point of occurring, remember that nothing is inevitable and immediately relax the muscle. Gradually, you will develop the habit of always being relaxed. For those with vocal or throat tics, the relaxation prevention may need to focus on respiration.

This involves monitoring the affected muscle to ensure that if tension build-up does occur, you can dispose of it quickly. This is particularly appropriate for tics and tensions. Using your awareness and relaxation training, you can verify that your muscle is relaxed before you enter a situation and check every five minutes or so just to make sure. If the tic occurs, despite all precautions to keep it relaxed, then immediately relax the muscles around the one affected. It will help if you keep completely still while doing this. Gradually, you will become more proficient, and you will be able to detect the tic or movement and relax it before it can be fully developed.

This exercise requires you to catch every tic and remember to relax the muscle throughout the day.

► Normalizing the Response

This approach to prevention depends on the type of tic or movement. The first point to establish is whether your tic is an exaggeration of a normal response. For example, excessive blinking might be caused by the person not realizing that he or she can blink using just the eyelid muscles. Likewise, a tension in the shoulders may have resulted from too much effort in an otherwise normal response. Are you moving your whole head when you need only move your eyes? Are your mouth movements exaggerated speech actions?

You will discover surplus effort from your own self-observation and from our evaluations of the risk situations that you have identified. If your blinking, or movement or tension takes place in situations where such a response would normally develop, then it is probably an exaggeration. Practice the action slowly and reduce the movement using the appropriate muscles. Watch what muscles other people use in the same response and copy them.

▶ Prevention Through a Competing Action

This is a technique developed by Nathan Azrin and colleagues and essentially it involves activating the muscle "antagonistic" to the muscle causing the twitch. Whatever direction your muscle is pulled by the tic or movement, you check this movement and deliberately contract the muscle in the opposite direction. This means waiting until the movement occurs, then implementing the "antagonist" action immediately. If your head tics to the left, you pull it to the right; or if your cheek tics upwards, you relax it downwards, thus competing with the tic and checking it. If you choose to use the competing muscle response you should follow the points below (we suggest here, however, that once you have checked the tic you immediately relax both muscles).

1. Choose a contraction that is socially acceptable.
2. Practice the response on its own for about 10 minutes a day before applying it to the tic.
3. Try to make the antagonist movement as small and as crisp as possible.
4. Make the competing response just intense enough to prevent the action taking off and no more.
5. Don't implicate superfluous muscles and do not strain.
6. If you realize you missed a tic, implement the competing action anyway – better late than never.
7. Try to implant the idea of the competing or antagonist action in your mind before you go into a situation so that you know automatically what to do.
8. Carry out and sustain the action for several minutes after tic onset.
9. Devise an antagonist action that is appropriate and does not attract attention.
10. Make sure you do not force the action and create more tension.
11. Only use the action to prevent tic onset, do not use it continuously to become another habit.
12. Plan the alternative action well in advance so that you know automatically what you must do in the situation and can immediately apply it.

This antagonistic contraction must be imperceptible and not excessively raise tension or, of course, become another tic. This method may be especially useful for long and violent tics which need to be contained. Table 4.4 gives examples of competing relaxing actions for different muscle groups.

▶ Restructuring Behavior

We have stressed in this manual that your movement is best seen in a wider context of how you are managing action, and we suggest that as well as concentrating on the movement itself, you look at the significance of any competing actions in order to find a competing response that involves an overall change to your action in the situation. This will often involve a change in posture and ideas about the high-risk situation, and involves a combination of physical and cognitive strategies.

If, in your evaluation, you realized that your expectancies in a certain situation were that others were judging you, and your underlying feeling was one of hostility, then with the cognitive restructuring of belief this evaluation can be altered to an expectation of friendliness – and you can adopt appropriate behavioral strategies to go with this feeling. Mathew, who had a head-turning tic, never engaged others in eye contact. By adopting the strategy of eye contact, he acted in accordance with his redefinition of the situation as friendly and developed at the same time an antagonist response, since he could not both make eye contact and move his head away. (See case example below.)

Mariette, who fiddled continuously with her fingers when watching television, found this was distracting her concentration, so she made sure that she sat still and, in particular, kept her hand occupied on her lap throughout her TV viewing. This activated a competing response but in the context of a change in approach to watching TV. (See case study below.)

The important rules for implementing cognitive-behavioral restructuring are:

1. Identify attitudes and expectancies you have towards the situation.
2. Establish the alternatives and more realistic attitudes and expectancies?
3. Implement the behavior that goes with these alternatives?
4. Ensure this new behavior an "antagonist" to the occurrence of the tic habit?

We hence encourage you with your therapist to script an alternative behavior in each high-risk tic activity that takes account of changes in thinking patterns, emotions and behavior. The new script of how to restructure behavior should be aimed at preventing tension build-up and, by definition, implementing strategies that are antagonistic to old tension-producing habits. The application of the method involves detailing in the script changes in planning, preparation, feedback, execution and evaluation of action, and is illustrated in the following examples. The new script should therefore contain details about: how I will plan and set goals differently; how I will approach the situation, posture, tension, movement; how I anticipate feeling in the situation; how I expect my behavior to be received by others; how I will judge and seek feedback on my actions; where I expect to feel tensions appropriate to the actions; the rhythm and control over my actions; which acts will be automated and which controlled; how I will evaluate overall performance and move onto the next task.

► Case Examples

Mathew

Mathew had a head tic and was constantly abruptly turning his head to the left. The tic was particularly obvious when he was in conversation and it had the effect of preventing him having eye contact with other people. By confronting his anticipation that he would be rejected, he came up with a different anticipation, namely that people would be content to return his look with a smile. He is now able to approach people without feeling that there is a reason to be prepared to be ignored, and he is more open in his encounters and appreciates the importance of facial expression and communication. His new way of approaching the situation includes maintaining an upright posture and addressing others face to face. Because he wishes to maintain visual fixation, he keeps his head straight and balances tension in his neck; by using this technique he is not pulled either way, and doesn't turn away when speaking. This new response is incompatible with the tic but goes along with his more adaptive cognitive-behavioral restructuring and redefinition of his activity.

Mariette

Mariette was in the habit of continually rubbing her fingers together when watching TV. She realized that the rubbing was more a distraction than an aid to listening. However, she also discovered that she felt uneasy just relaxing in front of the TV. For her, watching TV was a waste of time and she felt guilty when relaxing. However, she challenged this thought and replaced it with the alternative that periods of relaxation are important to good functioning. The alternative proved the more realistic approach for her needs and quality of life. Subsequently, she decided to allocate periods of time when she would only relax. In these periods, she made sure she sat comfortably in her sofa with her limbs and hands relaxed and in contact with the surface to make sure she rested calmly, and allowed herself to be absorbed in the TV program she was watching. Hence, relaxing and placing her hands comfortably on the sofa arms was incompatible with rubbing her fingers but, as in Mathew's case, it fitted into an overall cognitive-behavioral restructuring.

Marc

Marc had a simple tic affecting his left shoulder which would appear particularly when he was under pressure to complete his work. In these situations, he felt impatient and frustrated and his shoulder would ride up and down, contracted around his ear. However, Marc had always feared being seen as unproductive, despite no evidence or feedback to this effect. Hence, he would always be trying to do as much as possible as quickly as possible. When Marc challenged his way of thinking, he realized that his style of action actually made him nervous every time he needed to complete a task. Furthermore, it made him appear nervous and agitated in the eyes of others, plus, of course, making his tic onset more likely. Also, he wasted a lot of time worrying if he would accomplish all of his tasks. His alternative thought was that he would succeed in meeting his deadlines, since he always did so, and would do so more efficiently if he didn't prepare in such an intense fashion. He scheduled his assignments at a realistic rhythm with the revised and realistic expectation that he would complete each in a reasonable time. He worked particularly on relieving the tension in his arm, shoulders and neck, which seemed to form part of his drive to be always further ahead. He approached the job in a more upright sitting position, focusing on relaxing neck and shoulders while he concentrated, and was careful to limit his actions to dealing with the current task and dealing with other problems as they presented themselves one at a time, and not on the basis of anticipation with the feeling that he needed to rush ahead. Also, he carefully monitored his muscle activation prior to his writing or keying on the computer to ensure that he was not involving irrelevant muscles or movements.

▶ **Summary**

In summary, the procedure for cognitive-motor restructuring of behavior can be represented as:

Identify your anticipations in high-risk tic situations

↓

Discover more general beliefs underlying these anticipations

↓

Construct an alternative belief, which is less stressful, about the best way to act or organize

↓

Using the triple-column technique, test to find the belief that is most realistic

↓

Choose a set of behaviors and attitudes more suited to this new realistic belief

↓

Ensure that your tension level and muscle use reflect this new attitude in enactment of everyday activities

▶ **MAINTAINING THE NEW BEHAVIOR**

The new habit can be installed in a matter of a few weeks but we advise you to keep actively practicing for up to three months. It is particularly important to be especially vigilant during periods of high stress, since there is a tendency to revert back to earlier patterns of behavior at that time. Also, when new situations arise that are similar to old high-risk ones, but are novel versions, be careful to apply the strategies you have learned.

If you have several movement problems, it is advised that you tackle each problem one by one. Please address another movement when you feel you have mastered the first movement habit. We encourage you to draw a graph from your diary to monitor progress. You can compare the graph after the program (see Appendix 5) with your original self-observation. If you feel there is a greater than 90% improvement in your control of your problem in the targeted habit, then go on to the next habit, but continue practicing control of the first habit.

► Feedback

Feedback on your new performance is especially important to changing your habit since it rewards you for changing your habit and immediately tells you how well you did.

The first type of feedback is self-feedback. Ask yourself each day:

1. Is my problem worse or better? By how much?
2. By what degree has my control improved?
3. How confident am I that I will gain more control?
4. Do I feel overall more relaxed and comfortable?

Apart from your objective observations on the frequency of your problem, you can also note how your confidence about other aspects of your life has increased and whether this has led to more successful outcomes in your personal affairs and relations. Has your success in control of your muscle problem led to your changing other habits or lifestyles?

Another source of feedback is the comments of others around you, family, friends, associates. Often, people will give you their encouraging remarks unsolicited, but if not, try to get feedback from them, and their comments on how your appearance has changed.

Sensory feedback is also important. This involves getting direct physiological feedback from your new posture or movement about its new state. You may be able to check your relaxed state mentally or manually. Use the environmental surfaces around you to give you feedback on your posture and muscle state. Otherwise, keeping your muscles in contact with a third surface – perhaps another muscle, or a table top, or a pillow – can give feedback on relaxation. Small movements or tension in the feet and hands can be monitored by contact with a flat surface.

Remember the importance of all types of feedback in maintaining new brain and muscle patterns.

► What Not to Do

We have already noted in an earlier section that it is not a good idea to persevere with old coping strategies. The way *not* to try to prevent your response is by doing anything that will create more conflict or tension. There is sometimes a tendency during behavioral restructuring for people employing other antagonist actions to put *too* much physical force into it, out of keenness and desire to get ahead. Putting effort into changing your habit does not mean forcing it. The idea is to relax the tension and the *less tension* you apply, the more pleasantly and easily you acquire the new habit.

You must practice persistently and regularly in order to install the new habit. Doing it in an irregular way or once in a while is of no benefit. Your self-monitoring will help you realize that tic frequency and intensity vary from day to day according to activity and mood, so don't give up if you have a bad day; persist and you will succeed.

► CONCLUSIONS

Congratulations on successfully reducing the frequency, intensity of your tic and increasing your degree of control over your tic by implementing the strategies of the program and preventing its arrival. If you have not yet arrived at 100% control, it is important to identify why not. This may be a question of practice or it may mean modifying some strategies. Or again, maybe you did not have enough time in the program to cover all aspects of your tic behavior.

It is important that you persist with your new strategies. Persistence is the key to success and even if you have good or bad days, persistence in applying the strategies will eventually prove worth while and you will feel comfortable with your new way of thinking and acting. If you have problems remembering to practice, probably the best solution is to leave yourself notes or other reminders to prompt your memory. You will need to be vigilant about your practice for the next few months, but at a certain point it will just become a habit to not tic.

It is particularly important to be vigilant in applying the strategies during stressful moments or when you are tired, or when you are excited or on holiday or faced with an entirely new situation. It may be worth sitting down now and reflecting on any situations that might be likely to resemble your high-risk situations in order to be better prepared. If you do have a bad day and you find you have momentarily relapsed into a bad way of acting, do not despair, and ask yourself the following questions:

- What was the reason for my relapse?
- What strategies did I not employ?
- How can this knowledge help me to prevent relapse in the future?

If you have completed the program successfully serious relapses are unlikely, but if you feel that you may need a "refresher", you should always be ready to reread and re-enact strategies given in the program.

We advise that you deal thoroughly with one tic before progressing to another. But the application of the program to another tic or habit follows the same principles as the first application, and should be smoother given your prior experience. An important part of relapse prevention is giving yourself continuous feedback on your performance.

It is important you reward yourself for your efforts and remember to highlight what you have accomplished, not just what rests to do. Remember that the glass can be half-full or half-empty, but which you choose can affect your mood and optimism.

It may now also be a good idea to change other aspects of your life for the better, perhaps to quit smoking, take up exercises, begin a new hobby. It is important to get positive feedback for your new-found tension-free life, by perhaps exposing yourself to situations or activities that previously you may have avoided. Increase in confidence helps to avoid relapse. You can even seek opinions on your new habit from others you trust. Encouraging sympathetic remarks from close and trusted others provide good positive feedback.

At the same time, you must be aware of situations or states that might inadvertently lead you to put too much effort, or to adopt a tension-provoking posture. Also, even though you know you will function well in a situation, it could be that your anticipations are still out of synchrony with this fact and you anticipate worse than the reality, and, as we know, anticipation can produce tension. So, it is important to catch here any old automatic anticipations and modify the anticipation to be less tension-producing and more positive.

The type of events likely to lead to relapse are: fatigue; positive and negative stress; depression or just feeling sad; too occupied; ill; major environment or life changes; traumatizing event; alcohol; drugs; interpersonal conflict; all sentiments of insecurity. See all relapses as temporary rather than a catastrophe, and refer to the manual at the appropriate place if you feel unsure of a strategy. Define yourself more and more as someone who does not tic and is not a tic sufferer since most of your life is now non-tic.

Final Counsels

1. Be aware of your tension level at all times as well as your anticipations, particularly in difficult situations.
2. Be conscious of the continual coupling between thought, mood and action.
3. Continue regular application of strategies.
4. Be flexible in your approach to action, particularly a habitual action.
5. If you have a bad day, don't despair, consider what strategies you need to revise.

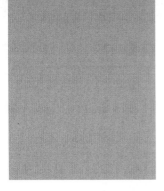

APPENDICES

*Appendices containing material to be answered by
the clients should be photocopied or downloaded. Clients should not
write their answers or comments directly on the pages
of the book.*

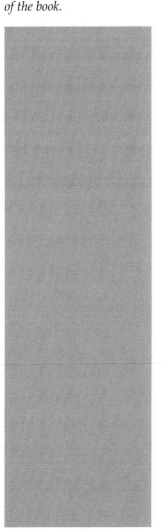

Appendix 1

QUESTIONNAIRES

Appendix 1a

TIC HISTORY/ASSESSMENT

- Description of tic: ....

  ....

- Anatomical site(s): ....

  ....

- Premonitory sensations: ....

  ....

- When tic began (date, age): ....

  ....

- Development of tics over time: ....

  ....

  ....

- Treatment sought so far: ....

  ....

  ....

- Medication/CBT: ....

  ....

- Other members of your family affected by tics: ....

  ....

- Tic frequency (estimate per day): ....

  ....

- Strategies you use to resist/control or otherwise deal with your tic now: ......

  ....

  ....

  ....

Appendix 1b

PERSONAL REACTION SCALE: IMPACT OF TICS ON LIFE

Name: .... Date: ....

The purpose of this questionnaire is to find out whether your tics have any effects on your mood, feelings or habits generally. Please insert "1" (= Yes) if you agree with the statement, and "0" (= No) if you disagree with it. Only insert "2" (= Maybe) if you are really not sure how you feel about the statement. Be sure to choose the answer that shows what you really feel about each statement, rather than how you think you should feel.

(0 = No; 1 = Yes; 2 = Maybe)

1. Because of the tics, I get tired more easily ....

2. I have started new hobbies and interests to keep my mind occupied because of this problem ....

3. I worry whether I will be able to put up with this problem for ever ....

4. I sometimes feel that my life is getting out of control because of the tics ....

5. I sometimes get annoyed having to suffer these tics ....

6. It is the way I think about the tics, not the tics themselves, that makes me upset ....

7. It makes me quite depressed thinking about having these tics ....

8. I am determined not to worry about these tics ....

9. Since having had these tics, I have lost some of my confidence ....

10. I worry that there is something seriously wrong with my body ....

11. Since my tics started, I am less independent than I used to be ....

12. I get more upset by little things since the start of my problem ....

13. Since my tics started, I find it harder to relax ....

14. I spend more time keeping busy since the start of the tics ....

15. I think that there is not much that can be done to control these tics ....

16. Since my problem started, I spend more time listening to the radio or watching TV ....

17. I think that most of my problems are caused by these tics ....

18. I think that a person has to learn to accept problems or difficulties that are encountered during life ....

19. I realize that it is preferable to look for a practical way to approach tics rather than find a perfect solution ....

20. I think I am a victim of the tics ....

21. Generally speaking, I think I am able to deal with the tics ....

22. I think I am incapable of organizing my life because of the tics ....

23. I would be happier if I could predict the arrival of the tics ....

24. Since the tics have started, I am more irritable with members of my family or my friends ....

25. I am more determined to succeed in life to the best of my abilities since my problem started ....

26. Since I have had this problem, I find that I am drinking more alcohol ....

27. Since the tics started, I feel that I cannot face up to daily problems like I used to ....

28. I am sure that certain people think that it is all in my head ....

29. Since the tics started, I have had to avoid strong feelings ....

30. Since the tics started, I have often felt exasperated or at the end of my tether ....

Appendix 1c

TENSION SCALE

		True	*False*
1.	I always feel tense	....	....
2.	I feel tenser in some muscles than in others	....	....
3.	Whenever I perform an activity, I feel a tension in parts of my body	....	....
4.	I am unable to relax completely	....	....
5.	I am aware that I tense unnecessarily when I perform an action	....	....
6.	Others have remarked that I look tense	....	....
7.	My tension is causing me other problems, like pain and immobility	....	....
8.	Even thinking of an activity or event can increase my tension level	....	....
9.	The tension drains my energy	....	....
10.	I don't seem to be able to live without tension	....	....
11.	I restrain my activities due to my tension	....	....
12.	It's not possible for me to function without tension	....	....

Appendix 1d

BELIEFS ABOUT TICS

		True	*False*
1.	Tics make me look interesting	....	....
2.	Tics are part of me	....	....
3.	I'm ambivalent about losing my tics	....	....
4.	If people don't like my tics, it's their problem	....	....
5.	Everybody has personal habits, so I'm no different	....	....
6.	Ticcing makes me feel good	....	....
7.	I function better because of my tics	....	....
8.	I feel I'm more of a character with my tics	....	....
9.	I'm not prepared to put effort into losing my tics	....	....
10.	My tics are special, they say something about me	....	....

Appendix 1e

STYLE OF PLANNING (STOP)

Below are listed examples of activities you are likely to encounter during the day. We ask you to indicate how you would anticipate dealing with these situations by marking a vertical line at right angles to the horizontal line in between the two extremes approaches to the problem.

If your approach most clearly ressembles the right option, place a vertical line as far as possible to the right; if it clearly ressembles the left, place your line to the far left. If your preference is towards one option but lies somewhere in between the two alternatives place your line at the appropriate point along the right or left section of the horizontal line.

If you would be equally likely to use both approaches with no preference then place the line midway.

1. You have five different jobs to do at home. Are you most likely to:

    ....|...................................

    Plan to start them   Plan to start one
    all at once   that you consider
                                                  most important

2. You are planning to relax for an hour and do nothing. Do you find this:

    ....|...................................

    Very difficult   Very easy

3. You are shopping in a supermarket and a person in front of you is slow and holding up the queue. Is your immediate reaction to feel:

    ....|...................................

    Very impatient   Very sympathetic

4. You want to raise a point and say something in a meeting. Do you:

    ....|...................................

    Plan all you want   Just start talking
    to say beforehand   and let your thoughts
                                                  follow on

---

5. When you are talking with another person, do you more often:

    ···|····································

    Adopt the mannerisms   Are not at all influenced
    of the other person   in your posture or tone of
                                                            voice by the other person

6. Do you find you overprepare for a task and put in more effort than is really
    required?

    ···|····································

    All the time   Never

7. When you carry out an assignment, do you:

    ···|····································

    Prepare well in   Wait until the last
    advance   minute to prepare

8. You are required to sit still for 15 minutes. Is this:

    ···|····································

    Impossible   No problem

9. When you are on your own, do you find yourself repeating words or phrases
    you have heard over and over to yourself?

    ···|····································

    Never   Very frequently

10. In general do you speak:

    ···|····································

    Faster than normal   Slower than normal

11. When planning your agenda for a day, do you:

    ···|····································

    Have a realistic idea of   Cram as much activity
    how much you can achieve   in as you can

12. Do you adequately plan time for your own leisure?

    ···|····································

    All the time   Never

13. Once you have set your mind on a plan, do you:

    ···|····································

    Find it easy to   Find it very difficult
    change to another   to accept change

14. You are under pressure from others to complete a task. Does this pressure:

    ···|····································

    Help in your   Make the planning
    planning   more difficult

15. Do you find when you concentrate on a job that:

....|....................................

You are frequently
distracted and your
mind wanders

You are able to screen
out distraction and keep
your mind firmly on the job

16. When you know others are watching you, do you more often assume that:

....|....................................

They will judge
you badly

They will judge
you well

17. You anticipate that some unfamiliar or unknown event is likely to occur. Do you:

....|....................................

Tense up immediately

Take it in your stride

18. Do you prefer:

....|....................................

Working to
a routine

Jobs involving
novel problems

19. Which is worse, when you anticipate:

....|....................................

Being bored

Being overstimulated

20. When doing an activity, are you more frequently:

....|....................................

Impatient to get
ahead and finish

Enjoying just
doing the job

21. If you could choose to project an image of yourself to friends, would you prefer this image be more often:

....|....................................

Efficient and
capable

Caring and
compassionate

22. Given that the same amount of work was expected in both cases, would you prefer a job that was:

....|....................................

Well structured

Left you free to
regulate your
own work

23. When estimating the length of time a job takes, do you more often:

....|....................................

Overestimate
how much you
can do

Underestimate
how much you
can do

24. Generally when deciding an important issue, are you more likely to:

. . . .|. . . . .

Take a long time   Make a decision
weighing up the   fairly quickly
pros and cons

25. You meet someone who is boring you. Do you most probably:

. . . .|. . . . .

Listen to them   Tell them right
anyway but feel   away you can't?
impatient   stop to talk

26. Do you feel you are forced to play a role and are not able to be yourself?

. . . .|. . . . .

Always   Never

27. Do you have a tendency to overcomplicate what to others seem straight forward plans?

. . . .|. . . . .

Always   Never

28. Do you find you get side tracked in the middle of doing a job and end up
doing unnecessary work?

. . . .|. . . . .

Always   Never

29. When planning a job do you imagine all sorts of unforeseen eventualities that
might happen and makes the job seem more difficult?

. . . .|. . . . .

Always   Never

30. When planning a job are you more likely to:

. . . .|. . . . .

Elaborate each   Stick with a
stage in detail   general idea of
beforehand   what is required

MOTIVATION QUESTIONNAIRE

		Yes	No
1.	Are you seeking to change your tic for yourself?	....	....
2.	Do you wish to please someone else?	....	....
3.	Does your tic/habit cause you distress in your daily life?	....	....
4.	Are there currently other major priorities to deal with in your life?	....	....
5.	Will you be experiencing other major life changes in the very near future?	....	....
6.	Do you understand and accept the rationale of the program so far?	....	....
7.	Do you feel ready to commit yourself to regular practice of exercises over 14 weeks?	....	....
8.	Are you waiting for a magic pill to eliminate your tic?	....	....
9.	Do you experience substantial benefits from ticcing?	....	....
10.	Do you believe that your tic is a permanent feature of yourself and that you will never get rid of it?	....	....

INCONVENIENCE REVIEW SHEET

- Please make a list here of all the inconveniences you have noted that the tic brings to your daily routine and which you wish to be rid of.

- These inconveniences can include avoidance of activities, fatigue from the tic, judgment of others or psychological effects such as feeling odd.

- Once you have made an exhaustive list of inconveniences, it is a good idea to reread it regularly to refresh your motivation and remind you of why you wish to eliminate your tic.

Inconveniences	Conveniences
....	....
....	....
....	....
....	....
....	....
....	....
....	....
....	....
....	....
....	....
....	....
....	....
....	....

- Are there any conveniences you see to keeping your tic? Perhaps you feel it makes you eccentric or it elicits sympathy? Be honest and ask yourself, are there any merits to having a tic? Bringing any benefits out into the open will help you better to evaluate your motivation to eliminate the tic. You may also profit from the awareness to ask if these are really benefits or just facts you've learned to live with.

- If you feel strongly that your tic is beneficial, clearly there may be little motivation to change it.

COPING STRATEGIES TO RESIST TICS THAT CREATE MORE TENSION

	Yes	No
• Holding tic in.	☐	☐
• Delaying tic.	☐	☐
• Disguising tic with another movement.	☐	☐
• Hiding tic with clothes, or wig or object (e.g., handbag).	☐	☐
• Avoiding situations for fear of tics.	☐	☐
• Mentally focusing on tic to keep it under control.	☐	☐
• Keeping whole body tense.	☐	☐
• Moving all the time.	☐	☐
• Stretching frequently.	☐	☐
• Adopting a posture to prevent onset.	☐	☐
• Tensing muscles on one side to counteract tic onset.	☐	☐

• Others:

....

....

....

....

....

Appendix 2

MANUAL WORKSHEETS

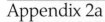

Appendix 2a

CHOOSING TO WORK ON ONE TIC AT A TIME

- Rate all the tics you are aware of in order of priority.
- The priority to deal with the tic should be based on its frequency, intensity and interference in life.
- A visible tic may have more priority that a less visible tic or one easily hidden.
- Make sure the tics are independent of one another, that is, they occur in different parts of the body and may occur at different times.
- Once you have chosen a tic, you should remain with this tic until you have finished the program, and feel you have a high degree of control. Only then progress to another tic.
- A complex tic may involve several muscle groups at the same time, or several sounds or phrases.

Priority	Description of tic	Motor	Phonic	Simple	Complex

MUSCLES INVOLVED

- Please write each one of your unwanted tics/habits in ascending order of difficulty. Register initially the tic/habit that seems to you to be the least problematic and finish by the tic/habit that seems to you most problematic.
- Identify the muscles involved in each of your unwanted tics/habits.

	Tic/habit	Muscles involved
1		
2		
3		
4		
5		

- Write here the first tic/habit you have chosen to work on.

  ....
  ....

Appendix 2c

PRACTICE MONITORING OF TIC FREQUENCY

▶ FREQUENCY

▶ 1. Day of Week

Date: ....

Hour: ....

Number of tics or individual movements: ....

Number of series: ....

▶ 2. Day of Weekend

Date: ....

Hour: ....

Number of tics or individual movements: ....

Number of series: ....

▶ 3. Entire Week

Date: ....

Hour: ....

Number of tics or individual movements: ....

Number of series: ....

Cognitive-Behavioral Management of Tic Disorders by K. O'Connor.
Copyright © 2005 John Wiley & Sons, Ltd.

HIGH-RISK SITUATIONS OR ACTIVITIES

Description of the situation or activity	General tension level (0–5)*	Intensity (0–5)*	Control (1–100)**

* 0 = none; 1 = barely; 2 = weak; 3 = moderate; 4 = strong; 5 = extremely strong
** 0 = none; 1–20 = very poor; 21–40 = weak control; 41–60 = moderate control; 61–80 = good to very good control; 81–100 = very good to perfect control

LOW-RISK SITUATIONS OR ACTIVITIES

Description of the situation or activity	General tension level (0–5)*	Intensity (0–5)*	Control (1–100)**

* 0 = none; 1 = barely; 2 = weak; 3 = moderate; 4 = strong; 5 = extremely strong
** 0 = none; 1–20 = very poor; 21–40 = weak control; 41–60 = moderate control; 61–80 = good to very good control; 81–100 = very good to perfect control

EVALUATION GRID FOR LOW- AND HIGH-RISK ACTIVITIES

Activities					
Low risk			High risk		
A	B	C	D	E	F

	A	B	C	D	E	F	
Likelihood of tic absent (1–3)							Likelihood of tic present (5–7)
In shape							Not feeling active enough
Doing							Watching
Relaxing							Attending
Calm							Preoccupied
Confidence in performance							Insecure

EVERYDAY ACTIONS AND PRINCIPAL MUSCLES INVOLVED

Standing up	Tension in legs, abdomen, buttocks.
Sitting down	Lean body forward and tense thighs, buttocks and abdomen until body lowered or lifted and back is straightened
Walking	Tension in feet, legs, and arm swing. Peel foot off the ground and pass over ankle of other foot, swing arms in opposition to leg
Talking	Face, eyes, mouth and hands gestures
Holding a telephone, or knife and fork	Tension in hand only
Picking up a suitcase/carrying shopping	Bend knees, tension in arm and shoulders and stomach
Typing/writing	Tension in fingers, and involved hand and eyes
Watching TV	Eyes
Sitting still doing nothing	No noticeable tension anywhere

THOUGHTS, FEELINGS AND BEHAVIORAL ACTIVITY

	Anticipatory thoughts	Emotions	Behavioral activity
Situation/Activity			
Situation/Activity			
Situation/Activity			

TRIPLE-COLUMN TECHNIQUE

Anticipations	Evidence justifying anticipations	Alternative more realistic anticipations

- Write down anticipation in first column.
- Write supporting anticipation in second column.
- Write alternative anticipation in third column.

Appendix 2j

CLOSE OTHER RATING: NOTES FOR EXTERNAL RATER

Thank you for agreeing to act as the external rater for: ....

Name: ....

As you know, ... is actually following a behavioral management program for tic disorder. The aim of the program is that the person learns, through practicing exercises, to control the tic problem. As an external rater in the process, your collaboration is extremely important.

Firstly, it is important to monitor and rate the person's tics from time to time throughout the program. This will help us to gain an independent evaluation of progress. In order to accomplish this monitoring, you will need to note the frequency and intensity of the tic for certain fixed periods throughout the day. It is important that .... is aware of your observation but that such observation is discrete, uncritical and not judgemental. You can use a counter to record the frequency of the person's tics if this helps your estimation, or you can make a mark on a piece of paper each time the tic occurs.

Throughout the treatment program, it is important for you to encourage .... in progress through making positive remarks such as "it's going well" or "you're really making an effort", particularly when he or she manages to control the tics or successfully completes an exercise. It is particularly important not to make negative remarks when the tic occurs, e.g., "oh no, you're ticcing yet again", as such remarks make the person more tense and are likely to increase ticcing. The therapist may ask for your cooperation to help in actively reinforcing aspects of the program. In this case, please follow the therapist's instructions. The therapist may also implicate you in other aspects of the program and request that you read some documents from the program to improve your knowledge.

Finally, you are clearly trusted and valued by .... or you would not have been chosen to act as an external evaluator. You probably know the person well and will recognize when support may be required. If there are difficult periods, or when you feel .... needs a reward to boost motivation or to be genuinely congratulated on accomplishments, you may be the person to arrange a treat. Please discuss this with the therapist.

Cognitive-Behavioral Management of Tic Disorders by K. O'Connor.
Copyright © 2005 John Wiley & Sons, Ltd.

Thank you for your collaboration. If you have queries about collaboration, please contact the therapist.

Close other rating: Observation record for tics of ....

PART ONE

The first part of the questionnaire concerns your general evaluation of the tics and your impressions and opinions concerning the problem.

1. How would you describe the principal problem?

    ....

    ....

    ....

    ....

2. Since when have you been aware of the problem?

    ....

    ....

    ....

    ....

3. How would you explain the problem?

    ....

    ....

    ....

    ....

4. Are you in agreement with the decision of .... to seek and follow the program through?

    ☐ Yes   ☐ No

5. Do you believe he/she will benefit from the program?

    ☐ Yes   ☐ No

    If yes, to what extent?

    | Extremely | Very much | A little | Not at all |

6. Are you ready to collaborate with the program?

    ☐ Yes   ☐ No

7. How do you presently help the person?

....

....

....

....

PART TWO

In order to monitor the tic efficiently, we need to decide on a unit of the tic to observe and a period for this observation (for example, one or two hours in an afternoon). Both the unit of the tic and the period must remain constant throughout the program. The tic unit should ideally be the tic chosen by .... with the therapist.

1. Description of tic unit.

....

....

....

....

2. Observation period (date and time), not less than one hour per day.

....

....

3. Number of tics counted, or number of series of tics counted.

....

4. Please note any other behavior or gestes associated with the tic habit.

....

....

....

....

5. Please note the intensity of the tic during the observation period (100 is the most intensity you have observed).

0	10	20	30	40	50	60	70	80	90	100

6. Duration of tic or tic series (please note in minutes).

....

7. To what extent do you find the tic annoying?
   (a) *For the person:*

   |_____|_____|_____|
   Extremely   Very much   A little   Not at all

   (b) *For you:*

   |_____|_____|_____|
   Extremely   Very much   A little   Not at all

8. Have you noticed other behaviors or problems generally associated with the tic/habit?

   ☐ Yes   ☐ No

   If yes, specify.

   ....
   ....
   ....
   ....

9. Does the tic/habit of .... have an impact on your life?

   ☐ Yes   ☐ No

   If yes, how?

   ....
   ....
   ....
   ....

10. Do you act differently or change your routine because of the tics/habits?

    ☐ Yes   ☐ No

    If yes, how?

    ....
    ....
    ....
    ....

Thank you.

Close other rating: Questionnaire for the external rater

Name: ....

Date: ....

Client name: ....

Relationship to the client: ....

1. According to you, has .... followed the program and
    practiced the exercises?

    ☐   Conscientiously
    ☐   More or less
    ☐   Not at all

2. Please note any improvement in the tic/habit due to the intervention. Please
    state the degree of improvement for each of the three aspects of the tic/habit.

    Intensity (force of the contraction on movement):

    |___|___|___|___|___|___|___|___|___|___|
    0   10   20   30   40   50   60   70   80   90   100

    Frequency:

    |___|___|___|___|___|___|___|___|___|___|
    0   10   20   30   40   50   60   70   80   90   100

    Duration of tic or series of tics :

    |___|___|___|___|___|___|___|___|___|___|
    0   10   20   30   40   50   60   70   80   90   100

3. Have you noticed any changes in other tics or muscles other than those in-
    volved?

    ☐ Yes   ☐ No

    If yes, specify.

    ....
    ....
    ....
    ....

4. Have you noticed any changes in the person's way of thinking or way of acting
    in everyday life?

    ☐ Yes   ☐ No

If yes, specify.

....

....

....

....

5. Globally, to what extent would you say the person has benefited from the program?

☐ Very much

☐ Substantially

☐ A little

☐ Not at all

Thank you for your collaboration.

Appendix 3

COGNITIVE TICS: SPECIAL CONSIDERATIONS

▶ **Phenomenology**

- **Cognitive or mental tics** are thoughts, phrases, urges, songs, words, scenes that intrude into consciousness, and are difficult to remove, so causing irritation to the person. They are not to be confused with **obsessions. Obsessions** are usually coherent doubts or images about aversive events or thoughts. **Mental tics** are neutral or pleasant or stimulating – at least initially. **Obsessions** are part of an obsession–compulsion sequence where an aversive thought leads on to bad consequences. **Mental tics** are sequences in themselves. The person does not report bad consequences related to mental tics, and one mental tic does not necessarily chain on to other mental tics, although, unlike obsessions, tics can be substituted.

▶ **Emotion**

- **Obsessions** are usually accompanied by anxiety. The goal in **mental tics** is generally to be stimulated or to relieve boredom or stress, not to increase or decrease anxiety. **Mental tics** persist because they meet the need for stimulation and also reinforce the need for stimulation. **Mental tics** will build on and encourage autostimulation, so they may become annoying or irritating to the person, but the emotion is more likely to be frustration rather than anxiety. In fact, mental tics have far more in common with motor and phonic tics than obsessions, and should be considered a mental form of the tense–release, frustration–action cycle producing tics, but where the background activity and muscle use relates to thinking.

▶ **Actions: Neutralization versus Tension Reduction**

- **Obsessions** lead to mental or physical neutralization. **Mental tics** simply repeat themselves with no neutralization, although they can lead the person to act. The action, however, is *in accordance* with the content of the tic, not, as in OCD neutralization, *against* the content of the obsession. **Mental tics** can be a signal for action. Sometimes a tic, like mentally repeating "big boobs", will lead to an action to try to touch "big boobs". This impulsive relationship between

Cognitive-Behavioral Management of Tic Disorders by K. O'Connor.
Copyright © 2005 John Wiley & Sons, Ltd.

mental tic and gesture is shown in Figure 5.1. The thought excites the action but it is the stimulation that is important, not the content of either mental or motor tic. The mental stimulation can easily be modified or substituted by a competing stimulation, since the intent of the action is often not to touch, but to release tension directed by the use of the mental content. Also, mental tics can themselves be substituted for by another mental tic or even a motor tic. An example here is a lady who counted the letters on billboards when driving, but was able to substitute this mental tic for a leg tic, which served the same tension-reducing purpose. Obsessions, of course, can rarely be substituted unless they touch the same personal theme.

- **Mental tics** are the same as physical tics in their role of stimulating and tension reduction. They also have an activity profile and occur as a consequence of ongoing state and activity. Although **mental tics** and **obsessions** are distinct, the person can accord importance to **mental tics** in the same way that a person accords importance to **obsessions**, and believe that he or she must follow through with an action or the level of tension will rise. Or the person may think that by repeating the action or thought, the need to repeat will eventually diminish. Of course, in reality, the person is actually reinforcing the tension by repeating the action (see Figure 7.5, p. 170). Examples of similar mental tics and obsessions are given in Table 5.1, p. 96.
- Just to make life doubly difficult, it is possible for a person to have both **mental tics** and **obsessions**. In this case, the two are still independent but one can lead to the other. The obsession may lead to frustration, which provokes the tic. Or the tics may be integrated into a superstitious obsession as lucky or unlucky, for example. However, in treatment, **mental tics** and **obsessions** are considered independently.

▶ Therapy for Mental Tics

- The characteristics of the mental tic are that it is stimulating by virtue of the form of the content, or associated features, or alliteration (e.g., "big girls got big boobs"), or shock value (e.g., "up and in his arse"), or since it presents a mental challenge (e.g., mentally counting sections on a blind, or mentally jumping over telegraph poles along the roadside), or because it generates a kind of autogenically induced agreeable sensation or association generated by repeating a favourite tune or text. However, in some cases, different mental tics within the same category can often be substituted just by suggestion. Mental tics may also be partially verbalized and can, of course, lead on to vocal or motor gestes.
- The diary, high-risk activity analysis and Kelly's grid will establish a profile together with evaluations associated with the **mental tic** and which provoke a need for tension release. Such background state and activity patterns of ticcing are addressed in the same way as other tics, but with the following additional strategies:
  - Slowing down the repetition of the **mental tic** can constitute a mental version of the discrimination exercises so that the tic loses its stimulant edge and the person understands how, by slowing down, there is control over its impact.

Literally slow down the thought process by prolonging each thought element and show how this decreases stimulation.

- Distance the person from the **mental tic** as a command to be acted on and see how many other alternative suitable thoughts can be substituted for the mental tic command to the same effect. By being distanced from the mental tic, the person can see that taking different perspectives on the mental tic can break the automatic link and calm the urge to repeat.
- As in the case of motor tics, the person can understand how repeating the tic maintains the reinforcing circle of activation and renews the need for stimulation met by the tic. Substituting the tic for another equally stimulating tic can illustrate the model and show that the precise content of the tic is less important that its stimulating impact.
- In the case of forbidden touching or other disruptive action following a **mental tic**, modify the action so that it bears less and less relation to the mental urge. Also, slow down and delay the action. Show the person that finally the content of the mental tic and action is only meaningful so far as it feeds a need for stimulation. The content is not meaningful in itself and does not need to be taken seriously. Rather, the level of sensorimotor activation triggering the need for the mental stimulation is the source of the problem.

Appendix 4

TIC-MONITORING DIARY

▶ Background to Self-monitoring Diary

There is currently no reliable way of objectively measuring tics as they occur. By their nature, tics are largely non-conscious and although it is possible that a micro detector such as a light-emitting diode, electromyogram or ultrasonic measure could objectively be located at the tic site, its very presence would affect tic onset either directly, by inhibiting or irritating the tic, or indirectly, by eliciting social discomfort at the sight of the measuring devices. In certain cases of other habit disorders, it is possible to gather indirect tangible evidence of the habit (e.g., hair, nails or signs of auto-mutilation). But such evidence in any event covers only some aspects of the habit.

The person is clearly well placed to monitor his or her own tic, but such a measure depends on the person's compliance and awareness. The *current daily tic diary* records frequency, intensity of sensation and degree of control over the tic on a daily basis in a specially prepared booklet. The person is trained in the use of the booklet and a unit of tic is defined at the beginning of the evaluation, together with a period during the day which is convenient for the person to record the tic occurrence. The rules are to keep the period and unit constant throughout the program. The diary can also form part of the awareness exercises which are part of habit reversal training since the person focuses on the muscle to detect occurrence.

▶ The Daily Tic Diary

The self-report diary serves three purposes. It trains the person in monitoring the tic, so providing data on otherwise inaccessible feelings of intensity of premonitory sensation and frequency of occurrence. At the same time, the person receives an awareness training in completing the booklet which may be part of a treatment program. Participants are frequently unaware of when the tic occurs and awareness training has itself been reported as an important treatment component (Wright & Miltenberger, 1987). Finally, completing the diary helps the person identify high- and low-risk situations for ticcing, which can then form the basis for a tic management hierarchy within a treatment protocol and also for revealing thoughts and emotions associated with ticcing (see later).

Cognitive-Behavioral Management of Tic Disorders by K. O'Connor.
Copyright © 2005 John Wiley & Sons, Ltd.

▶ Overview of the Dairy-keeping Procedure

The participants monitor their tic daily over a two-day period followed by a period of one and two weeks' practice and then continuously for the targeted period of time. Participant instructions are given on the instructional sheet. The first step is to establish awareness of the tic, then to monitor the tic initially for two days to establish the feasibility of monitoring, and to permit observation of the most frequent tic periods during the day to identify high- and low-risk situations. The person is introduced gradually to the maintenance of the diary. In the first instance, the person identifies the muscles implicated and the tic unit, using the format given in Appendices 2a and 2b. In Appendix 2c, the person notes the frequency over a two-day period and then over a full week. In Appendices 2d and 2e, high- and low-risk situations for tic onset are identified. Participants note, in the specially prepared booklet, the date and time of the tic occurrence, the frequency (total number of units per period), the intensity of the sensation to tic (none = 0, barely present = 1 to extremely strong = 5) and degree of control over the tic (none = 0 to perfect = 100). *Frequency* is defined in terms of agreed tic units. *Intensity* of sensation to tic is anchored to recent experience of the urge and the scale is subjectively calibrated according to an equivalence of the current rated intensity, with the greatest intensity (5) experienced in the last six months and the lowest intensity (1). In the absence of any detectable sensation associated with the tic, the rating is 0. Five distinct levels seem sufficient to identify gradations of intensity. People may become confused by use of finer gradation. Intensity refers to the strength of the sensation accompanying the tic. The initial aim in measuring intensity was to target the premonitory urge preceding or accompanying the tic. However, some participants report no or little separate premonitory sensation or they are unaware of the sensation, which, as Evers and van de Wetering (1994) suggest, may be absorbed in the muscle tension surrounding the tic-implicated muscle. In this case, the urge to tic overlaps with the tension in the tic muscle. Hence, the intensity of the sensation refers to any sensation in the area surrounding the tic muscle(s) consistently associated either before or during the tic onset. The instruction to the subject, however, is to gauge the intensity of the tic by sensation rather than extent of movement, degree of visibility or degree of experienced distress. The format of the continuous scale measuring *degree of control* (0–100) is generally well understood by participants who may be familiar with measuring degree in terms of percentage in other areas of life. Control is rated as the degree to which the person can resist or subvert or suppress the tic. However, degree of control may have a distinct meaning before and after behavior therapy. After therapy, control may mean ability to relax the muscle and not the tic, rather than hold or restrain the muscle in order to control and resist the tic. Degrees of control can be scaled according to categories of: very good to perfect, 81–100; good to very good, 61–80; moderate, 41–60; weak, 21–40; poor to very poor, 1–20; none at all, 0. An additional column is given in Appendices 2d and 2e for monitoring general body tension (this is separate from the tic sensation which may include local muscle tension). The reason for monitoring general tension is to help to identify tic periods since frequently they are associated with higher than normal general tension levels. After the person is more aware of the tic occurrence, this measure of a general tension can be dropped. A two-week supervised period using the diary forms in Appendix 6 improves trouble shooting, and prepares the person to fill in the diary, over the targeted time period. In the diary, the day is divided up into time periods from awakening until bedtime. The participant also notes very specifically the activity or activities undertaken at the time of the tic. Generalities are discouraged and the participant is asked to focus precisely on what he or she is doing/thinking at the time of the tic occurrence. Examples of the daily diary given in Appendix 6 should be photocopied and downloaded as often as necessary. They can be separated and compiled into small weekly booklets. The form includes the tic rating diary itself and a frontsheet defining tic, the tic unit, time period and participant identification. The daily diary training and use is discussed in more detail below.

▶ DAILY DIARY TRAINING AND USE

The daily monitoring training consists of seven phases:

1. **Identifying the muscles implicated in the simple or complex tic to be monitored.**
2. **Describing the form of the tic as precisely as possible, if necessary with the use of a mirror or video or close other to aid detection.**
3. **Choosing the tic unit and period in which the tic will be recorded, which must remain constant over the entire monitoring period.**
4. **Practice monitoring over two days and then over one week while identifying high- and low-risk profiles of situations associated with tic onset.**
5. **Continual recording of daily tic over two weeks' practice session under supervision.**
6. **Further continual recording of daily tic over the required or targeted treatment or other time period.**
7. **Plotting the tic frequency, intensity and control of the tic over the required time period.**

▶ Identifying Muscles to be Monitored

Awareness of the tic has to be developed to permit self-monitoring. Initially, participants are instructed on how to increase awareness by focusing on the implicated muscles and checking the focus regularly to detect any change in the level of tension. The criterion for tic occurrence is any abnormal involuntary contraction of the relevant muscle group that the participant feels to be either a partial or a complete tic sequence. In all cases, except eye blinks, the tics (once detected) are easily distinguished from other normal actions by virtue of their irregular, abrupt, spasmodic and uncontrolled nature. Abnormal eye blink tics are distinguished from normal blinks by the force of the contraction and the involvement of muscles other than the eyelid in the eye closure. If the tics occur very frequently and counting them is distracting, then participants are advised to make a mark on a piece of paper to record each tic occurrence and later to count the total.

Initially, the person is likely to detect the tic only after its onset. Here, the person needs to practice and focus more carefully on the tic-implicated muscle to detect onset earlier and earlier. The increased sensitivity of the detection threshold means that in all probability the frequency of tics recorded will appear to increase initially after training. This is why an initial practice period of two days is recommended. Awareness develops as the participant becomes more able to focus on the details of the tic and also becomes more comfortable at recording the tic occurrence.

▶ Describing the Form of the Tic

The sensations before, during and after the tic, and all the muscles implicated before, during and after the tic, need to be identified and described in the person's words. This can be accomplished through studied awareness exercises or with the aid of a muscle movement detector (e.g., a lightly placed hand, a mirror, an electromyogram (EMG) or a video or external observer).

Video and Audio Rating as an Aid to Tic Awareness

The video is recorded either in a formal two-way observation room or in a home environment. In the first part of the video, the person is filmed in a relaxing or neutral situation to acclimatize to the setting. The second part of the video is a re-creation of a high-risk tic situation. This is an attempt to stimulate a situation likely to produce tics. Establishing a high-risk situation in collaboration with the participant can generally be accomplished after the two-day initial monitoring exercise. Where possible, the high-risk situation is simulated physically (e.g., others watching the person; or being left waiting for someone). Where it is not possible to re-create the situation physically, we ask the person to imagine the risk situation until the tic is produced. A 10-minute recording is generally sufficient. The videos can be scored for frequency of simple tics or for complex tics. (However, the semi-voluntary nature of habit disorders makes them more susceptible to being fabricated or forced.) Also, a minority of those with habits or tics may feel the video inhibits their tic performance. The videos are then replayed (either at normal or slower speed) and used as feedback to reveal in more detail the form of the tic and to improve the client's awareness and a definition of the problem. Viewing the video permits most participants to examine and describe their tic in greater detail than previously. In the case of vocal tics, audio recording can be added, or recorded alone and played back in an identical manner to the video.

Close Other Participation as an Aid to Tic Monitoring (see Appendix 2j)

Where possible, a close other is recruited at the beginning of the study to act as a contingent positive reinforcer for the exercises practiced by the person during the program. The conditions of mutual support are spelled out in an initial communication and involve giving positive encouragement to complete the exercises and to avoid negative critical comments or gestures during ticcing. The close other then observes the person naturalistically over a period of time, prompting the person with an agreed non-compromising (if in public) code word when the tic arrives. The close other can also improve the degree of motivation and participation of the participant in the monitoring exercises through positive feedback and encouragement.

► Choosing the Tic "Unit" and Time Period

Where the participant has more than one tic, the principal tic causing most distress is identified. The unit sequence of the tic is either identified as a single tic or a series of identical tics in rapid succession if these tics cannot be separated.

A unit is a tic or series of tics targeted and noted in the diary at the beginning of the diary monitoring. It may, at one extreme, be an individual tic contraction monitored continuously over every period of the day. It may be a series of identical tics which follow rapidly one after another, where the person is not able to count accurately each individual tic in the series.

The diary is organized by date, time and situation. If the person is unable to continuously monitor the tic unit throughout the day, then convenience and tic situation will largely determine the targeted time period. For example, there is little point in monitoring the tic for an hour at the end of a day because this is a convenient time, if this situation/activity is least likely to provoke the tic.

Ideally, the person monitors the tic activity continuously throughout the day, noting all the situations. If this is not possible, then the period(s) chosen throughout the day should contain high-risk situations that are repeated on a regular basis. The time period of the situations obviously must be kept constant throughout the monitoring. The initial two-day practice period will help to establish a feasible time period with the participant.

Practice Monitoring and Situational Profile

The initial two-day practice monitoring period allows the person to experiment with recording tic units over a two-day period (preferably one weekday and one weekend day) and reporting on the feasibility of the exercise. The person also begins to note systematically when the tic is more or less likely to appear. These high- and low-risk periods can then be formalized in more detail, in discussion with the therapist/supervisor/close other, or by the person alone. The situations help in deciding the final monitoring period for the two-week practice period. Three high-risk and three low-risk situations are chosen in collaboration with the participant on the basis of the initial two-day diary ratings exercise (Appendices 2d and 2e). High-risk situations or activities are defined as three daily situations or activities when a strong uncontrollable tic or period of the tic is most likely to occur (Appendix 2d). Low-risk situations or activities are identified as three daily situations or activities when the tic is never or least likely to occur (Appendix 2e).

The high- and low-risk activities are described in as much concrete detail as possible. We have identified potential activities accompanying ticcing from our previous research in Table 1.4, p. 15. The importance of looking at background activity as well as just situation is that ultimately, for therapeutic purposes, tic onset is associated with background tension and, hence, the important factor is activity rather than situation. Activities help us to identify behavior better than bland descriptions such as "at home" or "working in the office". The personal agency in these situations should always be specified, e.g., "sitting down at home reading the paper" or "concentrating hard on writing a difficult report in the office". Once the activity has been identified in all its detail, then, if it is repeated often, it may be reported in short-hand in the diary. Other situational, sensory, behavioral factors associated with high-risk activities can also be noted to facilitate early warning detection.

The idea of a practice monitoring over two days is to explore the feasibility of monitoring over a trial period. After the tic unit and high-risk situations are identified, the person completes the actual tic diary for two weeks.

Complete the front sheet (Appendix 6), separate the daily diary sheets (photocopied or downloaded) and fold or staple them into a booklet. At the end of two weeks, subsequent problems arising during monitoring exercise over a longer period are solved with the aid of the guide below.

Trouble Shooting

Problem: Participant fills in diary retrospectively or several days at a time from memory.

Solution: Explore impediments to continuous monitoring: Is the person too occupied, too embarrassed? Does he or she consider that it makes no difference filling in the diary at the time or later?

Problem: Participant unilaterally changes target tic, or tic unit.

Solution: Perhaps the person has decided that another tic is more distressing than the targeted tic. The person may have awareness problems or wishes to minimize tic problem.

Problem: Participant completes diary for different time periods on consecutive days.

Solution: The time period chosen may not always be convenient and another time unit may need to be targeted. The person may not appreciate the importance of keeping the time period constant even if activities change.

Problem: Participant complains that diary is too aversive or too tiring to complete.

Solution: Participant may lack motivation or may be too distressed by recognition of tic problem. Explaining that awareness is an essential first step to control the tic may help. The person may also be investing more effort than necessary in completing the diary, e.g. filling in figures exactly in the middle of the box.

Reaction to Diary Monitoring

In a previous study of 105 participants (O'Connor et al., 2001b), diary keeping was reported to be aversive by a minority of cases and was stated explicitly as a reason for abandonment in four cases. On the other hand, the majority reported it to be beneficial in aiding awareness. In this study, despite the effort in preparing the participant and the time spent at each session with the participant checking the diary and discussing difficulties, 12 diaries were not completed adequately from a research point of view. The diaries were mostly from the waitlist group who had no further supervision for diary keeping after initial training. Reasons for discarding diaries from analysis were unreliability in monitoring periods, unilateral decision by participant to change the unit of tic or type of tic recorded (this most often happens after an improvement in the targeted tic), diary only partially completed, diary completed retrospectively, diary lost, diary containing too many missing days, illegibility.

▶ Further Recording over Required Time Period

The final time period will be chosen in accordance with the aims of the monitoring. The aims may be research, therapy or personal awareness. In any case, the sheets photocopied or downloaded from Appendix 6 can be organized into weekly booklets, which should be handed in at regular intervals to a supervisor, or a researcher if applicable to guarantee against loss. In any event, the tic diary should be carefully checked over by the supervisor/therapist/participant on a regular basis to avoid cumulative errors and to visibly reinforce the diary keeping. These ratings can then be entered as data points into a program such as Excel, or plotted by hand as a two-dimensional graph, with separate graphs for frequency, intensity and control on the x-axis and days of monitoring on the y-axis (see Figures A5.1–A5.4 on pp. 264–267).

▶ Plotting Tic Frequency, Intensity and Control

Illustrations of graphs from the daily diary plotted over different time periods are given in Appendix 5 along with tic descriptions and time units and time periods. Of note is the variation from day to day of tic occurrence, and the partial desynchrony between intensity, control and frequency. In research, the aim may be to look at similarities or differences over a number of clients. However, because of the wide variation in tic units, combining values across groups may only be meaningfully possible for intensity and control measures. For examining pre- and post-therapy changes, percentage differences in frequency may be a more reliable measure of change and will take account of initial values. The graphs can be averaged across days to show weekly trends (see Figures 6.2–6.5 on pp. 135, 140, 145 and 152).

On the other hand, the graphs may simply serve an instructional purpose on the nature of the tic. Demonstrating the ups and downs of the tic parameters over time and the variations in degree of control reassure the person about the "normality" of his or her experience of the variability of the problem. The situational/activity profile can also be elaborated for therapeutic or instructional purposes through expanding knowledge of other characteristics, thoughts, emotions, evaluations associated with tic onset (Appendix 2h).

▶   ADAPTING THE DIARY

Special considerations may be given to children and the elderly, where, for purposes of visibility or clarity, the diary may be enlarged physically or simplified conceptually by reducing the range and categories of scoring to suit abilities (e.g., binary categories [1, 0] for intensity or control). Alternative categories can also be identified in the child's terms, e.g., "a monster one", "a teeny one", for recording such things as intensity, or the diary could be animated in different colors to attract and sustain attention. Alternatively, the diary could be physically completed by a close other with the collaboration of the participant. The daily diary has, however, only been tested and developed on adult (16–65) participants.

Note that the tic diary can be modified for use with habit disorders. In this case, attention must be paid to appropriate habit disorder assessment procedures, and the emotions associated with premonitory urges may be more diverse. Mood may be an important component to monitor separately along with behavioral activity and tic frequency. The habit disorder is likely to occur less often than the tic, but be more variable and complex in its appearance. Hence, establishing the habit unit with the participant may require more time and attention and consequently awareness training may require a longer time.

▶   INSTRUCTIONS TO PERSON KEEPING THE DIARY

Over the time you have suffered from your involuntary motor habit, you have probably become accustomed to it. Perhaps you have even learned to live with the tic and ignore it. It is strongly likely that you have lost awareness of many of its features. Monitoring your tic not only helps you to become more aware of your problem but forms a first step to controlling it.

Self-monitoring requires you to focus on your tic in a way that you wouldn't do normally, and also at unusual times of the day. It requires effort and means that you must divide your attention between your activity and the tension in your muscle. However, we manage to divide our attention constantly between different jobs in life (for example, talking and watching) – it's all a question of practice. Some people are worried that focusing on the tic will make it worse or will make them unhappy if they realize how bad it is. This may happen initially or temporarily but the tic may also decrease as your focus becomes more regular. In any case, both knowledge and awareness are necessary in order to monitor it.

First of all, refer to Table 1.1 and identify your principal most distressing current tic. Now try to reproduce it voluntarily, consciously noting all the muscles implicated. This may seem awkward because typically the tic arrives involuntarily. Below, we will try to identify the moments when the tic is most likely and least likely to occur. Initially, you might have difficulty detecting when the tic muscle contracts. The best strategy is to focus on the region surrounding the implicated muscles. At first you may notice the tic only after its onset, but gradually through your focus you will be able to identify the exact muscles implicated, and also become aware when they first tense up.

You can use a mirror to feed back information on your muscle action or a trusted external observer might give you feedback at particular times, or you can lightly place your hand over the muscle and use the hand as an amplifier to help you to feel when it is active. If you have a video, you can tape yourself for 10 minutes and play it back (see video instructions). If you have a vocal tic, you can record on audiotape and play it back to help you to describe its features and become familiar with the sequence. The next practical step is to try out self-monitoring over a period of two days (Appendix 2c). The two-day period should ideally be a weekday and a weekend day to give variety and a change of environment.

During the two days, simply focus on the muscle and divide your attention between the tic and your everyday activity. At the same time, note situations and activities in which the tic is high or low risk (Appendices 2d and 2e). We ask you to count the number of individual or series of tics; to note exactly the muscles in which the tension occurs; to rate the intensity of the urge to tic; and to list high- and low-risk tic situations. Table 1.4 gives you some illustrations of these types of situations and activities from our previous research. Ticcing tends to be situation or activity specific. Although the situations are idiosyncratic across people, they do form a stable profile for any one individual. Finding your profile will help to direct you to discover other thoughts, emotions or behaviors associated with your tic onset, all of which can be recorded, as in Appendix 2h.

Monitoring the tic over a two-day period will also help you to decide how reasonable it is for you to monitor the tic every day and during how long a time period. Frequently, tics come in series and it is necessary to count a series as one unit. If the tics come quickly but not in a series, then on a piece of paper or with a portable counter you may need to note automatically the number of tics as they occur. If you decide, for example, to monitor the tic for just one time period during the day or at one specified situation, you need to be strict at always monitoring the tic within this time period. After monitoring successfully for two days, you can now monitor the tic for a full week. You should then be ready to monitor the tic over a trial two-week period using the formal daily diaries given in Appendix 6. Please photocopy or download them and combine seven into a weekly booklet along with the completed frontsheet. If you have difficulties keeping the diary, or time units, please refer to the trouble-shooting section or consult with your therapist or supervisor or close other who is helping you to monitor.

If necessary, you can repeat the two-week practice monitoring until you feel comfortable with the diary, the tic unit and the recording period.

You are now ready to start monitoring "for real" so you must decide on your monitoring period. The time period may be determined by the length of therapy or other interests, or simply your own interests. A minimum period of two months will permit recording of the waxing and waning of the tic as well as any systematic daily variations.

At the end of the monitoring period, you can enter the frequency, intensity and control figures into a calculator and compute a graph of the tic evolution over time. Examples of such plots are shown in Appendix 5. The plots give you visual feedback on your tic. You will surely note that your tic frequency and intensity vary a lot from day to day, and that the intensity, frequency and control do not always vary together. You can note your reactions to the graphs in the Reactions to Self-monitoring questionnaire in Appendix 6.

► Checklist for your Tic Diary

1. Identify the principal tic (refer to Table 1.1).
2. Detect and describe the tic through awareness training exercises and with the aid of voluntary contraction, video, audio or close other feedback, and enter in Appendix 2a.
3. Record the number of tics only over a trial two-day period (one weekday and one weekend day) and complete Appendix 2c.
4. At the same time, record at least three high- and three low-risk activities for tic onset, along with overall tension level, intensity and control ratings (see scale explanations in Appendices 2d and 2e).
5. Record other thoughts, emotions and behaviors associated with the three high-risk situations that may help you to anticipate and identify likely periods for tic onset (Appendix 2h).
6. If you feel unable to monitor tics throughout the day, decide on your target tic unit and daily recording time period. Record the unit and the time period, along with any other relevant comments, in the diary frontsheet in Appendix 6.
7. Cut out the front sheet and photocopy or download 14 daily diary sheets from Appendix 6. Fold or staple the front sheets and the front sheet into a portable booklet and keep the diary for two weeks.
8. After two weeks, review the program and any problems (either alone or with the therapist or collaborator if applicable). You can refer to the problem-solving and trouble-shooting section.
9. Either keep the diary for another two-week trial period if necessary, or combine other diaries over a longer time period following the procedure in Step 7.
10. At the end of the targeted time period, calculate graphs of frequency, intensity and control by hand or by computer to give visual feedback on tic evolution. Some graphs from a recent study are shown in Appendix 5 for illustration and comparison purposes.

Congratulations! You have completed an important tic-monitoring and awareness protocol. Please note your impressions of your tic and what you have learned from the monitoring exercise in the Reactions to Self-monitoring questionnaire in Appendix 6.

Appendix 5

GRAPHIC EXAMPLES FROM DAILY DIARIES

The four graphs in this appendix (Figures A5.1–A5.4) illustrate the form of the daily diary data over different time periods. The four cases were chosen to represent different types of tic/habit disorder as encountered in our clinic research program, and the use of different tic units to accommodate different monitoring capacities. The graphs illustrate the fluctuating nature and time course of tic/habit frequency. The range of tic frequency is quite variable while intensity and control tend to vary less continuously and resemble a step-like function with less gradation between levels. In the case of intensity, this restriction in range may be an artefact of the 0–5 score system. Three of the four graphs report some degree of control over the tic even in pre-treatment, but generally the control oscillates widely. But as frequency and intensity decrease, so control increases and stabilizes.

Figure A5.1(a)–(c) shows the frequency, intensity and degree of control plotted from the daily tic diary of a 37-year-old male diagnosed with Tourette's syndrome. The tic unit was a nodding movement combining head and neck in a forward jerk movement. As the tic frequency was once or more per minute, the diary was kept consistently for three 10-minute time periods every day during high-risk situations for 187 days, during, before and after behavioral treatment.

Figure A5.2(a)–(c) shows the frequency, intensity and degree of control for a 58-year-old female with multiple tics, diagnosed with Tourette's syndrome. The target tic contraction monitored in the diary was a tic involving contraction of jaw and mouth accompanied by a blowing noise. The daily frequency was low enough for the client to monitor the tic as a single unit continuously throughout the day, noting each individual occurrence of the tic. The diary was completed over a 124-day period before, during and after behavioral treatment.

Figure A5.3(a)–(c) shows the frequency, intensity and degree of control as rated by a 33-year-old female with a complex tic involving contraction of head, shoulder and neck to the left. The tic unit was monitored over three two-hour time periods per day over a period of 471 days before, during and after a behavioral treatment program.

Cognitive-Behavioral Management of Tic Disorders by K. O'Connor.
Copyright © 2005 John Wiley & Sons, Ltd.

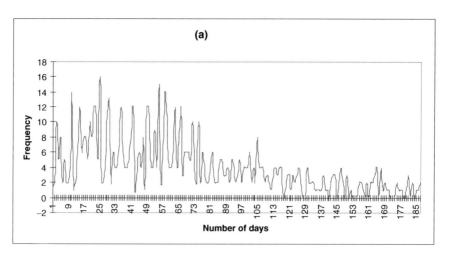

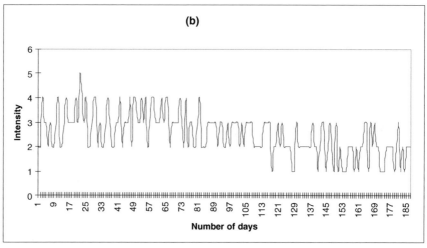

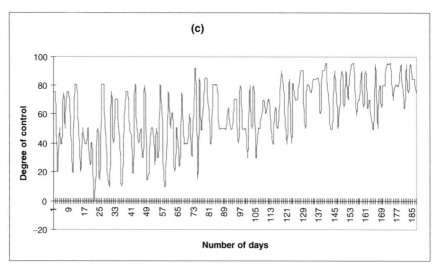

Figure A5.1 Graphic examples from daily diaries (Client #104)

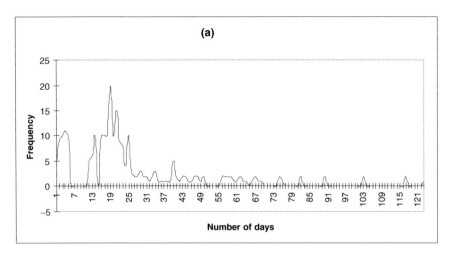

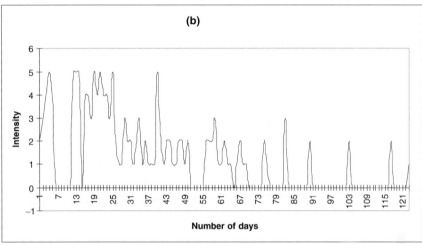

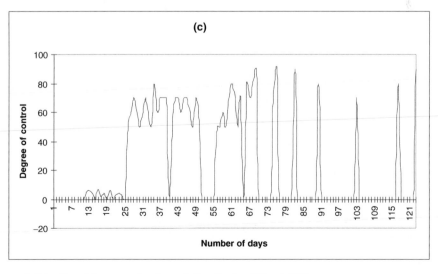

Figure A5.2 Graphic examples from daily diaries (Client #27)

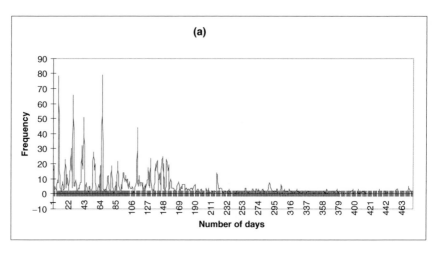

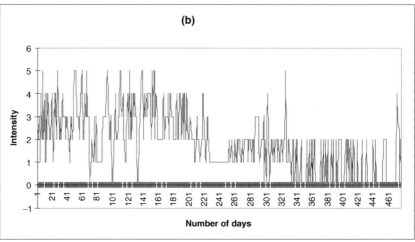

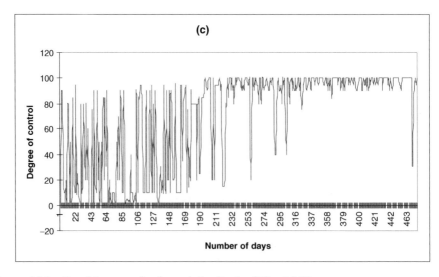

Figure A5.3 Graphic examples from daily diaries (Client #45)

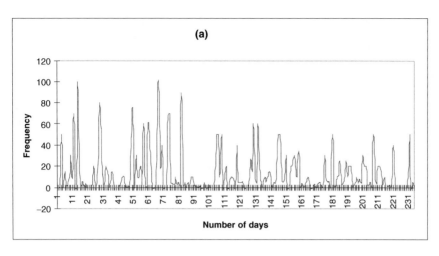

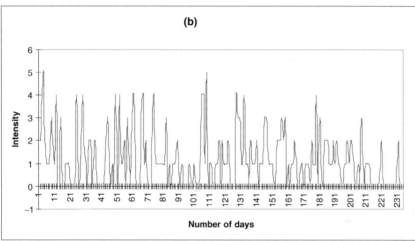

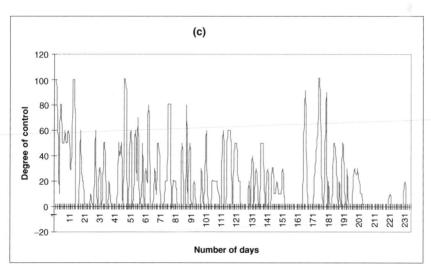

Figure A5.4   Graphic examples from daily diaries (Client #21)

Figure A5.4(a)–(c) shows frequency, intensity and degree of control ratings as recorded by a 40-year-old female with a hair-pulling habit disorder (trichotillomania). The unit was a single hair pulled with the left hand. The number of individual pulls were monitored continuously throughout the day, but for convenience the recording period was divided up into three four-hour periods and the diary was completed over 235 days.

Appendix 6

DAILY DIARY FORMS AND QUESTIONNAIRE

DAILY TIC DIARY
FRONT SHEET

Your identification: ....

Diary dates: ..... / ..... / ..... **to** ..... / ..... / .....

Targeted tic: ....

Description: ....

....

Tic unit is: ....

Tic recording period during the day is: ....

Abbreviations used in diary (e.g., for habitual situations/activities): ....

....

....

Other comments: ....

....

....

....

....

....

....

....

....

DAILY DIARY					
Date	Time	Frequency	Intensity (0–5)	Control (0–100%)	Situation/ Activity

To be photocopied as often as necessary for the treatment period.

► REACTIONS TO SELF-MONITORING TIC BEHAVIOR

In what ways are you more aware of your tic?

....
....
....

Did you find the self-monitoring difficult?

....
....
....

Do you now feel more comfortable or less comfortable with your tic?

....
....
....

Were you coping well with your tic before you self-monitored?

....
....
....

Are you better able to manage your tic because of the self-monitoring?

....
....
....

Has your attitude towards having your tic changed?

....
....
....

Did any aspects of the self-monitoring program require modification?

....
....
....

Appendix 7

TIC QUIZ

The following is a QUestion and answer Information exerciZe (QUIZ) to test your knowledge of tics. The answers, which your therapist will discuss with you, are given in a separate appendix.

1. Tics are involuntary reflexes over which I have no control.

    ☐ Totally agree   ☐ Disagree
    ☐ Partially agree   ☐ Totally disagree
    ☐ No opinion

2. Tics are caused entirely by neurological mechanisms.

    ☐ Totally agree   ☐ Disagree
    ☐ Partially agree   ☐ Totally disagree
    ☐ No opinion

3. The onset of my tic has nothing to do with how I think and feel.

    ☐ Totally agree   ☐ Disagree
    ☐ Partially agree   ☐ Totally disagree
    ☐ No opinion

4. Tic disorder is a very rare problem.

    ☐ Totally agree   ☐ Disagree
    ☐ Partially agree   ☐ Totally disagree
    ☐ No opinion

5. People with tics have other psychiatric problems.

    ☐ Totally agree   ☐ Disagree
    ☐ Partially agree   ☐ Totally disagree
    ☐ No opinion

6. Having tics means I'm badly behaved.

    ☐ Totally agree   ☐ Disagree

☐ Partially agree   ☐ Totally disagree

☐ No opinion

7. People judge me badly when they see my tic.

☐ Totally agree   ☐ Disagree

☐ Partially agree   ☐ Totally disagree

☐ No opinion

8. People with tics have less control over themselves than normal.

☐ Totally agree   ☐ Disagree

☐ Partially agree   ☐ Totally disagree

☐ No opinion

9. There is no cure for tics.

☐ Totally agree   ☐ Disagree

☐ Partially agree   ☐ Totally disagree

☐ No opinion

10. People with tics are less intelligent.

☐ Totally agree   ☐ Disagree

☐ Partially agree   ☐ Totally disagree

☐ No opinion

11. Tics are learned habits.

☐ Totally agree   ☐ Disagree

☐ Partially agree   ☐ Totally disagree

☐ No opinion

12. Tics release tension.

☐ Totally agree   ☐ Disagree

☐ Partially agree   ☐ Totally disagree

☐ No opinion

13. Tics are caused by stress.

☐ Totally agree   ☐ Disagree

☐ Partially agree   ☐ Totally disagree

☐ No opinion

14. People with tics are more nervous than others.

☐ Totally agree   ☐ Disagree

☐ Partially agree   ☐ Totally disagree

☐ No opinion

15. People with tics are more aggressive than others.

☐ Totally agree ☐ Disagree
☐ Partially agree ☐ Totally disagree
☐ No opinion

16. Vocal tics (making involuntary noises) are not the same as muscle tics.

☐ Totally agree ☐ Disagree
☐ Partially agree ☐ Totally disagree
☐ No opinion

17. My tics occur all the time.

☐ Totally agree ☐ Disagree
☐ Partially agree ☐ Totally disagree
☐ No opinion

18. The only way to deal with tics is to resist them or delay them or disguise them.

☐ Totally agree ☐ Disagree
☐ Partially agree ☐ Totally disagree
☐ No opinion

19. My tics mean my brain is not functioning properly.

☐ Totally agree ☐ Disagree
☐ Partially agree ☐ Totally disagree
☐ No opinion

20. Relaxation helps to control my tics.

☐ Totally agree ☐ Disagree
☐ Partially agree ☐ Totally disagree
☐ No opinion

21. If you hold in a tic and resist it, it will only come out later in another way since the pressure builds up.

☐ Totally agree ☐ Disagree
☐ Partially agree ☐ Totally disagree
☐ No opinion

22. My tics are a result of my tense lifestyle.

☐ Totally agree ☐ Disagree
☐ Partially agree ☐ Totally disagree
☐ No opinion

23. Anticipating and focusing on tics can provoke them.

☐ Totally agree   ☐ Disagree
☐ Partially agree   ☐ Totally disagree
☐ No opinion

24. Preventing my tics is better than controlling them.

☐ Totally agree   ☐ Disagree
☐ Partially agree   ☐ Totally disagree
☐ No opinion

25. Medication is the only way to control a tic.

☐ Totally agree   ☐ Disagree
☐ Partially agree   ☐ Totally disagree
☐ No opinion

26. Tics cannot be controlled, only delayed.

☐ Totally agree   ☐ Disagree
☐ Partially agree   ☐ Totally disagree
☐ No opinion

27. My tic will get worse as time goes by.

☐ Totally agree   ☐ Disagree
☐ Partially agree   ☐ Totally disagree
☐ No opinion

28. If I eliminate this tic, it will only be replaced by another in a different location.

☐ Totally agree   ☐ Disagree
☐ Partially agree   ☐ Totally disagree
☐ No opinion

29. Tics are a similar disorder to Parkinson's disease and Huntington's chorea.

☐ Totally agree   ☐ Disagree
☐ Partially agree   ☐ Totally disagree
☐ No opinion

30. A behavioral approach can help me to control my tics.

☐ Totally agree   ☐ Disagree
☐ Partially agree   ☐ Totally disagree
☐ No opinion

Thank you for completing the QUIZ. Your therapist will discuss the answer sheet with you.

FOLLOW-UP QUESTIONNAIRE

Client No: . . . .

Therapist: . . . .

Follow-up No.: . . . .

Date: . . . .

Time: . . . .

---

1. Have gains made in the program been maintained?

   Over last week

(a) Frequency	no. of units*											
(b) Control	0	10	20	30	40	50	60	70	80	90	100	
(c) Intensity	0	10	20	30	40	50	60	70	80	90	100	
(d) General level of tension	0	10	20	30	40	50	60	70	80	90	100	

   (tense)   (relax)

2. (a) If not maintained, why not?
   . . . .
   . . . .

   (b) What can be done to improve adherence? (Discuss with the person.)
   . . . .
   . . . .

3. (a) Which exercises is the person using on a regular basis? Specify.
   . . . .
   . . . .

   (b) Are they proving useful?
   . . . .
   . . . .

4. (a) Have the exercises been generalized to another tic or habit? If so specify.
   . . . .
   . . . .

---

* Check that unit has remained identical to the diary unit.

(b) Is the generalization successful?

....

....

5. Have there been any major changes in the person's:
    (a) life?

....

....

    (b) behavior?

....

....

    (c) emotional state?

....

....

    (d) physical condition?

....

....

    (e) medication or other intervention?

....

....

6. Has the change in tic/habit had any further impact on the person's quality
    of life? Specify.

....

....

7. How confident does the person feel that he or she will continue to progress
    in controlling the tic (0–100)? In controlling their tension level (0–100)?

....

....

8. (a) Does the person foresee any difficulties in continuing to keep or make
        further progress using the key strategies of the program (awareness, re-
        laxation, discrimination, style of action, competing response, cognitive
        restructuring, relapse prevention)? (Cover each strategy and note the
        response.)

....

....

....

....

....

    (b) Does the person feel that further information or coaching is needed? If
        so specify.

....

....

....

....

....

....

(c) Did you give specific coaching during the interview? If yes, specify.

....

....

9. Have others made positive/negative encouraging comments on the person's progress? Specify.

....

....

10. Any other comments by the person on progress or on the program?

....

....

....

....

....

....

Any evaluator comments on follow-up interview?

....

....

....

....

....

....

Date of next follow-up: _____

ANSWERS TO TIC QUIZ

1. Tics are usually considered semi-voluntary since people do have some control over the tics – they can usually resist or delay them. Some people can control their tics by adopting a calm attitude and controlling them mentally.

2. Although there is little evidence that any neurological deficit is involved, people with tics show higher than normal arousal, as shown by more active reflexes and brain chemical activity. However, this over-activation may be reversible, by behavioral or pharmacological therapy.

3. Tics are situational and seem mostly to arise when the person is involved in some but not other activities. Often the way we think or anticipate can produce a tic.

4. Although initially Tourette's syndrome was once considered to be very rare (affecting only 0.1% of the population), this figure has recently been revised to 1%. Some recent estimates put tic disorder at 8% and habit disorder at 20% of the population.

5. Tic disorder is classified as an impulsive disorder but there is no evidence of a direct link with other psychiatric disorders such as schizophrenia, depression or anxiety. Sometimes, people with tics will also have other problems, but this comorbidity is independent of the tics. Children, for example, frequently suffer from hyperactivity.

6. Although tics are classified as impulsive disorders, this does not mean that the sufferer is impulsive in the normal way. It's just a general diagnostic category and also includes habits such as hair pulling or nail biting.

7. Adult people will generally habituate to someone who has tics. Particularly if the person is in a supportive environment, people will just accept the tics as a familiar part of the person. Obviously, if the tic is directly disturbing to others (e.g., loud noise), it may continue to provoke irritation. People with tics do, nonetheless, tend to suffer from self-image problems and are concerned with how they look. Paradoxically, sometimes the strategies used to hide or disguise the tic attract more attention than the tic, since these strategies can appear bizarre.

8. Tics appear to be out of control especially when they appear in series, but there is no evidence that people with tics are more out of control than anyone else

---

in other respects. In fact, tics tend to arise in specific situations, and the rest of the time the person is in control.

9. Tics do occasionally spontaneously remit, especially in children, but rarely in adults. Their intensity and frequency can, however, wax and wane. But cognitive-behavior therapy and medication have shown some degree of success in alleviating the problem.

10. There is no evidence that people with tics are less intelligent or less educated than people with other problems. In fact, most people with tics function well in everyday life, and lead normal lives.

11. The cause of tics is unknown but there is evidence that specific tics, despite their reflex nature, are learned habits which developed when the person was young. In this respect, they are similar to other habit disorders such as hair pulling, skin scratching or nail biting, which can be acquired in childhood.

12. Muscle tension, particularly at tic-affected sites, is a common problem in people with tics, and ticcing does seem to temporarily relieve tension but unfortunately this tense–release cycle increases chronic tension in the long run.

13. Tics are not caused by stress. In fact, attentional stress may reduce tics. There is evidence that tics may be on a continuum with complex habits such as hair pulling, fingernail biting or scratching. Such habits have features in common with tics, and may be worse when mood is worse but they are not caused by stress.

14. People with tics are not more nervous than usual despite the label "nervous tics". There is no consistent evidence that people with tics suffer more from anxiety. Tics are not the same as obsessions or compulsions.

15. Tics are linked sometimes to frustration since people get frustrated by their tics. In children with a severe form of tic disorder, such as Tourette's syndrome, this frustration is sometimes associated with rage syndrome. There was a claim in psychoanalysis that tics represent repressed hostility, but this idea is no longer considered valid or relevant to treatment.

16. Vocal tics are also associated with tension. Vocal reflexes, like motor reflexes, release tension. Vocal tics are similar to muscle tics and treatable in the same way.

17. It might seem that your tics occur all the time, particularly if you are focused on them. Tic frequency can vary from a few to several hundred tics per day, but usually there is a pattern which makes them worse at some times and better at other times of the day.

18. You may think by repressing your tics you are helping yourself, but you are actually increasing tension which paradoxically is more likely to produce tics.

19. It is unclear if people with tics process information differently from others or that their brain functions differently, but they may have difficulty planning actions optimally, perhaps due to their use of inefficient strategies.

20. True. One of the overall aims of our program is to deal with overall motor activation and teaching relaxation is part of the intervention aimed to reduce overall activation.

21. There is no evidence that tics work like a hydraulic pressure system needing to lift off steam. If the urge to tic persists, it is because overall tension level has not been addressed, so the background activation producing the tic is still there at source. Learning to control and regulate high activation will naturally eliminate the need to tic.

22. Everyday activities build up tension levels, in particular activities where the person is attempting too much and putting in more effort than necessary.

23. There is some evidence that anticipating a tic can make onset more likely. This may be because the person is preparing for the tic and reacting to it prematurely, so creating tension.

24. Regulating actions, thoughts and emotions can reduce tension and over-activation, so preventing the tic. Conversely, trying to fight or reverse the tic may cause more tension.

25. Neuroleptic and muscle relaxant medications have been shown useful in re-ducing tic frequency and intensity, but rarely to zero. They probably act on neurochemical pathways involved in motor activation. But behavioral exer-cises offer a viable alternative way of controlling activation.

26. It is possible to prevent tic occurrence completely if the central activation level is controlled. Delaying a tic is not a recommended strategy because it is not addressing the source of the problem and leads you to believe tic onset is inevitable.

27. Tics wax and wane over time but usually, if they are not treated, they will never disappear completely and may indeed worsen or generalize to other body parts at different times of life.

28. Reducing overall level of activation and tension will prevent tic substitution. Replacing one tic by another does not address the central problem.

29. There is no consistent evidence that the same brain structures deficient in neurological and motor neuron disorders are also affected in tic disorder. All, of course, involve movement mechanisms in the brain, but not in the same way. Tics will not lead on to a worse motor or brain disorder.

30. Evidence is accumulating from small-scale studies that a behavioral program can aid the control of tics. In our recent study, 60% of people with tics bene-fited from the current program and maintained gain at two-year follow-up. A behavioral approach is different from other psychoanalytic approaches in that it emphasizes managing behavior in the here and now, not dwelling on the past.

REFERENCES

Abernethy, B. (1988). Dual-task methodology and motor skills research: Some applications and methodological constraints. *Journal of Human Movement Studies*, **14**, 101–132.

Abernethy, B., Neal, R. & Konig, P. (1994). Visual-perceptual and cognitive differences between expert, intermediate and novice snooker players. *Applied Cognitive Psychology*, **8**, 185–211.

Allen, A.J., Leonard, H.L. & Swedo, S.E. (1995). Case study: A new infection-triggered, autoimmune subtype of pediatric OCD and Tourette's syndrome. *Journal of the American Academy of Child and Adolescent Psychiatry*, **34** (3), 307–311.

Allen, K.D. (1998). The use of an enhance simplified habit-reversal procedure to reduce disruptive outbursts during athletic performance. *Journal of Applied Behavior Analysis*, **31**, 489–492.

Alsobrook, J.P. & Pauls, D.L. (2002). A factor analysis of tic symptoms in Gilles de la Tourette's syndrome. *American Journal of Psychiatry*, **159** (2), 291–296.

American Psychiatric Association (1994). *Diagnostic and statistical manual of mental disorders*, 4th edn, revised. Washington, DC: American Psychiatric Press.

Anderson, G.M., Leckman, J.F. & Cohen, D.J. (1999). Neurochemical and neuropeptide systems. In: J.F. Leckman & D.J. Cohen (eds), *Tourette's syndrome. Tics, obsessions, compulsions. Developmental psychopathology and clinical care* (pp. 261–281). New York: John Wiley & Sons.

Anderson, M.T., Vu, C., Derby, K.M., Goris, M. & McLaughlin, T.F. (2002). Using functional analysis procedures to monitor medication effects in an outpatient and school setting. *Psychology in the Schools*, **39**, 73–76.

Anholt, G., Emmelkamp, P. & Cath, D. (2002). How specific are the automatic obsessional cognitions of OCD spectrum patients? A comparative study with the aid of the OBQ. Presented at the *32nd Congress of the EABCT*, Maastricht, The Netherlands (September 18–21).

Azrin, N.H. & Nunn, R.G. (1973). Habit reversal: A method of eliminating nervous habits and tics. *Behaviour Research and Therapy*, **11**, 619–628.

Azrin, N.H. & Nunn, R.G. (1977). *Habit control in a day*. New York: Simon & Schuster.

Azrin, N.M. & Peterson, A.L. (1988a). Habit reversal for the treatment of Tourette syndrome. *Behavior Research and Therapy*, **26** (4), 347–351.

Azrin, N.H. & Peterson, A.L. (1988b). Behavior therapy for Tourette's syndrome and tic disorders. In: D.J. Cohen, R.D. Bruun & J.F. Leckman (eds), *Tourette's syndrome and tic disorders: Clinical understanding and treatment* (Chap. 16; pp. 238–255). New York: John Wiley & Sons.

Azrin, N.H. & Peterson, A.L. (1989). Reduction of an eye tic by controlled blinking. *Behavior Therapy*, **20**, 467–473.

Azrin, N.H. & Peterson, A.L. (1990). Treatment of Tourette syndrome by habit reversal: A waiting-list control group comparison. *Behavior Therapy*, **21**, 305–318.

Baker, B., Kleven, S., Turnbull, S. & Dickinson, J. (1988). Transfer of training and task compatibility. *Journal of Human Movement Studies*, **14**, 133–143.

Barr, C.L. & Sandors, P. (1998). Current status of genetic studies of Gilles de la Tourette syndrome. *Canadian Journal of Psychiatry*, **43** (4), 351–357.

Beck, A.T. (1970). *Depression*. Philadelphia: University of Pennsylvania Press.

Bergin, A., Waranch, H.R., Brown, J., Carson, K. & Singer, H.S. (1998). Relaxation therapy in Tourette syndrome: A pilot study. *Pediatric Neurology*, **18** (2), 136–142.

Bernstein, N. (1967). *The co-ordination and regulation of movements.* Oxford: Pergamon Press.

Bernstein, D.A. & Borkovec, T.D. (1973). *Progressive relaxation training.* Champaign, IL: Research Press.

Berthiaume, C., Turgeon, L. & O'Connor, K. (2004). L'évaluation et le traitement psychologique du trouble obsessionnel-compulsif chez les enfants et les adolescents: Découvertes récentes. *Journal de Thérapie Comportementale et Cognitive,* **14** (1), 35–46.

Berthier, M.L., Kulisevsky, J., Gironell, A. & Heras, J.-A. (1996). Obsessive-compulsive disorder associated with brain lesions: Clinical phenomenology, cognitive function, and anatomic correlates. *Neurology,* **47** (2), 353–361.

Beuter, A., Larocque, D. & Glass, L. (1989). Complex oscillations in a human motor system. *Journal of Motor Behavior,* **21** (3), 277–289.

Biswal, B., Ulmer, J.L., Krippendorf, R.L., Harsch, H.H., Daniels, D.L., Hyde, J.S. & Haughton, V.M. (1998). Abnormal cerebral activation associated with a motor task in Tourette syndrome. *American Journal of Neuroradiology,* **19** (8), 1509–1512.

Black, J.L., Lamke, G.T. & Walikonis, J.E. (1998). Serologic survey of adult patients with obsessive-compulsive disorder for neuron-specific and other autoantibodies. *Psychiatry Research,* **81** (3), 371–380.

Bliss, J. (1980). Sensory experiences of Gilles de la Tourette syndrome. *Archives of General Psychiatry,* **37** (12), 1343–1347.

Blowers, G.H. & O'Connor, K.P. (1996). *Personal construct psychology in the clinical context.* Ottawa: University of Ottawa Press.

Bornstein, R.A. (1990). Neuropsychological performance in children with Tourette's syndrome. *Psychiatry Research,* **33** (1), 73–81.

Bornstein, R.A. (1991a). Neuropsychological performance in adults with Tourette syndrome. *Psychiatry Research,* **37**, 229–236.

Bornstein, R.A. (1991b). Neuropsychological correlates of obsessive characteristics in Tourette syndrome. *Journal of Neuropsychiatry and Clinical Neuroscience,* **3**, 157–162.

Bornstein, R.A., Baker, G.B., Bazylewich, T. & Douglass, A.B. (1991). Tourette syndrome and neuropsychological performance. *Acta Psychiatrica Scandinavica,* **84** (3), 212–216.

Brasic, J.R. (2001). Clinical assessment of tics. *Psychological Reports,* **89** (1), 48–50.

Brasic, J.R. & Bronson, B. (2001). Tardive dyskinesia. In: D.H. Jacobs, F. Talavera, N. Galvez-Jimenez, S.R. Benbadis & N.Y. Lorenzo (eds), *EMedicine Journal,* **2** (6). Online at: http://www.emedicine.com/neuro/topic362.htm.

Brett, P.M., Curtis, D., Robertson, M.M. & Gurling, H.M.D. (1995). Exclusion of the 5-HT-sub (1A) serotonin neuroreceptor and tryptophan oxygenase genes in a large British kindred multiply affected with Tourette's syndrome, chronic motor tics, and obsessive-compulsive behavior. *American Journal of Psychiatry,* **152** (3), 437–440.

Brisebois, H., O'Connor, K.P., Brault, M., Robillard, S. & Loiselle, J. (2001). Situational cues in chronic tic and habit disorders. Presented at *World Congress of Behavioural and Cognitive Therapies (WCBCT).* Vancouver, Canada, July 17–21.

Bruggeman, R., Buitelaar, J.K., Gericke, G.S., Hawkridges, S.M., Temlett, J.A. (2001). Risperidone versus pimozide in Tourette's disorder: A comparative double-blind parallel-group study. *Journal of Clinical Psychiatry,* **62**, 50–56.

Brunia, C.H.M. (1980). What is wrong with legs in motor preparation? Motivation, motor and sensory processes of the brain. *Progress in Brain Research,* **54**, 232–236.

Brunia, C.H.M. & Damen, E.J. (1988). Distribution of slow brain potentials related to motor preparation and stimulus anticipation in a time estimation task. *Electroencephalography and Clinical Neurophysiology,* **69** (3), 234–243.

Brunia, C.H.M. & Vuister, F.M. (1979). Spinal reflexes as indicator of motor preparation in man. *Physiology and Psychology,* **7** (4), 377–380.

Brunia, C.H.M., Scheirs, J.G.M. & Haagh, S.A.V.M. (1982). Changes of Achilles tendon reflex amplitudes during a fixed foreperiod of four seconds. *Psychophysiology,* **19**, 63–70.

Budman, C.L., Bruin, R.D., Park, K.S., Lesser, M. & Olson, M. (2000). Explosive outbursts in children with Tourette's Disorder. *Journal of the American Academy of Child and Adolescent Psychiatry,* **39** (10), 1270–1276.

Bullen, J.G. & Helmsley, D.R. (1983). Sensory experience as a trigger in Gilles de la Tourette's syndrome. *Journal of Behavior Therapy and Experimental Psychiatry,* **14**, 197–201.

Busatto, G.F., Zamignani, D.R., Buchpiguel, C.A., Garrido, G.E., Glabus, M.F., Rocha, E.T., Maia, A.F., Rosario-Campos, M.C., Campi Castro, C., Furuie, S.S., Gutierrez, M.A., McGuire, P.K. & Miguel, E.C. (2000). A voxel-based investigation of regional cerebral blood flow abnormalities in obsessive-compulsive disorder using single photon emission computed tomography (SPECT). *Psychiatry Research*, **99** (1), 15–27.

Carpenter, L.L., Leckman, J.F., Scahill, L. & McDougle, C.J. (1999). Pharmacological and other somatic approaches to treatment. In: J.F. Leckman & D.J. Cohen (eds), *Tourette's syndrome. Tics, obsessions, compulsions. Developmental psychopathology and clinical care* (pp. 370–398). New York: John Wiley & Sons.

Carr, J.E. (1995). Competing responses for the treatment of Tourette syndrome and tic disorders. *Behaviour Research and Therapy*, **33**, 455–456.

Carr, J.E., Taylor, C.C., Wallander, R.J. & Reiss, M.L. (1996). A functional analytic approach to the diagnosis of a transient tic disorder. *Journal of Behavior Therapy and Experimental Psychiatry*, **27** (3), 291–297.

Casey, B.J., Tottenham, N. & Fossella, J. (2002). Clinical, imaging, lesion, and genetic approaches toward a model of cognitive control. *Developmental Psychobiology*, **40**, 237–254.

Castellanos, F.X., Fine, E.J., Daysen, D., Marsh, W.L., Rapoport, J.L. & Hallett, M. (1996). Sensorimotor gating in boys with Tourette's syndrome and ADHD: Preliminary results. *Biological Psychiatry*, **39**, 33–41.

Cath, D.C., Hoogduin, C.A.L., van de Wetering, B.J.M., van Woerkom, C.A.M., Roos, R.A.C. & Rooymans, H.G.M. (1992a). Tourette syndrome and obsessive-compulsive disorder. An analysis of associated phenomena. In: T.N. Chase, A.J. Friedhoff & D.J. Cohen (eds), *Advances in neurology* (Vol. 58, pp. 33–41). New York: Raven Press.

Cath, D.C., Spinhoven, P., Hoogduin, C.A.L., Landman, A.D., van Woerkom, T.C.A.M., van de Wetering, B.J.M., Roos, R.A.C. & Rooijmans, H.G.M. (2001a). Repetitive behaviors in Tourette's syndrome and OCD with and without tics: What are the differences? *Psychiatry Research*, **101**, 171–185.

Cath, D.C., Spinhoven, P., Landman, A.D. & van Kempen, G.M.J. (2001b). Psychopathology and personality characteristics in relation to blood serotonin in Tourette's syndrome and obsessive-compulsive disorder. *Journal of Psychopharmacology*, **15** (2), 111–119.

Cath, D.C., Spinhoven, P., van de Wetering, B.J.M., Hoogduin, C.A.H., Landman, A.D., van Woerkom, T.C.A.M., Roos, R.A.C. & Rooijmans, H.G.M. (2001c). The relationship between types and severity of repetitive behaviors in Gilles de la Tourette's disorder and obsessive-compulsive disorder. *Journal of Clinical Psychiatry*, **611** (7), 505–513.

Cath, D.C., Spinhoven, P., van Woerkom, T.C.A.M., van de Wetering, B.J.M., Hoogduin, C.A.L., Landman, A.D., Roos, R.A.C. & Rooijmans, H.G.M. (2001d). Gilles de la Tourette's syndrome with and without obsessive-compulsive disorder compared with obsessive-compulsive disorder without tics: Which symptoms discriminate? *Journal of Nervous and Mental Disease*, **189**, 219–228.

Cath, D.C., van de Wetering, B.J.M., van Woerkom, T.C.A.M., Hoogduin, C.A.L., Roos, R.A.C., Rooijmans, H.G.M. (1992b). Mental play in Gilles de la Tourette syndrome and obsessive-compulsive disorder. *British Journal of Psychiatry*, **161**, 542–545.

Caudill, D., Weinberg, R. & Jackson, A. (1983). Psyching up and track athletes: A preliminary investigation. *Journal of Sport Psychology*, **5**, 231–235.

Chambertin, C.J. & Magill, R.A. (1992). The memory representation of motor skills: A test of schema theory. *Journal of Motor Behavior*, **24** (4), 309–319.

Channon, S., Flynn, D. & Robertson, M.M. (1992). Attentional deficits in Gilles de la Tourette syndrome. *Neuropsychiatry, Neuropsychology and Behavioral Neurology*, **5**, 170–177.

Channon, S., Pratt, P. & Robertson, M.M. (2003). Executive function, memory, and learning in Tourette's syndrome. *Neuropsychology*, **17** (2), 247–254.

Chappell, P.B., Riddle, M.A., Scahill, L., Lynch, K.A., Schultz, R., Arnsten, A., Leckman, J.F. & Cohen, D.J. (1995). Guanfacine treatment of comorbid attention-deficit hyperactivity disorder in Tourette's syndrome: Preliminary clinical experience. *Journal of the American Academy of Child and Adolescent Psychiatry*, **34**, 1140–1146.

Chee, K. & Sachdev, P. (1997). A controlled study of sensory tics in Gilles de la Tourette syndrome and obsessive-compulsive disorder using a structured interview. *Journal of Neurology, Neurosurgery and Psychiatry*, **62** (2), 188–192.

Christensen, G.A., Ristvedt, S.L. & Backenzie, T.B. (1993). Identification of trichotillomania cue profiles. *Behavioral Research and Therapy*, **31** (3), 315–320.

Clark, D.A. (2004). *Cognitive-behavioral therapy for OCD*. New York: Guilford Press.

Clarke, M.A., Bray, M.A. & Kehle, T.J. (2001). A school-based intervention designed to reduce the frequency of tics in children with Tourette's syndrome. *School Psychology Review*, **30** (1), 11–22.

Clemenz, B.A., Farber, R.H., Lam, M.N. & Swerdlow, N.R. (1996). Ocular motor responses to unpredictable and predictable smooth pursuit stimuli among patients with obsessive-compulsive disorder. *Journal of Psychiatry and Neuroscience*, **21** (1), 21–28.

Coffey, B.J., Biederman, J., Geller, D.A., Spencer, T.J., Kim, G.S., Bellordre, C.A., Frazier, J.A., Cradock, K. & Magovcevic, M. (2000). Distinguishing illness severity from tic severity in children and adolescents with Tourette's syndrome. *Journal of the American Academy of Child and Adolescent Psychiatry*, **39** (5), 1–6.

Cohen, J.C., Bruun, R.D. & Leckman, J.F. (1988). *Tourette's syndrome and tic disorders: Clinical understanding and treatment*. New York: John Wiley & Sons.

Cohen, D.J., Leckman, J.F. & Shaywitz, B.A. (1992). The Tourette syndrome and other tics. In: J.F. Leckman & D.J. Cohen (eds), *Clinical guide to child psychiatry* (pp. 3–26). New York: Raven Press.

Coles, M.E., Frost, R.O., Heimberg, R.G. & Rhéaume, J. (2003). "Not just right experiences": Perfectionism, obsessive-compulsive features and general psychopathology. *Behaviour Research and Therapy*, **41** (6), 681–700.

Comings, D.E. (1990). *Tourette syndrome and human behavior* (828 pp.). CA: Hope Press.

Comings, D. & Comings, B. (1984). Tourette syndrome and attention deficit disorder with hyperactivity – are they due to the same gene? *Journal of the American Academy of Child and Adolescent Psychiatry*, **23**, 138–146.

Commander, M., Corbett, J., Prendergast, M. & Ridley, C. (1991). Reflex tics in two patients with Gilles de la Tourette syndrome. *British Journal of Psychiatry*, **159**, 877–879.

Corbett, J.A. (1976). The nature of tics and Gilles de la Tourette syndrome. In: F. Abuzzahab & F. Anderson (eds), *Gilles de la Tourette's syndrome* (Vol. 1, pp. 26–32). St Paul, Minnesota: Mason.

Costello, E.J. & Angold, A. (1988). Scales to assess child and adolescent depression: Checklists, screens, and nets. *Journal of the American Academy of Child and Adolescent Psychiatry*, **27**, 726–737.

Cui, R.Q., Egkner, A., Huter, D., Lang, W., Lindinger, G. & Deecke, L. (2000a). High resolution spatiotemporal analysis of the contingent negative variation in simple or complex motor tasks and a non-motor task. *Clinical Neurophysiology*, **111**, 1847–1859.

Cui, R.Q., Huter, D., Egkher, A., Lang, W., Lindinger, G. & Deecke, L. (2000b). High resolution DC-EEG mapping of the Bereitschaftspotential preceding simple or complex bimanual sequential finger movement. *Experimental Brain Research*, **134**, 49–57.

de Groot, C.M. & Bornstein, R.A. (1994). Obsessive characteristics in subjects with Tourette's syndrome are related to symptoms in their parents. *Comprehensive Psychiatry*, **35** (4), 248–251.

de Groot, C.M., Janus, M.-D. & Bornstein, R.A. (1995). Clinical predictors of psychopathology in children and adolescents with Tourette syndrome. *Journal of Psychiatric Research*, **29** (1), 59–70.

Dean, J.T., Nelson, E. & Moss, L. (1992). Pathologic hair pulling: A review of the literature and case reports. *Comprehensive Psychiatry*, **33** (2), 84–91.

Deepak, K.K. & Behari, M. (1999). Specific muscle EMG biofeedback for hand dystonia. *Applied Psychophysiology and Biofeedback*, **24** (4), 267–280.

de la Tourette, G. (1885). Etude sur une affection nerveuse caracterisee par de l'incoordination motrice accompagnee d'echolalia et de coprolalia, *Archives Neurologie* (Paris), **9**, 19–42, 158–200.

Dietrich, A. (2004). Neurocognitive mechanisms underlying the experience of flow. *Consciousness and Cognition*.

Dion, Y. (2004). Medication. Oral presentation at the *Annual Conference of Quebec Gilles de la Tourette Foundation*. Louis-H. Lafontaine Hospital, Montreal (September).

Dion, Y., Annable, L., Sandor, P. & Chouinard, G. (2002). Risperidone in the treatment of Tourette's syndrome: A double-blind placebo-controlled trial. *Journal of Clinical Psychopharmacology*, **22**, 31–39.

Duggal, H.S. & Haque Nizamie, S. (2002). Bereitschaftspotential in tic disorders: A preliminary observation. *Neurology (India)*, **50**, 487–489.

Eapen, V., O'Neill, J., Gurling, H.M. & Robertson, M.M. (1997). Sex of parent transmission effect in Tourette's synrome: Evidence for earlier age at onset in maternally transmitted cases suggests a genomic imprinting effect. *Neurology*, **48** (4), 934–937.

Eapen, V., Pauls, D.L. & Robertson, M.M. (1993). Evidence for autosomal dominant transmission in Tourette's syndrome: United Kingdom cohort study. *British Journal of Psychiatry*, **162**, 593–596.

Enoch, J.M., Schreier, H.A. & Barroso, L. (1995). Visual field defects in psychiatric disorders: Possible genetic implications. *Biological Psychiatry*, **37** (4), 275–277.

Ernst, M., Zametkin, A.J., Jons, P.H., Matochik, J.A., Pascualvaca, D. & Cohen, R.M. (1999). High presynaptic dopaminergic activity in children with Tourette's disorder. *Journal of the American Academy of Child and Adolescent Psychiatry*, **38** (1), 86–94.

Evers, R.A.F. & van de Wetering, B.J.M. (1994). A treatment model for motor tics based on a specific tension-reduction technique. *Journal of Behavior Therapy and Experimental Psychiatry*, **25**, 255–260.

Eysenck, H.J. & Eysenck, S.B.G. (1980). *Manual of the Eysenck Personality Questionnaire*. London: Hodder & Stoughton.

Eysenck, H.J. & Thompson, W. (1966). The effects of distraction on pursuit rotor learning, performance and reminiscence. *British Journal of Psychology*, **57** (1, 2), 99–106.

Factor, S.A. & Molho, E.S. (1997). Adult-onset tics associated with peripheral injury. *Movement Disorders*, **12** (6), 1052–1055.

Fahn, S. (1993). Motor and vocal tics. In: R. Curlan (ed.), *Handbook of Tourette's syndrome and related tic and behavioural disorders*. New York: Dekker.

Fahn, S., Marsden, C.D. & Caine, D.B. (1987). Classification and investigation of dystonia. In: C.D. Marsden & S. Fahn (eds), *Movement Disorders*, vol. 2. London: Butterworths.

Fallon, T. Jr & Schwab-Stone, M. (1992). Methodology of epidemiological studies of tic disorders and comorbid psychopathology. In: T.N. Chase, A.J. Friedhoff & D.J. Cohen (eds), *Advances in Neurology* (Vol. 58, pp. 43–52). New York: Raven Press.

First, M.B., Frances, A. & Pincus, H.A. (1995). DSM-IV criteria for Tourette's: Reply. *Journal of the American Academy of Child and Adolescent Psychiatry*, **34** (4), 402.

Fisk, A.D. & Rogers, W.A. (1988). The role of situational context in the development of high-performance skills. *Human Factors*, **30** (6), 703–712.

Friedman, A., Campbell Polson, M. & Dafoe, C.G. (1988). Dividing attention between the hands and the head: Performance trade-offs between rapid finger tapping and verbal memory. *Journal of Experimental Psychology: Human Perception and Performance*, **14** (1), 60–68.

Frost, R.O., Marten, P., Lahart, C. & Rosenblate, R. (1990). The dimensions of perfectionism. *Cognitive Therapy and Research*, **14** (5), 449–468.

Frost, R.O., Rhéaume, J. & Novara, C. (2002). Perfectionism. In: R.O. Frost & G. Steketee (eds), *Cognitive approaches to obsessions and compulsions: Theory, assessment, and treatment*. Oxford, UK: Elsevier.

Fuata, P. & Griffiths, R.A. (1992). Cognitive behavioural treatment of a vocal tic. *Behaviour Change*, **9** (1), 14–18.

Gaffney, G.R., Sieg, K. & Hellings, J. (1994). The MOVES: A self-rating scale for Tourette's syndrome. *Journal of Child and Adolescent Psychopharmacology*, **4**, 269–280.

Garcia-Colera, A. & Semjen, A. (1988). Distributed planning of movement sequences. *Journal of Motor Behavior*, **20** (3), 341–367.

Garvey, M.A., Perlmutter, S.J., Allen, A.J., Hamburger, S., Lougee, L., Leonard, H.L., Witowski, M.E., Dubbert, B. & Swedo, S.E. (1999). A pilot study of penicillin prophylaxis for neuropsychiatric exacerbations triggered by streptococcal infections. *Biological Psychiatry*, **45** (12), 1564–1571.

George, M.S., Trimble, M.R., Costa, D.C., Robertson, M.M., Ring, H.A. & Ell, P.J. (1992). Elevated frontal cerebral blood flow in Gilles de la Tourette syndrome: A 99Tcm-HMPAO SPECT study. *Psychiatry Research*, **45** (3), 143–151.

George, M.S., Trimble, M.R., Ring, H.A., Sallee, F.R. & Robertson, M.M. (1990). Obsessions in obsessive-compulsive disorder with and without Gilles de la Tourette's syndrome. *American Journal of Psychiatry*, **150** (1), 93–97.

Georgiou, N., Bradshaw, J.L., Phillips, J.G., Cunnington, R. & Rogers, M. (1997). Functional asymmetries in the movement kinematics of patients with Tourette's syndrome. *Journal of Neurology, Neurosurgery and Psychiatry*, **63**, 188–195.

Gerlsma, C., Emmelkamp, P.M.G. & Arrindell, W.A. (1990). Anxiety, depression, and perception of early parenting: A meta-analysis. *Clinical Psychology Review*, **10**, 251–277.

Giedd, J.N., Rapoport, J.L., Leonard, H.L., Richter, D. & Swedo, S.E. (1996). Case study: Acute basal ganglia enlargement and obsessive-compulsive symptoms in an adolescent boy. *Journal of the American Academy of Child and Adolescent Psychiatry*, **35** (7), 913–915.

Gilbert, D.L., Batterson, J.R., Sethuraman, G. & Sallee, F.R. (2004). Tic reduction with risperidone versus pimozide in a randomized, double-blind crossover trial. *Journal of the American Academy of Child and Adolescent Psychiatry*, **43** (2), 206–214.

Gioia, G.A., Isquith, P.K., Guy, S.C. & Kenworthy, L. (2000). *Behavior rating inventory of executive function*. Odessa, FL: Psychological Assessment Resources.

Gironell, A., Rodriguez-Fornells, A., Kulisevsky, J., Pascual, B., Riba, J., Barbanoj, M. & Berthier, M. (2000). Abnormalities of the acoustic startle reflex and reaction time in Gilles de la Tourette syndrome. *Clinical Neurophysiology*, **111**, 1366–1371.

Goetz, C.G., Tanner, C.M., Wilson, R.S. & Shannon, K.M. (1987). A rating scale for Gilles de la Tourette's syndrome: Description, reliability, and validity. *Neurology*, **37**, 1542–1544.

Goh, A.M.Y., Bradshaw, J.L., Bradshaw, J.A. & Georgiou-Karistianis, N. (2002). Inhibition of expected movements in Tourette's syndrome. *Journal of Clinical and Experimental Neuropsychology*, **24** (8), 1017–1031.

Goldberg, D.P. (1972). *The detection of psychiatric illness by questionnaire: A technique for the identification and assessment of non-psychotic psychiatric illness*. London: Oxford University Press.

Goldenberg, J.N., Brown, S.B. & Weiner, W.J. (1994). Coprolalia in younger patients with Gilles de la Tourette syndrome. *Movement Disorders*, **9** (6), 622–625.

Greene, R.W. (2001). *The explosive child*, 2nd edition (336 pp.). NY: First Quill edition.

Griesemer, D.A. (1997). Pergolide in the management of Tourette syndrome. *Journal of Child Neurology*, **12**, 402–403.

Grondin, C. & O'Connor K.P. (2001). Community Group Support Workshop. Federation of Quebec Associations for parents of people suffering mental illness, Annual meeting, Quebec City, Canada (June 14–15).

Grover, C. & Craske, B. (1992). Perceiving tongue position. *Perception*, **21**, 661–670.

Hadley, N.H. (1984). *Fingernail biting. Theory, research and treatment*. New York: Spectrum Publications, Inc.

Hafner, R.J. (1988). Obsessive-compulsive disorder: A questionnaire survey of a self-help group. *International Journal of Social Psychiatry*, **34**, 310–315.

Hagin, R.A., Beecher, R., Pagano, G. & Kreeger, H. (1982). Effects of Tourette syndrome on learning. *Advances in Neurology*, **35**, 323–328.

Harcherik, D.F., Leckman, J.F., Detlor, J. & Cohen, D.J. (1984). A new instrument for clinical studies of Tourette's syndrome. *Journal of the American Academy of Child Psychiatry*, **23** (2), 153–160.

Heaton, R.K., Chelune, G.J., Talley, J.L., Kay, G.G. & Curtiss, G. (1993*). Wisconsin Card Sorting Test Manual. Revised and expanded*. Psychological Assessment Resources, Inc.

Hicks, R.A., Conti, P.A. & Bragg, H.R. (1990). Increases in nocturnal bruxism among college students implicate stress. *Medical Hypotheses*, **33**, 239–240.

Hoekstra, R.J., Visser, S. & Emmelkamp, P.M.G. (1989). A social learning formulation of the etiology of obsessive-compulsive disorders. In: P.M.G. Emmelkamp, W.T.A.M. Everaerd, F. Kraaimaat & M.J.M. van Son (eds), *Fresh perspectives on anxiety disorders*. Amsterdam: Swets & Zeitlinger.

Hollander, E. (1993). Obsessive-compulsive spectrum disorders: An overview. *Psychiatric Annals*, **23**, 355–358.

Hollander, E. & Benzaquen, S.D. (1997). The obsessive-compulsive spectrum disorders. *International Review of Psychiatry*, **9**, 99–109.

Hollander, E., Schiffman, E., Cohen, B., Rivera-Stein, M.A., Rosen, W., Gorman, J.M., Fyer, A.J., Papp, L. & Liebowitz, M.R. (1990). Signs of central nervous system dysfunction in obsessive-compulsive disorder. *Archives of General Psychiatry*, **47**, 27–32.

Hollins, M. & Goble, A.K. (1988). Perception of the length of voluntary movements. *Somatosensory Research*, **5** (4), 335–348.

Holzer, J.C., Goodman, W.K., Price, L.H., Bear, L., Leckman, J.F. & Heninger, G.R. (1994). Obsessive-compulsive disorder with and without a chronic tic disorder: A comparison of symptoms in 70 patients. *British Journal of Psychiatry*, **164**, 469–473.

Hood, K.K., Baptista-Neto, L., Beasley, P.J., Lobis, R., Pravdova, I. (2004). Case study: Severe self-injurious behavior in comorbid Tourette's disorder and OCD. *Journal of the American Academy of Child and Adolescent Psychiatry*, **43** (10), 1298–1303.

Hoogduin, C.A.L. (1986). On the diagnosis of obsessive-compulsive disorder. *American Journal of Psychotherapy*, **40** (1), 36–51.

Hoogduin, K., Verdellen, C. & Cath, D. (1997). Exposure and response prevention in the treatment of Gilles de la Tourette's syndrome: Four case studies. *Clinical Psychology and Psychotherapy*, **4** (2), 125–135.

Hugo, F., van Heerden, B., Zungu-Dirwayi, N. & Stein, D.J. (1999). Functional brain imaging in obsessive-compulsive disorder secondary to neurological lesions. *Depression and Anxiety*, **10** (3), 129–136.

Hyde, T.M. & Weinberger, D.R. (1995). Tourette's syndrome: A model neuropsychiatric disorder. *Journal of the American Medical Association*, **273** (6), 498–501.

Itard, J.M.G. (1825). Mémoire sur quelques fonctions involontaires des appareils de la locomotion, de la préhension et de la voix. *Archives of General Medicine*, **8**, 385–407.

Jacobson, E. (1938). *Progressive relaxation*. Chicago: University of Chicago Press.

Jaegers, S.M.H.J., Peterson, R.F., Dantuma, R., Hillen, B., Geuze, R. & Schellekens, J. (1989). Kinesiologic aspects of motor learning in dart throwing. *Journal of Human Movement Studies*, **16**, 161–171.

Jagger, J., Prusoff, B.A., Cohen, D.J., Kidd, K.K., Carbonari, C.M. & John, K. (1982). The epidemiology of Tourette's syndrome: A pilot study. *Schizophrenia Bulletin*, **8** (2), 267–278.

Jahanshahi, M. & Marsden, C.D. (1989). Motor disorders. In: G. Turpin (ed.), *Handbook of clinical psychophysiology* (pp. 555–583). London: John Wiley & Sons.

Jankovic, J. (1997). Phenomenology and classification of tics. *Neurological Clinics of North America*, **15**, 267–275.

Johannes, S., Weber, A., Muller-Vahl, K.R., Kolbe, H., Dengler, R. & Münte, T.F. (1997). Event-related brain potential show changed attentional mechanisms in Gilles de la Tourette syndrome. *European Journal of Neurology*, **4**, 152–161.

Johannes, S., Wieringa, B.M., Nager, W., Muller-Vahl, K.R., Dengler, R. & Munte, T.F. (2001). Electrophysiological measures and dual-task performance in Tourette syndrome indicate deficient divided attention mechanisms. *European Journal of Neurology*, **8** (3), 253–260.

Johannes, S., Wieringa, B.M., Nager, W., Muller-Vahl, K.R., Dengler, R. & Munte, T.F. (2002). Excessive action monitoring treatment of Tourette syndrome. *Journal of Neurology*, **249** (8), 961–966.

Jones, K.M., Swearer, S.M. & Friman, P.C. (1997). Relax and try instead: Abbreviated habit reversal for maladaptive self-biting. *Journal of Applied Behavior Analysis*, **30**, 697–699.

Jones, L.A. (1988). Motor illusions: What do they reveal about proprioception? *Psychological Bulletin*, **103** (1), 72–86.

Jourden, F.J., Bandura, A. & Banfield, J.T. (1991). The impact of conceptions of ability on self-regulatory factors and motor skill acquisition. *Journal of Sport and Exercise Psychology*, **8**, 213–226.

Kahn, F.J., Huart, F. & Monod, H. (1988). Variation of the maximum maintenance time of an isometric contraction in the presence of a second contraction. *Ergonomics*, **31** (9), 1287–1298.

Kane, M.J. (1994). Premonitory urges as "attentional tics" in Tourette's syndrome. *Journal of the American Academy of Child and Adolescent Psychiatry*, **33** (6), 805–808.

Karoly, P. (1993). Mechanisms of self-regulation: A system's view. *Annual Reviews of Psychology*, **44**, 23–52.

Karp, B.I., Porter, S., Toro, C. & Hallett, M. (1996). Simple motor tics may be preceded by a premotor potential. *Journal of Neurology, Neurosurgery and Psychiatry*, **61**, 103–106.

Kaufman, J., Birmaher, B., Brent, D., Rao, U., Flynn, C., Moreci, P., Williamson, D. & Ryan, N. (1997). Schedule for affective disorders and schizophrenia for school age children present and lifetime version (K-SADS-PL): Initial reliability and validity data. *Journal of the American Academy of Child and Adolescent Psychiatry*, **36** (7), 980–988.

Kay, M., Guernsey de Zapien, J., Altamirano Wilson, C. & Yoder, M. (1993). Evaluating treatment efficacy by triangulation. *Social Science and Medicine*, **36** (12), 1545–1554.

Keele, S.W. (1968). Movement control in skilled motor performance. *Psychological Bulletin*, **70** (6, Part 1), 387–403.

Kelso, J.A.S. (1994). The informational character of self-organized co-ordination dynamics. *Human Movement Science*, **13**, 393–413.

Kent, L. & Craddock, N. (2003). Is there a relationship between attention deficit hyperactivity disorder? *Journal of Affective Disorders*, **73**, 211–221.

Kerbeshian, J. & Burd, L. (2003). Tourette syndrome and prognosis in autism. *European Child and Adolescent Psychiatry*, **12**, 103.

Kimura, K., Imanaka, K. & Kita, I. (2002). The effects of different instructions for preparatory muscle tension on simple reaction time. *Human Movement Science*, **21**, 947–960.

King, R.A., Scahill, L., Vitulano, L.A., Schwab-Stone, M., Tercyak, K.P. Jr & Riddle, M.A. (1995). Childhood trichotillomania: Clinical phenomenology, comorbidity, and family genetics. *Journal of the American Academy of Child and Adolescent Psychiatry*, **34** (11), 1451–1459.

Kleinsasser, B.J., Misra, L.K., Bhatara, V.S. & Sanchez, J.D. (1999). Risperidone in the treatment of choreiform movements and aggressiveness in a child with "PANDAS". *South Dakota Journal of Medicine*, **52** (9), 345–347.

Knell, E.R. & Comings, D.E. (1993). Tourette's syndrome and attention-deficit hyperactivity disorder: Evidence for a genetic relationship. *Journal of Clinical Psychiatry*, **54** (9), 331–337.

Knowlton, B.J., Mangels, J.A. & Squire, L.R. (1996). A neostriatal habit learning system in human. *Science*, **273**, 1399–1402.

Kornhuber, H.H. (1978). Cortex, basal ganglia and cerebellum in motor control. In: W.A. Cobb & H. Van Duijn (eds), *Contemporary clinical neurophysiology*. Amsterdam: Elsevier.

Kornhuber, H.H. & Deecke, L. (1977). Cerebral potentials and the initiation of voluntary movement. In: J.E. Desmedt (ed.), *Attention, voluntary contraction and event-related cerebral potentials*. Basel: Karger.

Kraemer, H.C., Noda, A. & O'Hara, R. (2004). Categorical versus dimensional approaches to diagnosis: Methodological challenges. *Journal of Psychiatric Research*, **38**, 17–25.

Kugler, P.N. & Turvey, M.T. (1990). *Information, natural law, and the self-assembly of rhythmic movement*. London: Erlbaum.

Kurlan, R. (1992). Tourette syndrome in a special education population. Hypotheses. *Advances in Neurology*, **58**, 75–81.

Kurlan, R. (2001). How to treat ADHD in patients with Tourette syndrome. Presented at the *International Symposium on Tourette Syndrome and Other Neurodevelopmental Disorders*. Toronto, Canada (May).

Lamberg, L. (2003). ADHD often undiagnosed in adults: Appropriate treatment may benefit work, family, social life. *Journal of the American Medical Association*, **290**, 1565–1567.

Lang, A.E., Consky, E. & Sandor, P. (1993). "Signing tics" – insights into the pathophysiology of symptoms in Tourette's syndrome. *Annals of Neurology*, **33** (2), 212–215.

Lawson, J.S., Marshall, W.L. & McGrath, P. (1979). The social self-esteem inventory. *Educational and Psychological Measurement*, **39**, 803–811.

Leckman, J.F. & Chittenden, E.H. (1990). Gilles de la Tourette's syndrome and some forms of obsessive-compulsive disorder may share a common *genetic* diathesis. *Encéphale*, **16** (Spec. No. 1), 321–323.

Leckman, J.F. & Cohen, D.J. (1999). *Tourette's syndrome: Developmental psychopathology and clinical care*. New York: John Wiley & Sons.

Leckman, J.F., Grice, D.E., Barr, L.C., de Vries, A.L.C., Martin, C., Cohen, D.J., McDouble, C.J., Goodman, W.K. & Rasmussen, S.A. (1994/1995). Tic-related vs non-tic-related obsessive compulsive disorder. *Anxiety*, **1**, 208–215.

Leckman, J.F., Riddle, M.A., Hardin, M.T., Ort, S., Swartz, K.L., Stevenson, J. & Cohen, D.J. (1989). The Yale Global Tic Severity Scale (YGTSS): Initial testing of a clinical-rated scale of tic severity. *Journal of the American Academy of Child and Adolescent Psychiatry*, **28**, 566–573.

Leckman, J.F., Sholomskas, D., Thompson, W.D., Belanger, A. & Weissman, M.M. (1982). Best estimate of lifetime psychiatric diagnosis: A methodological study. *Archives of General Psychiatry*, **39** (10), 879–883.

Leckman, J.F., Walker, D.E. & Cohen, D.J. (1993). Premonitory urges in Tourette's syndrome. *American Journal of Psychiatry*, **150** (1), 98–102.

Leckman, J.F., Zhang, H., Vitale, A., Lahnin, F., Lynch, K., Bondi, C., Kim, Y.-S. & Peterson, B.S. (1998). Course of tic severity in Tourette syndrome: The first two decades. *Pediatrics*, **102** (1), 14–19.

Leclerc, J. (2004). Les crises de rage. Conference presented at *Association Québécoise du Syndrome de la Tourette*, Montreal.

Leonard, H.L., Lenane, M.C., Swedo, S.E., Rettew, D.C., Gershon, E.S. & Rapoport, J.L. (1992). Tics and Tourette's disorder: A 2- to 7-year follow-up of 54 obsessive-compulsive children. *American Journal of Psychiatry*, **149** (9), 1244–1251.

Leplow, B. (1990). Heterogenity of biofeedback training effects in spasmodic torticollis: A single-case approach. *Behaviour Research and Therapy*, **28** (4), 359–365.

Leuthold, H. & Jentzsch, I. (2002). Distinguishing neural sources of movement preparation and execution. An electrophysiological analysis. *Biological Psychology*, **60**, 173–198.

Lewis, P.A. & Miall, R.C. (2003). Distinct systems for automatic and cognitively controlled time measurement: Evidence from neuroimaging. *Currrent Opinion in Neurobiology*, **13**, 1–6.

Lohr, J.B. & Wisniewski, A. (1987). *Movement disorders: A neuropsychiatric approach*. New York: John Wiley & Sons.

Lougee, L., Perlmutter, S.J., Nicolson, R., Garvey, M.A. & Swedo, S.E. (2000). Psychiatric disorders in first-degree relatives of children with pediatric autoimmune neuropsychiatric disorders associated with streptococcal infections (PANDAS). *Journal of the American Academy of Child and Adolescent Psychiatry*, **39** (9), 1120–1126.

Lussier, F. & Flessas, J. (2001). *Neuropsychologie de l'enfant. Troubles développementaux et de l'apprentissage*. Paris: Dunod.

Mahone, E.M., Cirino, P.T., Cutting, L.E., Cerrone, P.M., Hagelthorn, K.M., Hiemenz, J.R., Singer, H.S. & Denckla, M.B. (2002). Validity of the behavior rating inventory of executive function in children with ADHD and/or Tourette syndrome. *Archives of Clinical Neuropsychology*, **17** (7), 643–662.

Mansuetto, C.S., Goldfinger Golomb, R., McCombs Thomas, A. & Townsley Stemberger, R.M. (1999). A comprehensive model for behavioral treatment of trichotillomania. *Cognitive and Behavioral Practice*, **6**, 23–43.

Marlatt, G.A. & Gordon, J.R. (1985). Relapse prevention. In: P. Davidson & S. Davidson (eds), *Behavior medicine*. New York: Brunner.

Marsden, C.D., Harrison, M.J.G. & Bundey, S. (1976). Natural history of idiopathic torsion dystonia. In: R. Eldridge & S. Fahn (eds), *Advances in neurology*, Vol. 14. New York: Raven Press.

Mason, A., Banerjee, S., Eapen, V., Zeitlin, H. & Robertson, M.M. (1998). The prevalence of Tourette syndrome in a mainstream school population. *Developmental Medicine and Child Neurology*, **40**, 292–296.

McConville, B.J. & Norman, A.B. (1992). Nicotine potentiation of haloperidol in reducing tic frequency in Tourette's disorder: Reply. *American Journal of Psychiatry*, **149** (3), 418.

McKinlay, B.D. & Dixon, M.J. (2001). What makes a tic tick? Motoric disinhibition and the incidental associations theory of tic formation. Paper presented at the *International Symposium on Tourette's Syndrome and other Neurodevelopmental Disorders*. Toronto, Canada, (May 31–June 2).

McMahon, W.M., van de Wetering, B.J., Filloux, F., Betit, K., Coon, H. & Leppert, M. (1996). Bilineal transmission and phenotypic variation of Tourette's disorder in a large pedigree. *Journal of the American Academy of Child and Adolescent Psychiatry*, **35** (5), 672–680.

Meyer, D.E., Abrams, R.A., Kornblum, S., Wright, C.E. & Smith, J.E.K. (1988). Optimality in human motor performance: Ideal control of rapid aimed movements. *Psychological Review*, **95** (3), 340–370.

Michaels, C.F. (1988). S-R compatibility between response position and destination of apparent motion: Evidence of the detection of affordances. *Journal of Experimental Psychology: Human Perception and Performance*, **14** (2), 231–240.

Miele, G.M., Tilly, S.M., Frist, M. & Frances, A. (1990). The definition of dependence and behavioural addictions. *British Journal of Addiction*, **85** (11), 1421–1423.

Miguel, E.C., Coffey, B.J., Baer, L., Savage, C.R., Rauch, S.L. & Jenike, M.A. (1995). Phenomenology of intentional repetitive behaviors in obsessive-compulsive disorder and Tourette's disorder. *Journal of Clinical Psychiatry*, **56** (6), 246–255.

Miltenberger, R.G., Fuqua, R.W. & McKinley, T. (1985). Habit reversal with muscle tics: Replication and component analysis. *Behavior Therapy*, **16**, 39–50.

Miltenberger, R.G., Fuqua, R.W. & Woods, D.W. (1998). Applying behavior analysis to clinical problems: Review and analysis of habit reversal. *Journal of Applied Behavior Analysis*, **31**, 447–469.

Müller, N., Putz, A., Kathman, N., Lehle, R., Günther, W. & Straube, A. (1997). Characteristics of obsessive-compulsive symptoms in Tourette's syndrome, obsessive-compulsive disorder, and Parkinson's disease. *Psychiatry Research*, **70**, 105–114.

Müller, N., Putz, A., Straube, A. & Kathmann, N. (1995). Obsessive-compulsive disorder and Gilles de la Tourette syndrome: Differential diagnosis of organic and psychogenic symptoms. *Nervenarzt*, **66** (5), 372–278.

Müller, N., Riedel, M., Zawta, P., Günther, W. & Straube, A. (2002). Comorbidity of Tourette's syndrome and schizophrenia – biological and physiological parallels. *Progress in Neuro-Psychopharmacology and Biological Psychiatry*, **26** (7), 1245–1258.

Müller, S.V., Johannes, S., Wieringa, B., Weber, A., Müller-Vahl, K., Matzke, M., Kolbe, H., Dengler, R. & Münte, T.F. (2003). Disturbed monitoring and response inhibition in patients with Gilles de la Tourette syndrome and co-morbid obsessive compulsive disorder. *Behavioural Neurology*, **14**, 29–37.

Muller-Vahl, K.R., Berding, G., Brucke, T., Kolbe, H., Meyer, G.J., Hundeshagen, H., Dengler, R., Knapp, W.H. & Emrich, H.M. (2000). Dopamine transporter binding in Gilles de la Tourette syndrome. *Journal of Neurology*, **247** (7), 514–520.

Nomoto, F. (1989). Tourette's syndrome. *Journal of Mental Health*, **35**, 63–70.

Obeso, J., Rothwell, J. & Marsden, C.J. (1981). Simple tics in Gilles de la Tourette's syndrome are not prefaced by a normal premovement EEG potential. *Journal of Neurology, Neurosurgery and Psychiatry*, **44** (8), 735–738.

Obsessive Compulsive Cognitions Working Group (1997). Cognitive assessment of obsessive-compulsive disorder. *Behaviour Research and Therapy*, **35** (7), 667–682.

O'Connor, K.P. (1980). Applications of the CNV in psychophysiology. In: P. Venables & I. Martin (eds), *Techniques in psychophysiology* (pp. 396–430). Chichester: John Wiley & Sons.

O'Connor, K.P. (1989). Individual differences and motor systems. In: T. Ney & A. Gale (eds), *Smoking and human behaviour* (pp. 141–170). Chichester: John Wiley & Sons.

O'Connor, K.P. (2001). Clinical and psychological features distinguishing obsessive compulsive and chronic tic disorders. *Clinical Psychology Review*, **21** (4), 631–660.

O'Connor, K.P. (2002). A cognitive-behavioral/psychophysiological model of tic disorders. *Behaviour Research and Therapy*, **40**, 1113–1142.

O'Connor, K.P. (in press). Contrasting Tourette's Syndrome and tic disorders with OCD. In: J.S. Abramovitz & A.C. Moats (eds), *Handbook of Controversial Issues in Obsessive Compulsive Disorder*. Kluwer Academic Press.

O'Connor, K.P. & Gareau, D. (1994). *Tics et problèmes de tension musculaire*. Quebec: Sogides.

O'Connor, K.P. & Langlois, R. (1998). Changes in self-efficacy and craving during smoking reduction. Do smokers feel more confident in quitting after first reducing? *Clinical Psychology and Psychotherapy*, **5**, 145–154.

O'Connor, K.P. & Lapierre, G.D. (1994). *The traffic light test*. Montreal: Stelate Systems.

O'Connor, K.P., Aardema, F. & Brisebois, H. (2001a). Validation of a style of planning action (STOP) as a discriminator between tic disorder, obsessive-compulsive disorder and generalized anxiety. Presented at *World Congress of Behavioral and Cognitive Therapy*. Vancouver, Canada (July).

O'Connor, K.P., Borgeat, F., Stip, E., Brault, M., Loiselle, J. & Robillard, S. (1997a). A clinical and experimental study of simple and complex tic disorder. Rapport de la subvention RS-930675, *FRSQ*.

O'Connor, K.P., Brault, M., Loiselle, J., Robillard, S., Borgeat, F. & Stip, E. (2001b). Evaluation of a cognitive-behavioral program for the management of chronic tic and habit disorders. *Behavior Research and Therapy*, **39**, 667–681.

O'Connor, K.P., Brault, M., Robillard, S. & Loiselle, J. (2003). Behavioral activity associated with onset in chronic tic and habit disorders. *Behavior Research and Therapy*, **41**, 241–249.

O'Connor, K.P., Brault, M., Robillard, S., Loiselle, J., Dubord, J., Stip, E. & Borgeat, F. (2001c). Does behavior therapy modify motor performance in chronic tic disorder? Presented at *World Congress of Behavioral and Cognitive Therapy*. Vancouver, Canada (July).

O'Connor, K.P., Gareau, D. & Blowers, G.H. (1993). Changes in construals of tic-producing situations following cognitive and behavioral therapy. *Perceptual and Motor Skills*, **77**, 776–778.

O'Connor, K.P., Gareau, D. & Blowers, G. (1994). Personal constructs amongst chronic tic sufferers. *British Journal of Clinical Psychology*, **13** (2), 151–158.

O'Connor, K., Gareau, D. & Borgeat, F. (1995). Muscle control in chronic tic disorders. *Biofeedback and Self-Regulation*, **20** (2), 111–121.

O'Connor, K.P., Gareau, D. & Borgeat, F. (1997b). A comparison of behavioral and cognitive-behavioral management of tic disorders. *Clinical Psychology and Psychotherapy*, **4** (2), 105–117.

O'Connor, K.P., Lavoie, M., Robert, M., Dubord, J., Stip, E. & Borgeat, F. (in press). Brain–behavior relations during motor processing in chronic tic and habit disorder. *Cognitive and Behavioral Neurology*.

O'Connor, K.P., Loyer, M., Lesage, A. & Robillard, S. (1998). *The prevalence of tic disorders in a community sample*. Centre de recherche Fernand-Seguin (unpublished document).

O'Connor, K.P., Robert, M., Dubord, J. & Stip, E. (2000). Automatic and controlled processing in chronic tic disorders. *Brain and Cognition*, **43**, 349–352.

O'Connor, K.P., Serawaty, M. & Stip, E. (1999). Simple and complex motor processing in chronic tic disorders. *Brain and Cognition*, **40** (1), 211–215.

Onofrj, M., Paci, C., D'Andreamatteo, G. & Toma, L. (2000). Olanzapine in severe Gilles de la Tourette syndrome: A 52-week double-blind cross-over study vs low-dose pimozide. *Journal of Neurology*, **247**, 443–446.

Orvaschel, H. & Puig-Antich, J. (1987). *Schedule for Affective Disorders and Schizophrenia for School-age Children: Epidemiologic 4ᵗʰ Version*. Ft Lauderdale, FL: Nova University, Center for Psychological Study.

Orvaschel, H., Puig-Antich, J., Chambers, W., Tabrizi, M.A. & Johnson, R. (1982). Retrospective assessment of prepubertal major depression with the Kiddie-SADS-e. *Journal of the American Academy of Child and Adolescent Psychiatry*, **21** (4), 392–397.

Osman, A., Hornblum, S. & Meyer, D. (1990b). Response times in a countermanding paradigm. *Journal of Experimental Psychology*, **16** (1), 183–198.

Osman, A., Kornblum, S. & Meyer, D.E. (1990a). Does motor programming necessitate response execution? *Journal of Experimental Psychology, Human Perception and Performance*, **16** (1), 183–198.

Ost, L.-G. (1987). Applied relaxation: Description of a coping technique and review of controlled studies. *Behaviour Research and Therapy* **25**, 397–409.

Parraga, H.C., Parraga, M.I., Spinner, L.R., Kelly, D.P. & Morgan, S.L. (1998). Clinical differences between subjects with familial and non-familial Tourette's syndrome: A case series. *International Journal of Psychiatry in Medicine*, **28** (3), 341–351.

Patterson, R.M. & Little, S.C. (1943). Spasmodic torticollis. *Journal of Nervous and Mental Disease*, **98**, 571–599.

Pauls, D.L. (1992). The genetics of obsessive compulsive disorder and Gilles de la Tourette's syndrome. *Psychiatric Clinics of North America*, **15** (4), 759–766.

Pauls, D.L. (2001). Is Tourette syndrome inherited? Presented at the *International Symposium on Tourette Syndrome and Other Neurodevelopmental Disorders*. Toronto, Canada (May).

Pauls, D.L. & Hurst, C.R. (1996). *Schedule for Tourette and other behavioural syndromes (adult form)*. The Yale family/genetic study self-report questionnaire for tics, obsessive-compulsiveness, attentional difficulties, impulsivity and motor hyperactivity. New Haven, CT: Child Study Center, Yale University School of Medicine.

Pauls, D.L., Alsobrook, J.P. II, Goodman, W., Rasmussen, S. & Leckman, J.F. (1995). A family study of obsessive-compulsive disorder. *American Journal of Psychiatry*, **152** (1), 76–84.

Pauls, D.L., Raymond, C.L., Stevenson, J.M. & Leckman, J.F. (1991). A family study of Gilles de la Tourette syndrome. *American Journal of Human Genetics*, **48** (1), 154–163.

Pélissier, M.-C. & O'Connor, K.P. (2004). Cognitive-behavioral treatment for trichotillomania, targeting perfectionism. *Clinical Case Studies*, **3** (1), 57–69.

Peterson, A.L. & Azrin, N.H. (1992). An evaluation of behavioral treatments for Tourette syndrome. *Behavior Research and Therapy*, **30** (2), 167–174.

Peterson, A.L. & Azrin, N.A. (1993). Behavioral and pharmacological treatment for Tourette's syndrome: A review. *Applied and Preventive Psychology*, **2**, 231–242.

Peterson, A.L., Campise, R.L. & Azrin, N.H. (1994). Behavioral and pharmacological treatments for tic and habit disorders: A review. *Developmental and Behavioral Pediatrics*, **15** (6), 430–441.

Peterson, B. (2001). Brain imaging of Tourette syndrome. Presented at the *International Symposium on Tourette Syndrome and Other Neurodevelopmental Disorders*. Toronto, Canada (May 31–June 2).

Peterson, B.S. & Cohen, D.J. (1998). The treatment of Tourette's syndrome: Multimodal, developmental intervention. *Journal of Clinical Psychiatry*, **59**, 62–72.

Peterson, B.S., Leckman, J.F., Arnsten, A., Anderson, G.M., Staib, L.H., Gore, J.C., Bronen, R.A., Malison, R., Scahill, L. & Cohen, D.J. (1999). Neuroanatomical circuitry. In: J.F. Leckman & D.J. Cohen (eds), *Tourette' syndrome. Tics, obsessions, compulsions. Developmental psychopathology and clinical care* (pp. 230–260). New York: John Wiley & Sons.

Peterson, B., Thomas, P., Kane, M., Scahill, L., Zhang, H., Bronen, R., King, R., Leckman, J. & Staib, L. (2003). Basal ganglia volumes in patients with Gilles de la Tourette's syndrome. *Archives of General Psychiatry*, **60**, 415–424.

Peterson, B.S., Zhang, H., Anderson, G.M. & Leckman, J.F. (1998). A double-blind, placebo-controlled, crossover trial of an antiandrogen in the treatment of Tourette's syndrome. *Journal of Clinical Psychopharmacology*, **18** (4), 324–331.

Phillips, M.L., Marks, I.M., Senior, C., Lythgoe, D., O'Dwyer, A.M., Meehan, O., Williams, S.C., Brammer, M.J., Bullmore, E.T. & McGuire, P.K. (2000). A differential neural response in obsessive-compulsive disorder patients with washing compared with checking symptoms to disgust. *Psychological Medicine*, **30** (5), 1037–1050.

Piacentini, J., Shaffer, D., Fisher, P., Schwab-Stone, M., Davies, M. & Gioia, P. (1993). The Diagnostic Interview Schedule for Children-Revised Version (DISC-R): III. Concurrent criterion validity. *Journal of the American Academy of Child and Adolescent Psychiatry*, **32** (5), 658–665.

Podivinsky, F. (1968). Torticollis. In: P.K. Vinken & G.W. Bruyn (eds), *Handbook of clinical neurology: Diseases of the basal ganglia* (Vol. 6, pp. 567–603). North-Holland: Elsevier.

Purdon, C. (1999). Thought suppression and psychopathology. *Behaviour Research and Therapy*, **37**, 1029–1054.

Rachman, S. & Hodgson, R. (1980). *Obsessions and compulsions*. New York: Prentice Hall.

Randolph, C., Hyde, T.M., Gold, J.M., Goldberg, T.E. & Weinberger, D.R. (1993). Tourette's syndrome in monozygotic twins: Relationship of tic severity to neuropsychological function. *Archives of Neurology*, **50**, 725–728.

Rapoport, J.L. (1990). Obsessive compulsive disorder and basal ganglia dysfunction. *Psychological Medicine*, **20**, 465–469.

Rasmussen, S.A. & Eisen, J.L. (1992). The epidemiology and differential diagnosis of obsessive-compulsive disorder. *Journal of Clinical Psychiatry*, **53** (Suppl.), 4–10.

Rauch, S., Beer, L., Cosgrove, G.R. & Jenike, M.A. (1995). Neurosurgical treatment of Tourette's syndrome: A critical review. *Comprehensive Psychiatry*, **36**, 141–156.

Regeur, L., Pakkenberg, B., Fog, R. & Pakkenberg, H. (1986). Clinical features and long-term treatment with pimozide in 65 patients with Gilles de la Tourette's syndrome. *Journal of Neurology, Neurosurgery and Psychiatry*, **49**, 791–795.

Reich, W. (2000). Diagnostic Interview for Children and Adolescents (DICA). *Journal of the American Academy of Child and Adolescent Psychiatry*, **39** (1), 59–66.

Rektor, I., Bares, M. & Kubova, D. (2001). Movement-related potentials in the basal ganglia: A SEEG readiness potential study. *Electroencephalography and Clinical Neurophysiology*, **112**, 2146–2153.

Rektor, I., Louvel, J. & Lamarche, M. (1998). Intracerebral recording of potentials accompanying simple limb movements: A SEEG study in epileptic patients. *Electroencephalography and Clinical Neurophysiology*, **107**, 277–286.

Rettew, D.C., Cheslow, D.L., Rapoport, J.L., Leonard, H.L., Lenane, M.C., Black, B. & Swedo, S.E. (1991). Neuropsychological test performance in trichotillomania: A further link with obsessive-compulsive disorder. *Journal of Anxiety Disorders*, **5**, 225–235.

Rhéaume, J., Freeston, M.H., Dugas, M.J., Letarte, H. & Ladouceur, R. (1995). Perfectionism, responsibility and obsessive-compulsive symptoms. *Behavior Research and Therapy*, **33** (7), 785–794.

Richards, E.H. (1992). Nicotine gum in Tourette's disorder. *American Journal of Psychiatry*, **149** (3), 417.

Roane, H.S., Piazza, C.C., Cercone, J.J. & Grados, M. (2002). Assessment and treatment of vocal tics associated with Tourette's syndrome. *Behavioral Modification, 26*, 482–498.

Robertson, M.M. (2000). Tourette syndrome, associated conditions and complexities of treatment. *Brain*, **123**, 425–462.

Robertson, M. (2001). Diagnosing Tourette syndrome. Is it a common disorder? Presented at the *International Symposium on Tourette Syndrome and Other Neurodevelopmental Disorders*. Toronto, Ontario (May).

Robertson, M.M. & Eapen, V. (1992). The pharmacologic controversy of CNS stimulants in Gilles de la Tourette syndrome. *Clinical Neuropharmacology*, **15**, 408–425.

Robertson, M.M. & Eapen, V. (1996). The national hospital interview schedule for the assessment of Gilles de la Tourette syndrome. *International Journal of Methods in Psychiatric Research*, **6** (4), 203–226.

Robertson, M.M. & Gourdie, A. (1990). Familial Tourette's syndrome in a large British pedigree associated psychopathology, severity, and potential for linkage analysis. *British Journal of Psychiatry*, **156**, 515–521.

Robertson, M.M. & Stern, J.S. (1998). Tic disorders: New developments in Tourette syndrome and related disorders. *Current Opinion in Neurology*, **11** (4), 373–380.

Robertson, M.M. & Stern, J.S. (2000). Gilles de la Tourette Syndrome: Symptomatic treatment based on evidence. *European Child and Adolescent Psychiatry*, **9** (1), 160–175.

Robertson, M.M., Banerjee, S., Kurlan, R., Cohen, D.J., Leckman, J.F., McMahon, W., Pauls, D.L., Sandor, P. & van de Wetering, B.J.M. (1999). The Tourette syndrome Diagnostic Confidence Index: Development and clinical associations. *Neurology*, **53**, 2108–2112.

Robertson, M.M., Trimble, M.R. & Lees, A.J. (1989). Self-injurious behaviour and the Gilles de la Tourette syndrome: A clinical study and review of the literature. *Psychological Medicine*, **19**, 611–625.

Rosenberg, L.A., Brown, J. & Singer, H.S. (1994). Self-reporting of behavior problems in patients with tic disorders. *Psychological Reports*, **74** (2), 653–654.

Roy, C., O'Connor, K.P. & Stravynski, A. (2002). La phobie sociale: Une comparaison entre deux modèles d'activation de la réponse physiologique, comportementale et subjective. Conference presented at: *Colloque sur l'apport de la technologie à l'évaluation et à l'intervention psychologique*. Université du Québec à Montréal (March).

Sachdev, P.S., Chee, K.Y. & Aniss, A.M. (1997). The audiogenic startle reflex in Tourette's syndrome. *Biological Psychiatry*, **41** (7), 796–803.

Salkovskis, P.M. & Clark, D.M. (1993). Panic disorder and hypochondriasis. Special Issue: Panic, cognition and sensations. *Advances in Research and Therapy*, **15**, 23–48.

Sallee, F.R. & Spratt, E.G. (1998). Tics and Tourette's disorder. In: T.H. Ollendick & M. Hersen (eds), *Handbook of child psychopathology*, 3rd edition (pp. 337–353). New York: Plenum Press.

Sallee, F.R., Nesbitt, L., Jackson, C., Sine, L. & Sethuraman, G. (1997). Relative efficacy of haloperidol and pimozide in children and adolescents with Tourette's disorder. *American Journal of Psychiatry*, **154**, 1057–1062.

Sanberg, P.R., Silver, A.A., Shytle, R.D., Philipp, M.K., Cahill, D.W., Fogelson, H.M. & McConville, B.J. (1997). Nicotine for the treatment of Tourette's syndrome. *Pharmacology and Therapeutics*, **74** (1), 21–25.

Sarason, I.G., Johnson, J.H. & Siegel, J.M. (1978). Assessing the impact of life changes: Development of the life experiences survey. *Journal of Consulting and Clinical Psychology* **46** (5), 932–946.

Savelsbergh, G.J.P. & Whiting, H.T.A. (1988). The effect of skill level, external frame of reference and environmental changes on one-handed catching. *Ergonomics*, **31** (11), 1655–1663.

Schmidt, R. (1988). Motor and action perspectives on motor behaviour. In: O. Meijer & K. Roth (eds), *Motor behavior*. North-Holland: Elsevier.

Scholz, O.B., Ott, R. & Sarnoch, H. (2001). Proprioception in somatoform disorders. *Behaviour Research and Therapy*, **39**, 1429–1438.

Schultz, R.T., Carter, A.S., Scahill, L. & Leckman, J.F. (1999). Neuropsychological findings. In: J.F. Leckman & D.J. Cohen (eds), *Tourette's syndrome – tics, obsessions, compulsions. Developmental psychopathology and clinical care*. New York: John Wiley & Sons.

Schut, A.J., Pincus, A.L., Castonguay, L.G., Bedics, J., Walling, F., Yanni, G. & Truckor, D. (1997). Attachment and interpersonal problems in non-clinical hair pulling. Paper presented at the *31st Annual Convention of the Association for the Advancement of Behavior Therapy*, Miami Beach, Florida.

Scott, B.L. & Jankovic, J. (1996). Delayed-onset progressive movement disorders after static brain lesions. *Neurology*, **46**, 68–74.

Scotti, J.R., Schulman, D.E. & Hojnacki, R.M. (1994). Functional analysis and unsuccessful treatment of Tourette's syndrome in a man with profound mental retardation. *Behavior Therapy*, **25** (4), 721–738.

Seligman, A. (1991). *Echolalia*. California: Hope Press.

Shapiro, E. & Shapiro, A.K. (1986). Semiology, nosology and criteria for tic disorders. *Revue Neurologique (Paris)*, **142** (11), 824–832.

Shapiro, A.K. & Shapiro, E. (1992). Evaluation of the reported association of obsessive-compulsive symptoms or disorder with Tourette's disorder. *Comprehensive Psychiatry*, **33** (3), 152–165.

Shapiro, E.S., Shapiro, A.K., Fulop, G., Hubbard, M., Mandeli, J., Nordlie, J. & Phillips, R. (1989). Controlled study of haloperidol, pimozide, and placebo for the treatment of GTS. *Archives of General Psychiatry*, **46**, 722–730.

Shapiro, A.K., Shapiro, E.S., Young, J.G. & Feinberg, T.E. (1988). *Gilles de la Tourette syndrome*. New York: Raven Press.

Sheehy, M.P. & Marsden, C.D. (1982). Writer's cramp – a focal dystonia. *Brain*, **105**, 461–480.

Shiffrin, R.M. & Schneider, W. (1977). Controlled and automatic human information processing: II. Perceptual learning, automatic attending, and a general theory. *Psychological Review*, **84**, 127–190.

Shytle, R.D., Silver, A.A., Sheehan, K.H., Wilkinson, B.J., Newman, M., Sanberg, P.R. & Sheehan, D. (2003). The Tourette's disorder scale (TODS): Development, reliability, and validity. *Assessment*, **10**, 273–287.

Silverstein, S.M., Como, P.G., Palumbo, D.R., West, L.L. & Osborn, L.M. (1995). Multiple sources of attentional dysfunction in adults with Tourette's syndrome: Comparison with attention deficit-hyperactivity disorder. *Neuropsychology*, **9** (2), 157–164.

Smith, S.J.M. & Lees, A.J. (1989). Abnormalities of the blink reflex in Gilles de la Tourette syndrome. *Journal of Neurology, Neurosurgery and Psychiatry*, **52**, 895–898.

Snider, L.A. & Swedo, S.E. (2003). Post-streptococcal-autoimmune disorders of the central nervous system. *Current Opinion in Neurology*, **16**, 359–265.

Spencer, T., Biederman, J., Harding, M., Wilens, T. & Faraone, S. (1995). The relationship between tic disorders and Tourette's syndrome revisited. *Journal of the American Academy of Child and Adolescent Psychiatry*, **34** (9), 1133–1139.

Speilberger, C.D., Gorsuch, R.L. & Lushene, R.E. (1970). *The state-trait anxiety inventory (test manual)*. Palo Alto: Consulting Psychologist Press.

Stanley, M.A., Prather, R.C., Wagner, A.L., Davis, M.L. & Swann, A.C. (1993). Can the Yale-Brown Obsessive Compulsive Scale be used to assess trichotillomania? A preliminary report. *Behavioral Research and Therapy*, **31** (2), 171–177.

Stanne, M.B., Johnson, D.W. & Johnson, R.T. (1999). Does competition enhance or inhibit motor performance? A meta analysis. *Psychological Bulletin*, **125**, 133–154.

Stip, E., O'Connor, K.P., Lecours, A.R., Prud'homme, P. & Elie, R. (1999). Coprolalia and decreased motor inhibition in Tourette's disorder: Evidence from a lexical decision task. *Brain and Cognition*, **40** (1), 262–264.

Sukhodolosky, D.G., Scahill, L., Zhang, H., Peterson, B.S., King, R.A., Lombroso, P.J., Katsovich, L., Findley, D. & Leckman, J.F. (2003). Disruptive behavior in children with Tourette's syndrome: Association with ADHD comorbidity, tic severity, and functional impairment. *Journal of the American Academy of Child and Adolescent Psychiatry*, **42** (1), 98–105.

Summerfeldt, L.J., Hood, K., Antony, M.M., Richter, M.A. & Swinson, R.P. (2004). Impulsivity in obsessive-compulsive disorder: Comparisons with other anxiety disorders and within tic-related subgroups. *Personality and Individual Differences*, **36**, 539–553.

Summerfeldt, L.J., Richter, M.A., Antony, M.M. & Swinson, R.P. (1999). Symptom structure in obsessive-compulsive disorder: A confirmatory factor analytic study. *Behaviour Research and Therapy*, **37**, 297–311.

Swedo, S.E. & Leonard, H.L. (1994). Childhood movement disorders and obsessive-compulsive disorder. *Journal of Clinical Psychiatry*, **55** (Suppl.), 32–37.

Swedo, S.E., Leonard, H.L., Garvey, M., Mittleman, B., Allen, A.J., Perlmutter, S., Lougee, L., Dow, S., Zamkoff, J. & Dubbert, B.K. (1998). Pediatric autoimmune neuropsychiatric disorders associated with streptococcal infections: Clinical description of the first 50 cases. *American Journal of Psychiatry*, **155** (2), 264–271.

Thibault, G., O'Connor, K., Stip, E, & Lavoie M.E. (2004). Event-related potentials and resources allocation anomaly in chronic tic disorders. *International Journal of Psychophysiology*, **54** (1–20), 155.

Thibert, A.L., Day, H.I. & Sandor, P. (1995). Self-concept and self-consciousness in adults with Tourette syndrome. *Canadian Journal of Psychiatry*, **40**, 35–39.

Tiffany, S. (1990). A cognitive model of drug uses and drug use behavior. Role of automatic and non-automatic processes. *Psychological Review*, **97** (2), 147–168.

Tijssen, M.A.J., Brown, P., Morris, H.R. & Lees, A. (1999). Late onset startle induced tics. *Journal of Neurology, Neurosurgery and Psychiatry*, **67**, 782–784.

Tourette Syndrome Classification Study Group (1993). Definitions and classification of tic disorders. *Archives of Neurology*, **50**, 1013–1016.

Trifiletti, R.R. & Packard, A.M. (1999). Immune mechanisms in pediatric neuropsychiatric disorders. Tourette's syndrome, OCD, and PANDAS. *Child and Adolescent Psychiatry Clinic of North America*, **8** (4), 767–775.

Tryon, W.W. (1993). The role of motor excess and instrumented activity measurement in attention deficit hyperactivity disorder. *Behavior Modification*, **17** (4), 371–406.

Tulen, J.H., van de Wetering, B.J. & Boomsma, F. (1998). Autonomic regulation during rest and mental load in Gilles de la Tourette syndrome. *Psychological Reports*, **83** (2), 515–529.

Turgeon, L., O'Connor, K. & Marchand, A. (1998). Recollections of parent–child relationships in OCD outpatients compared to panic disorder outpatients and normal controls. *World Congress of Behavioral and Cognitive Therapies (WCBCT)*, Acapulco, Mexico.

Turpin, G. (1983). The behavioral management of tics disorders: A critical review. *Advances in Behavior Research and Therapy*, **5**, 203–245.

Turvey, M.T., Shaw, R.E. & Mace, W. (1978). Issues in the theory of action: Degrees of freedom, coordinate structures and coalitions. In: J. Requin (ed.), *Attention and performance*, VII (pp. 557–595). Hillsdale, NJ: Erlbaum.

van Donkelaar, P. & Franks, I.M. (1991). Preprogramming vs on-line control in simple movement sequences. *Acta Psychologica*, **77**, 1–19.

van Woerkom, T.C., Roos, R.A.C. & van Dijk, J.G. (1994). Altered attentional processing of background stimuli in Gilles de la Tourette syndrome: A study in auditory event-related potentials evoked in an oddball paradigm. *Acta Neurologica Scandinavica*, **90** (2), 116–123.

Verdellen, C.W.J., Keijsers, G.P.J., Cath, D.C. & Hoogduin, C.A.L. (2004). Exposure with response prevention versus habit reversal in Tourette's syndrome: A controlled study. *Behaviour Research and Therapy*, **42**, 501–511.

Verdellen, C., Keijsers, G., Hoogduin, C. & Cath, D. (2002). Habit reversal versus exposure with response prevention in Tourette's syndrome: Outline of the results of a randomized, comparative study. Submitted to *32nd Congress of the EABCT*. Maastricht, The Netherlands (September).

Vogel, P.A., Stiles, T.C. & Nordahl, H.M. (1997). Recollections of parent–child relationships in OCD outpatients compared to depressed outpatients and healthy controls. Paper presented at the *Anxiety Disorders American Association*, New Orleans.

Walters, A.S., Boudwin, J., Wright, D. & Jones, K. (1988). Three hysterical movement disorders. *Psychological Reports*, **62**, 979–985.

Watson, T.S. & Sterling, H.E. (1998). Brief functional analysis and treatment of a vocal tic. *Journal of Applied Behavior Analysis*, **31**, 471–474.

Weimer, W. (1977). Motor theories of mind. In: R. Shaw & J. Bransford (eds), *Perceiving, acting and knowing: Toward an ecological psychology* (pp. 270–322). Hillsdale, NJ: Erlbaum.

Welner, Z., Reich, W., Herjanic, B., Jung, K.G. & Amado, H. (1987). Reliability, validity, and parent/child agreement studies of the Diagnostic Interview for Children and Adolescents (DICA). *Journal of the American Academy of Child and Adolescent Psychiatry*, **26** (5), 649–653.

Wilhelm, S., Deckersbach, T. & Coffey, B. (2001). Habit reversal for Tourette's disorder. Presented at *World Congress of Behavioral and Cognitive Therapies*, Vancouver, Canada (July).

Wilhelm, S., Deckersbach, T., Coffey, B.J., Bohne, A., Peterson, A.L. & Baer, L. (2003). Habit reversal versus supportive psychotherapy for Tourette's disorder: A randomized controlled trial. *American Journal of Psychiatry*, **160**, 1175–1177.

Wilkinson, B.J., Newman, M.B., Shytle, R.D., Silver, A.A., Sanberg, P.R. & Sheehan, D. (2001). Family impact of Tourette's syndrome. *Journal of Child and Family Studies*, **10** (4), 477–483.

Wojcieszek, J.M. & Lang, A.E. (1995). Gestes antagonistes in the suppression of tics: "Tricks for tics". *Movement Disorders*, **10** (2), 226–228.

Woods, D.W. & Miltenberger, R.G. (1995). Habit reversal: A review of applications and variations. *Journal of Behavior Therapy and Experimental Psychiatry*, **26** (2), 123–131.

Woods, D.W. & Miltenberger, R.G. (2001). *Tic disorders, trichotillomania, and other repetitive behavior disorders. Behavioral approaches to analysis and treatment*. Boston: Kluwer Academic Publishers.

Woods, D.W., Miltenberger, R.G. & Flach, A.D. (1996a). Habits, tics, and stuttering: Prevalence and relation to anxiety and somatic awareness. *Behavior Modification*, **20** (2), 216–225.

Woods, D.W., Miltenberger, R.G. & Lumley, V.A. (1996b). Sequential application of major habit-reversal components to treat motor tics in children. *Journal of Applied Behavior Analysis*, **29** (4), 483–493.

Woods, D.W., Twohig, M.P., Flessner, C.A. & Roloff, T.J. (2003). Treatment of vocal tics in children with Tourette syndrome: Investigating the efficacy of habit reversal. *Journal of Applied Behavior Analysis*, **36**, 109–112.

Woods, T.S., Watson, T.S., Wolfe, E., Twohig, M.P. & Friman, P.C. (2001). Analyzing the influence of tic-related talk on vocal and motor tics in children with Tourette's syndrome. *Journal of Applied Behavior Analysis*, **34**, 353–356.

Wright, K.M. & Miltenberger, R.G. (1987). Awareness training in the treatment of head and facial tics. *Journal of Behaviour Therapy and Experimental Psychiatry*, **18** (3), 269–274.

Yudofsky, S.C. & Hales, R.E. (eds) (1992). *The American Psychiatric Press Textbook of Neuropsychiatry*. Washington, DC: American Psychiatric Press Inc.

Zapella, M. (2002). Early-onset Tourette syndrome with reversible autistic behaviour: A dysmaturational disorder. *European Child and Adolescent Psychiatry*, **11**, 18–23.

Ziemann, U., Paulus, W. & Rothenberger, A. (1997). Decreased motor inhibition in Tourette's disorder: Evidence from transcranial magnetic stimulation. *American Journal of Psychiatry*, **154**, 1277–1284.

Zuellig, A.R., Newman, M.G., Kachin, K.E. & Constantino, M.J. (1997). Differences in parental attachment profiles in adults diagnosed with generalized anxiety disorder, panic disorder, or non-disordered. Poster presented at the *31st Conference of the Association for Advancement of Behavior Therapy*, Miami Beach, Florida.

INDEX

Page numbers in **bold** indicate major treatment of a subject.
Figures and tables are denoted by the prefixes F and T respectively, e.g. F1.2, T7.1.

Printed and bound by CPI Group (UK) Ltd, Croydon, CR0 4YY

17/04/2025

14658906-0001